To my daughter, Cara B. Jones,
and others aspiring to become a surgeon.
Pursue your dream. With compassion,
curiosity, commitment, and grit, you can make it.
— Daniel B. Jones

To my children Ishani and Shalin, the Harvard medical students,
and the BIDMC surgical residents and fellows — all of whom
are voracious daily learners — and who inspire me to help shift
the learning curve. Welcome to a career in surgery - the best
profession in the world!
— Alok Gupta

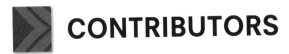

CONTRIBUTORS

Mohamad Rassoul Abu-Nuwar, MD
Clinical Fellow, Minimally Invasive & Bariatric Surgery
Harvard Medical School
Beth Israel Deaconess Medical Center
Boston, Massachusetts

Souheil W. Adra, MD, FACS, FASMBS
Director
Metabolic and Weight Loss Surgery
Chief
Harvard Medical Faculty Physicians
Surgery
Beth Israel Deaconess Hospital-Milton
Milton, Massachusetts

Heidee Albano, BSN, RN, CNOR
Clinical Advisor, West Campus
Operating Room
Transplant, Robotics, General,
MIS, Bariatrics, ACS, Plastics /
Reconstructive, GU and GYN
Beth Israel Deaconess Medical Center
Boston, Massachusetts

Seema P. Anandalwar, MD, MPH
Research Fellow, Surgery
Beth Israel Deaconess Medical Center
Boston, Massachusetts

Lorenzo Anez-Bustillos, MD, MPH
Resident
Department of Surgery
Harvard Medical School
Beth Israel Deaconess Medical Center
Boston, Massachusetts

Meredith A. Baker, MD
Resident
Department of Surgery
Harvard Medical School
Beth Israel Deaconess Medical Center
Boston, Massachusetts

Courtney Barrows, MD
Resident
Department of Surgery
Harvard Medical School
Beth Israel Deaconess Medical Center
Boston, Massachusetts

Myles D. Boone, MD, MPH
Anesthesiology
Dartmouth-Hitchcock Medical Center
Lebanon, New Hampshire

Gabriel Brat, MD, MPH
Assistant professor, Surgery
Beth Israel Deaconess Medical Center
Boston, Massachusetts

Alfred E. Buxton, MD
Josephson Ben-Haim Professor of
Medicine
Cardiovascular Division
Harvard Medical School
Beth Israel Deaconess Medical Center
Boston, Massachusetts

Mark P. Callery, MD
Professor, Surgery
Beth Israel Deaconess Medical Center
Boston, Massachusetts

Gabrielle E. Cervoni, MD
Resident Physician
Department of Surgery
Beth Israel Deaconess Medical Center
Boston, Massachusetts

Jane Cheng, MD, FACC, FHRS
Professor, Medicine
Cardiovascular Division
University of Minnesota
Minneapolis, Minnesota

Andrew D. Chung, MD, FRCPC
Beth Israel Deaconess Medical Center
Boston, Massachusetts

Michael N. Cocchi, MD
Assistant Professor of Emergency
Medicine
Harvard Medical School
Senior Medical Director, Critical Care
Quality
Beth Israel Deaconess Medical Center
Boston, Massachusetts

Carly D. Comer, MD
General Surgery Resident
Department of Surgery
Beth Israel Deaconess Medical
Center
Boston, Massachusetts

Kirsten Dansey, MD
Clinical Fellow, Surgery
Beth Israel Deaconess Medical Center
Boston, Massachusetts

William R. Deterling, BSBA
Director of Revenue Cycle
Department of Surgery
Beth Israel Deaconess Medical
Center
Harvard Medical Faculty Physicians
Boston, Massachusetts

Christopher Digesu, MD
Surgical Resident PGY5
Department of Surgery
Beth Israel Deaconess Medical Center
Boston, Massachusetts

Molly J. Douglas, MD
Acute Care Surgeon
University of Arizona College of
Medicine
Tucson, Arizona

Mariam F. Eskander, MD
General Surgery Resident
Beth Israel Deaconess Medical Center
Boston, Massachusetts

Amy R. Evenson, MD, MPH
Assistant Professor of Surgery
Harvard Medical School
Surgeon, Transplant Surgery
Beth Israel Deaconess Medical Center
Boston, Massachusetts

Ann Marie Feinstein, RN, BSN, CWOCN
Beth Israel Deaconess Medical Center
Boston, Massachusetts

Erika K. Fellinger, MD, FACS
Director CHA Endoscopy Training,
Department of Surgery
General and Minimally Invasive Surgery,
Cambridge Health Alliance
Clinical Instructor, Harvard University
Boston, Massachusetts

Emilie B.D. Fitzpatrick, MD
General Surgery
William Beaumont Army Medical Center
El Paso, Texas

Sidhu P. Gangadharan, MD, MHCM
Chief, Division of Thoracic Surgery and
Interventional Pulmonology
Beth Israel Deaconess Medical Center
Associate Professor of Surgery Harvard
Medical School
Boston, Massachusetts

Denise W. Gee, MD
Assistant Professor
Harvard Medical School
Massachusetts General Hospital
Boston, Massachusetts

Abraham Geller, MD
Clinical Fellow, Surgery
Massachusetts General Hospital
Boston, Massachusetts

Brian C. Goh, MD, PhD
Resident Physician
Harvard Combined Orthopaedic
Residency Program
Department of Orthopaedic Surgery
Massachusetts General Hospital
Boston, Massachusetts

Charlotte L. Guglielmi, MA, BSN, RN, CNOR
Clinical Manager, Perioperative
Education
Beth Israel Deaconess Medical Center
Boston, Massachusetts

Alok Gupta, MD
Assistant Professor
Harvard Medical School
Division of Acute Care Surgery
Beth Israel Deaconess Medical Center
Boston, Massachusetts

Priya S. Gupta, MD, MPH
Instructor in Medicine
Division of General Internal Medicine
Harvard Medical School / Massachusetts
General Hospital
Boston, Massachusetts

Jordan R. Gutweiler, MD, FACS
Instructor in Surgery
Harvard Medical School
Mount Auburn Hospital
Cambridge, Massachusetts

Allen D. Hamdan, MD
Physician
Department of Vascular Surgery
Beth Israel Deaconess Medical Center
Boston, Massachusetts

Daniel A. Hashimoto, MD, MS
Associate Director of Research,
Surgical AI & Innovation Laboratory
General Surgery Resident
Department of Surgery
Massachusetts General Hospital
Boston, Massachusetts

Rashi Jhunjhunwala, MD, MA
General Surgery PGY-3 Resident
Beth Israel Deaconess Medical
Center
Boston, Massachusetts

Sayuri P. Jinadasa, MD, MPH
Chief Surgical Resident
Beth Israel Deaconess Medical Center
Boston, Massachusetts

Cara B. Jones
Columbia University
New York, New York

Daniel B. Jones, MD, MS
Professor of Surgery
Harvard Medical School
Vice Chair of Surgery
Beth Israel Deaconess Medical Center
Boston, Massachusetts

Stephanie B. Jones, MD
Associate Professor of Anaesthesia
Harvard Medical School
Vice Chair, Education
Department of Anesthesia, Critical Care
and Pain Medicine
Beth Israel Deaconess Medical
Center
Boston, Massachusetts

Mojdeh S. Kappus, MD
Clinical Assistant Professor
Department of Surgery
Jacobs School of Medicine &
Biomedical Sciences
University at Buffalo
Buffalo, New York

Daniel Kaufman, MD
Resident
Department of Urology
Lahey Hospital and Medical Center
Burlington, Massachusetts

Jeffrey R. Keane, JR., BSN, RN, CNOR
Unit Based Educator
Perioperative Services
Beth Israel Deaconess Medical Center
Boston, Massachusetts

Daniel O. Kent, MD
Resident Physician
Research Administrative Resident
Department of Surgery
Harvard Medical School
Beth Israel Deaconess Medical Center
Boston, Massachusetts

Michael S. Kent, MD
Associate Professor of Surgery at
Harvard Medical School
Division of Thoracic Surgery and
Interventional Pulmonology
Department of Surgery
Beth Israel Deaconess Medical Center
Boston, Massachusetts

Tara S. Kent, MD, MS
Associate Professor
Department of Surgery
Harvard Medical School / Beth Israel
Deaconess Medical Center
Boston, Massachusetts

Ruslan Korets, MD
Assistant Professor
Division of Urology
Harvard Medical School
Beth Israel Deaconess Medical Center
Boston Massachusetts

Cindy M. Ku, MD
Instructor in Anaesthesia
Harvard Medical School
Associate Residency Program Director
Department of Anesthesia, Critical
Care, and Pain Medicine
Beth Israel Deaconess Medical Center
Boston, Massachusetts

Julia Larson, BS
Clinical Research Coordinator
Department of Anesthesia, Critical Care
and Pain Medicine
Beth Israel Deaconess Medical Center
Boston, Massachusetts

Stella J. Lee, MD
Clinical Fellow in Orthopaedic Surgery
Harvard Medical School
Boston, Massachusetts

Robin B. Levenson, MD
Department of Radiology
Harvard Medical School
Beth Israel Deaconess Medical Center
Boston, Massachusetts

Sarah Maben, MD
Anesthesia and Critical Care Fellow
Beth Israel Deaconess Medical Center
Boston, Massachusetts

Lucy C. Martinek, MD
Trauma and Acute Care Surgeon
Marshfield Clinic Health System
Marshfield, Wisconsin

Nisha Narula, MD
Surgery Chief Resident
Department of Surgery
Harvard Medical School
Beth Israel Deaconess Medical Center
Boston, Massachusetts

Brian Minh Nguyen, MD
General Surgeon
Southern California Permanente
Medical Group
Kaiser Permanente San Diego
San Diego, California

Kerry L. O'Brien, MD
Assistant Professor
Department of Pathology
Harvard Medical School
Medical Director Blood Bank
Beth Israel Deaconess Medical Center
Boston, Massachusetts

Brian O'Gara, MD, MPH
Instructor, Harvard Medical School
Beth Israel Deaconess Medical Center
Department of Anesthesia, Critical
Care, and Pain Medicine
Boston, Massachusetts

Stephen R. Odom II, MD
Physician, Surgical Critical Care
Beth Israel Deaconess Medical Center
Boston, Massachusetts

Therese Pare, RN, BSN, CWOCN
Beth Israel Deaconess Medical Center
Boston, Massachusetts

Charles S. Parsons, MD
Instructor in Surgery
Department of Surgery
Harvard University
Boston, Massachusetts

Sylvester A. Paulasir, MD
Surgeon
Memorial Hospital Jacksonville
Jacksonville, Florida

Alison M. Pease, MD
Resident Physician
Department of Surgery
Beth Israel Deaconess Medical Center
Boston, Massachusetts

Blaine T. Phillips, MD, MPH
General Surgery Resident Physician,
PGY-1
Beth Israel Deaconess Medical Center
Boston, Massachusetts

Jordan Pyda, MD, MPH
Clinical Fellow in Surgery
Harvard Medical School
Resident Physician in General Surgery
Beth Israel Deaconess Medical Center
Boston, Massachusetts

Nakul Raykar, MD, MPH
Resident
Department of Surgery
Beth Israel Deaconess Medical Center
Boston, Massachusetts

Kortney Robinson, MD, MPH
General Surgery Resident PGY-4
Department of Surgery
Harvard Medical School
Beth Israel Deaconess Medical Center
Boston, Massachusetts

Edward K. Rodriguez, MD, PhD
Associate Professor of Orthopaedic
Surgery
Harvard Medical School
Boston, Massachusetts

Kelsey Romatoski, BA
Medical Student
Rush Medical College
Chicago, Illinois

Debra J. Savage, MSN, RN, CNOR
PNEP Peri-Operative Educator
Beth Israel Deaconess Medical Center
Boston, Massachusetts

Steven D. Schwaitzberg, MD, FACS
Professor and Chairman
Department of Surgery
Professor of Biomedical Informatics
Jacobs School of Medicine and
Biomedical Sciences
University at Buffalo
The State University of New York

Stephanie K. Serres, MD, PhD
General Surgery Resident
Beth Israel Deaconess Medical Center
Boston, Massachusetts

David J. Shim, MD, PhD
Cardiac Electrophysiology Fellow
Cardiovascular Division, Harvard
Medical School, Beth Israel Deaconess
Medical Center
Boston, Massachusetts

Madhu Siddeswarappa, MD, MRCS (Glasgow)
Instructor in Surgery
Harvard Medical School
Department of Surgery
Beth Israel Deaconess Medical Center
General Surgeon at Beth Israel
Deaconess Hospital
Plymouth, Massachusetts

Peter A. Soden, MD
Clinical Fellow
Beth Israel Deaconess Medical Center
Boston, Massachusetts

Peter L. Steinberg, MD
Assistant Professor
Division of Urology
Harvard Medical School
Beth Israel Deaconess Medical
Center
Boston, Massachusetts

Alessandra Storino, MD
General Surgery Resident
Department of Surgery
Harvard Medical School and Beth Israel
Deaconess Medical Center
Boston, Massachusetts

Nicholas E. Tawa, JR, MD, PhD
Assistant Professor of Surgery
Beth Israel Deaconess Medical Center
Boston, Massachusetts

Bijan J. Teja, MD, MBA
Clinical Fellow, Harvard Medical School
Anesthesia Resident
Beth Israel Deaconess Medical Center
Boston, Massachusetts

Stephanie Therrien, BSc
Practice Manager
Division of Minimally Invasive and
Bariatric Surgery
Beth Israel Deaconess Medical Center
Boston, Massachusetts

Jacqueline E. Wade, MD
Clinical Fellow
Beth Israel Deaconess Medical Center
Boston, Massachusetts

Ammara Watkins, MD
Clinical Fellow,
Beth Israel Deaconess Medical Center
Boston, Massachusetts

Omar Yusef Kudsi, MD, MBA, FACS
Surgeon
Good Samaritan Medical Center
Brockton, Massachusetts

Wei Wei Zhang, MD
Acute Care Surgery and Critical Care
Fellow
Department of Surgery
Harvard Medical School and Beth Israel
Deaconess Medical Center
Boston, Massachusetts

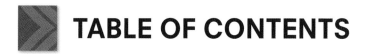

TABLE OF CONTENTS

SECTION I: WORK ON THE WARDS

SECTION IV: SCUT

SECTION V: OPERATING ROOM

SECTION VI: OUTSIDE OF THE HOSPITAL

SECTION VII: CODE OF CONDUCT

VIDEO CONTENTS

ACKNOWLEDGMENTS

Special thanks to the residents and faculty of the Department of Surgery at the Beth Israel Deaconess Medical Center for your insights and written contributions. Also, thanks to the staff of the Carl J Shapiro Simulation and Skills Center, Darren Tavernelli, Mike McBride, David Fobert and Brian Nguyen for assistant in filming tasks and procedures.

— Daniel B. Jones

FOREWORD

In composing this foreword for *The Surgery Boot Camp Manual: A Multimedia Guide for Surgical Training*, I was transported back to my first few months as a surgical intern. I remember how overwhelmed I felt not only by the profound responsibility for the lives and well-being of patients, but also by my limited knowledge of the tasks required to navigate and succeed in caring for patients within the very complex environment of a busy clinical service. Medical school had provided me with a strong foundation for the world I was entering, yet I still did not feel wholly prepared to perform the many essential tasks that were now expected of me. As I was often reminded by my senior residents, I was just a "diamond in the rough." There was no doubt in my mind that the learning curve ahead would be a steep one.

In 2012, the Department of Surgery at Beth Israel Deaconess Medical Center established the *Surgical Boot Camp* program for fourth-year Harvard Medical School students— one of the first such programs in the nation— as a transitional experience from medical school to surgical residency. During our journey in life, we not too infrequently find ourselves between "what was" and "what's next." A corridor in space and time which has been referred to as *liminal space*, derived from the Latin word *limen*, meaning threshold—a place between the familiar and the unknown. It is a place where all the transformation takes place. Where we leave our old world behind, but are not yet sure of our new reality. Transitions and changes are uncomfortable and anxiety provoking. Much as we try to compartmentalize change, they effect all aspects of our life— relationships, family, and our career. Transitions are best navigated if they are approached intentionally and within a community, rather than going at it alone. This guide will tie you to our own community of educators and learners at Beth Israel Deaconess Medical Center.

It would be difficult to find two more dedicated and innovative educators to co-edit this book and assemble a wide group of outstanding Harvard faculty and residents to contribute to this comprehensive and practical guide. Daniel Jones, MD, MS, Chief of Bariatric and Minimally Invasive Surgery, is the editor or coeditor of dozens of books and textbooks and a dedicated teacher and mentor to scores of residents. Alok Gupta, MD, Director of our Surgical Critical

Care Fellowship, served as the founding Director of the Harvard Surgical Boot Camp Program and continues to lead this very popular course.

In well-organized sections, contributors share their expertise and advice on a variety of topics that range from preparing for the operating room to troubleshooting Foley catheters and central-line placement, acquiring the fundamentals of laparoscopic surgery, appreciating the importance of work-life balance, and embracing a moral code that guides the pursuit of professionalism in all aspects of one's career.

Over the past 500 years, the Latin term vade mecum or "go with me" has been used as a reference to invaluable manuals or guidebooks sufficiently compact to be carried in a deep pocket. I am fully confident that *The Surgery Boot Camp Manual* will provide you an invaluable surgical vade mecum as you navigate your own transition as a "diamond in the rough" toward a highly successful career in the field of surgery.

Elliot L. Chaikof, MD, PhD

PREFACE

Welcome to *The Surgery Boot Camp Manual: A Multimedia Guide for Surgical Training*! This resource is primarily intended for fourth-year medical students who will soon become surgical interns. However, the content presented here is still both appropriate and beneficial to a vast array of healthcare professionals at various stages of surgical training. This includes medical students who will soon complete their surgical clerkship, junior surgical residents who want to review their recently acquired skillset, and midlevel practitioners who find themselves working in the surgical field. Similarly, this resource is applicable to all of the surgical subspecialties and can also benefit those who are practicing in other procedurally oriented disciplines such as procedural dermatology, interventional radiology, and emergency medicine.

Although medical school adequately prepares students for residency from a fund-of-knowledge and global perspective, there is often a deficit when it comes to technical and procedural abilities required at the next level. Interns show up to residency proficient in their foundational pillars (eg, obtaining a medical history, conducting a thorough yet focused physical examination, devising a differential diagnosis, and establishing a management plan), but structured education and curricula for skills beyond this are either lacking in thoroughness or missed entirely. Unsurprisingly, the areas of medicine that demand a unique hands-on skillset frequently see interns overwhelmed when residency expectations have not been met by their 4 years of medical education. This is undoubtedly frustrating for both residency programs and the fourth-year medical students who will soon be joining their ranks.

With surgical interns often lacking proficiency and confidence when it comes to the practical, procedural, and technical skills required of them at the next level, medical schools around the country have aimed to fill this void over the last decade by implementing surgical boot camp courses to graduating fourth-year medical students. These programs have been largely successful. As a result, boot camp courses in other disciplines, such as obstetrics and gynecology, emergency medicine, and even internal medicine, have followed suit in an attempt to improve the preparedness of their own fourth-year medical students. This manual and multimedia guide aims to mitigate this educational deficiency and improve the pragmatic readiness of incoming surgical interns just as these in-person boot camp courses have done over the last decade.

Dr. Alok Gupta, one of the leaders of our editorial team and a trauma surgeon and surgical intensivist at Beth Israel Deaconess Medical Center (BIDMC) in Boston, Massachusetts, was one of the first surgical educators in the country to identify the need to improve the educational process for fourth year medical students during their transition to surgical residency. In order to rectify this educational deficiency, he started one of the nation's first surgery boot camp courses in 2010 at Harvard Medical School (HMS), nearly a decade before the American College of Surgeons (ACS), the Association of Program Directors in Surgery (APDS), and the Association for Surgical Education (ASE) acknowledged the importance of enhancing the preparedness of surgical interns and began development of their own Resident Prep Curriculum.[1] Since the inception of Dr. Gupta's surgery boot camp course, its innovative curriculum has served as a model for over 75 other medical schools across the country as they attempt to design and standardize their own residency preparatory courses at their respective institutions.

Although Dr. Gupta's course was quite effective in preparing his own students, he realized that there was no formal resource to accompany his own boot camp course or the others that had been implemented across the country. Furthermore, he realized that such a text would not only greatly benefit his students and those enrolled in boot camp courses at other institutions, but it would also benefit those medical students who did not have access to surgery boot camp courses. In order to fix this problem, Dr. Gupta recruited Dr. Daniel B. Jones, Professor of Surgery at HMS and both the Vice Chair of Surgery, Technology, and Innovation and the Chief of the Division of Bariatric and Minimally Invasive Surgery at BIDMC, to help with the production of this resource as the other leader of our editorial team. Dr. Gupta sought Dr. Jones because of both his experience as a past president of the ASE and his dedication to medical student and surgical education throughout the entirety of his career. He also boasts an impressive record of producing innovative mediums for delivering medical education. Therefore, having Dr. Jones as other senior editor for *The Surgery Boot Camp Manual: A Multimedia Guide for Surgical Training* means that our audience is getting the best in medical education and the first medical text that is accompanied by its own video library with exciting videos on how to perform basic skills and procedures.

The appropriateness of the partnership between Dr. Gupta and Dr. Jones in delivering this resource is highlighted by the fact that a few years after Dr. Gupta started his boot camp course and was still actively improving upon its

---

[1]American College of Surgeons. *ACS/APDS/ASE Resident Prep Curriculum*. American College of Surgeons; 2019. https://www.facs.org/education/program/resident-prep. Accessed July 16, 2019.

curriculum, Dr. Jones was simultaneously helping design a study through the ACS and ASE to assess the efficacy of medical student simulation-based skills curriculum.[2] As a result, while Dr. Gupta was busy advancing the educational experience of fourth-year medical students who were soon going to become interns and junior residents, Dr. Jones was focusing his efforts on assessing the educational experience of less experienced surgeons-in-training during their surgical clerkships. This broad audience of medical students, interns, and junior residents, which Dr. Jones and Dr. Gupta have spent countless hours educating, just so happens to be the audience for this manual.

How will *The Surgery Boot Camp Manual: A Multimedia Guide for Surgical Training* help you as you embark upon your transition to and journey through residency? In order to answer this, we should first briefly provide some context for Dr. Gupta's boot camp course and its evolution over the years. Dr. Gupta's surgery boot camp course is a fully immersive, month-long course that enhances the preparedness of medical students who will soon be entering into their surgical residency. His course was so successful that, soon after the commencement of his course, similar courses at HMS-affiliated hospitals for other disciplines outside of general surgery soon materialized as well. These different courses had different philosophies. Those for internal medicine were primarily aimed at ensuring that all the vital knowledge learned in medical school was, indeed, solidified. This differed from the philosophy of Dr. Gupta's surgical boot camp course, which aimed to teach students all the information they were *not* formally taught during their 4 years of medical school. The teaching philosophy of *The Surgery Boot Camp Manual: A Multimedia Guide for Surgical Training* assimilates that of Dr. Gupta's surgical boot camp course: to teach what was not taught during medical school with similar teaching modalities to what is offered by Dr. Gupta's course at HMS. This is not to say that this resource will not also recapitulate and reinforce information you learned throughout medical school, as it certainly will. What this resource does is shift the learning curve from internship to the fourth year of medical school, as we see great value in educating you on skills and procedures that have not historically been mandatory to master prior to residency training.

The material provided through this multimedia resource is the embodiment of Dr. Gupta's surgical boot camp course at HMS. It is adapted from his high-yield curriculum that has been offered to HMS students for nearly a decade. Under the dedicated stewardship of Dr. Gupta, the content of this course has

[2]Glass CC, Acton RD, Blair PG, et al. American College of Surgeons/Association for Surgical Education medical student simulation-based surgical skills curriculum needs assessment. *Am J Surg.* 2014;207(2):165-169.

been validated by continuous assessment and feedback from his students during this time and has resulted in this course being the highest rated elective at HMS since its inception. Meanwhile, the content of this manual has been delivered to you in a way that only Dr. Jones can execute with his years of experience pioneering innovative ways to improve and standardize medical student and surgical resident curricula. In fact, it was the innovative mind of Dr. Jones to pair online educational videos to the procedural chapters provided throughout text. Together, Dr. Gupta and Dr. Jones were able to effectively collaborate and create the perfect resource for surgical trainees who find themselves in medical school or the early stages of residency.

With *The Surgery Boot Camp Manual: A Multimedia Guide for Surgical Training*, we have made every effort to deliver this comprehensive, in-person course to you to allow you to prepare yourself at your own pace, wherever you find yourself in your surgical training. In fact, this resource represents the collective effort of over 3000 hours of work from numerous surgeons and surgeons-in-training.

The authors of this book include attending surgeons, surgical residents, fourth-year medical students, and even experts from other departments. Each of our authors was carefully selected for a specific reason: there are some topics that are better taught by residents than by attendings. For example, we have a chapter written by an attending on "How an *attending* would want you to prepare for the operating room." This chapter *should* be written by an attending. Similarly, we recruited the expertise of both an attending anesthesiologist and transfusion medicine pathologist to help write our chapter on "blood transfusions." These are the healthcare professionals that you are most likely to consult as an intern when dealing with blood transfusion complications and, therefore, these individuals were most qualified to author this chapter. Similarly, our chapter on "How to be a successful intern" is not a topic that you want an attending to write, so we recruited a chief resident to draft this content instead. Furthermore, we only recruited authors who are extremely passionate about teaching and only those who are either experts in their corresponding field and/ or have vast experience upon which to draw upon when writing about a given topic. The editorial team achieved this same level of diversity as well by including surgeons at various levels of training. This was intentional and ensured the presence of unique perspectives, from both the teacher and the trainee, during the editing process so that our content was pertinent, focused, and appropriate to your level of training.

This is the first resource to bring this increasingly popular medical school course and deliver it in a form that is accessible to all students. It has taken years to assemble, and the editorial team is proud of the effort that went into its production. Although *The Surgery Boot Camp Manual: A Multimedia Guide for Surgical Training* cannot replace the value of an in-person boot camp course, it can serve as a great supplement to this experience and can also help prepare soon-to-be surgical interns who do not have access to these courses.

As an associate editor of *The Surgery Boot Camp Manual: A Multimedia Guide for Surgical Training* and recently matriculated PGY-1 who is now just finishing the first month of my internship, I have already found my experiences in helping create this resource to be invaluable when it comes to my preparedness on the floor and within in the operating room. It is my hope that you will find this text and online video library as beneficial as I have as you continue your surgical training.

Blaine T. Phillips, MD, MPH
General Surgery Resident, PGY-1
Beth Israel Deaconess Medical Center
Clinical Fellow in Surgery
Harvard Medical School
Boston, Massachusetts

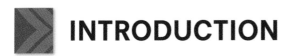

INTRODUCTION

BLAINE T. PHILLIPS, MD, MPH | DANIEL B. JONES, MD, MS

OVERVIEW

For those of you who have recently completed your journey through medical school and are now moving on to residency, we offer you our congratulations! Your years of hard work and perseverance have been rewarded with the opportunity to join in what we believe to be the most rewarding profession—that of a surgeon. As you embark upon the next phase of your medical careers as surgical residents, you are most likely experiencing a number of paradoxical emotions—excitement and fear, relief and apprehension, and pride and humility. The job of a surgeon is arduous and strenuous work with significant psychological and physiological demands. It will require efficient data collection, impeccable judgment, and flawless decision-making. With that said, it is also intellectually stimulating, endlessly rewarding, and addictively challenging.

As soon-to-be surgical interns, we are certain that you are questioning your preparedness for the great responsibility that will soon be placed upon your shoulders. Within months, you will be entrusted with the lives of patients. While this is true, we want to reassure you that you will *not* be alone as you start your career as medical professionals. First, the institutions that you will soon join as house staff will provide you with an environment where you will be supervised when making tough and important decisions and one where you will be supported as you tackle the challenges of a surgical residency. Second, there will be numerous materials that will help prepare you as you make this transition from medical school to residency. *The Surgery Boot Camp Manual: A Multimedia Guide for Surgical Training* is one of those materials and will serve as a valuable and easily accessible resource for you.

EXPECTATIONS

Assimilating into the unique, complex, and often intimidating environment of the operating room, and even that of the bedside of the surgical patient, can be a daunting task for those who are inexperienced or unprepared. In order to truly excel as surgical interns, hard work and dedication are required. Surgical interns are expected to demonstrate mastery of a variety of technical skills, function as an efficient member of the team, practice compassion while interacting with patients, and demonstrate self-motivation as an adult learner. They should always be driven to grow and improve. Our aim is to provide our audience with information, practical advice, and technical instructions to ease the medical school to residency transition and to maximize your potential for success. We will accomplish through a comprehensive and holistic approach when discussing the different characteristics that make a surgical intern a proficient one.

Among the aforementioned requirements needed for success as an intern, self-motivation as an adult learner is absolutely essential to your continued progress and will largely impact both how much you get out of this resource and how well you navigate through residency and grow as a surgeon. Whether you are about to begin your surgical clerkship, starting your intern year, or looking for opportunities for review the skills you learned during your internship, your dedication to improving your craft will predominantly depend upon your willingness to learn day-in and day-out—no matter how difficult it is during the day to find time to study or how exhausted you are when you return home after a long day at the hospital. The same concept applies to this resource and how much you will benefit from its use. This multimedia guide will provide the greatest benefit when it is not only utilized during initial acquisition of technical skills and procedures prior to their clinical implementation, but also when it is used to review what was may have been observed or performed in the clinical setting on any given day. Remember that practice makes perfect, especially when that practice is reinforced.

We acknowledge the challenges facing medical students, interns, and junior residents when it comes to finding the time and energy to study while simultaneously working long and tiring shifts in the hospital. As a result, we have intentionally made sure *The Surgery Boot Camp Manual: A Multimedia Guide for Surgical Training* is as user-friendly as possible. In order to facilitate this, we have designed this text to be small enough to fit into one of your white coat pockets to ensure easy accessibility while working on the floor. Additionally, this text and its corresponding video library, which includes step-by-step demonstrations of common procedures and basic technical skills, can also be accessed by any device connected to the internet. Our hope is that this ease of accessibility will help you view this multimedia guide as one of your primary resources, both during your time in the hospital and while you are studying at home.

CONTENT

Although surgical boot camp courses often provide their material though different modalities, such as didactics, simulation sessions, and technical skills training, we obviously cannot offer all of this here. Therefore, our challenge was to figure out a way to best transform the in-person surgical boot camp experience into one that you can engage in autonomously, without it being dependent upon the direct assistance and supervision of attending instructors. *The Surgery Boot Camp Manual: A Multimedia Guide for Surgical Training* accomplished this by engaging the reader with an online video library of technical skills and common bedside procedures. Our manual also provided clinical pearls at the end of each chapter. This latter feature will reinforce key teaching points and will also help you retain the information provided.

The chapters in this book will serve as the "didactic" component found in surgical boot camp courses. Chapters will be self-explanatory in their goals and objectives. We will not directly provide content on surgical pathology, such as pancreatitis or abdominal aortic aneurysms. However, pathology *will* be discussed when it is necessary to understand the information and training provided. We will have chapters that teach you how to write orders. We will have chapters that teach you how to tie knots. We will have chapters that teach you how to recognize different instruments in the operating room and how to decide between them based upon the next step in a procedure and the anatomy that is presented to you (eg, when to use a DeBakey versus an Adson). Most chapters will follow the same format and be focused in their delivery. However, some chapters will take on a more original approach if we feel the teaching points are more effectively communicated with this methodology or without bulleted concepts or enumerated instructions. For example, procedural chapters will be different in format from chapters introducing you to the operating room and to the surgical wards.

"Simulation sessions" provided in surgical boot camp courses are a valuable learning tool. Although it is next to impossible to perfectly replicate the environment that you will find yourself in when a patient is coding or hypotensive, simulation sessions can provide a similar environment with high emotional valence without risk to patients while providing valuable learning experiences. Although we are unable to mimic simulation sessions in real time, *The Surgery Boot Camp Manual: A Multimedia Guide for Surgical Training* teaches you the key point you must know for common—and potentially emergent—beside procedures through both text and our online video library. Some of the procedures you will learn include chest tube placement, open cricothyroidotomy,

Foley catheter placement, bag mask ventilation, and intubation, just to mention a few. With all this said, however, leadership and closed-loop communication can only best be practiced with in-person simulation sessions at your respective institutions to supplement the content presented here.

Finally, we will teach you technical skills, such as open suturing, knot tying, and basic laparoscopic technique. Again, these skills will be taught through a combination of text from individual chapters and from our online video library. What you get out of the skills component of this book will be based solely on the time and effort you invest, which goes back to our emphasis on self-motivation as an adult learner. Mastery of these skills will pay dividends for your progression and development during residency because attendings and senior residents trust junior residents who demonstrate proficiency with their technical skills. The same can be applied to proficiency demonstrated with procedures. In the end, being "interested" is great, but being engaged, competent, and skilled is even better.

Overall, *The Surgery Boot Camp Manual: A Multimedia Guide for Surgical Training* takes a novel approach by providing step-by-step instructions along with video demonstrations of fundamental skills and procedures utilized at both the bedside and operative settings. This educational tool is intended to be used as a practice and study guide, as well as a bedside and online manual. Students can read about specific areas of interest, watch demonstration videos that supplement the text, and practice skills that they anticipate will be needed in their upcoming clinical rotations. It can also be used as a quick reference to review step-by-step instructions for unanticipated procedural opportunities that may arise on the ward. It is also worth noting that links to these videos can be found within the content in the online version of the text, and icons for this video supplementation are also found in the corresponding locations within the hard copy of the manual. ▶

CONCLUSION

For those of you with internship on the near horizon, you will soon take the Hippocratic Oath as you officially join the medical profession. For those of you who have previously sworn to fulfill its covenant, you know the gravity of its tenets as you have already assumed responsibility for your very own patients. In either case, we know that you have made great sacrifices to get to where you are on your journey to become a medical professional. As your journey continues to unfold, you will continue to make sacrifices. You will miss important family and life events. You will lose sleep. *But*, you will make these sacrifices without hesitation as you take care of patients when they most need your care and attention, whether that is on the floor, the intensive care unit, or the operating room.

As an intern and junior resident, you will make educated guesses on diagnoses with incomplete information. You will make decisions on treatment plans with less and less supervision as you progress through residency. Eventually, you ascend to the point of ultimate responsibility, and on that day, your patients will look down at their hospital armbands and see your last name printed as their attending surgeon. When that day comes, your patients will expect no deviation from the tightrope of clinical perfection that is associated with our profession.

You will make errors. Some of them will be minor. Others, unfortunately, may be fatal. Be strong, and most of all, remember to learn from these errors and be honest about them with your patients and their families. You will make do with what you have, whether that is a limited-resource environment on an international medical mission or the uncomfortable plastic mattress in the hospital on-call room. You will eventually make up for educational debt. You will most likely never make up for lost hours of sleep. You will make countless small checkboxes each and every day for the foreseeable future. You will make multiple trips to see that patient that you are really worried about after her complicated postoperative course. You will make lifelong friends over the course of your residency and career. In the end, our advice to you is to take care of yourself, embrace the relationships you make, and take care of your patients and of one another.

Internship will require that you recalibrate your mind each and every day so that you can maximally focus on the task at hand. However, while you should prepare for each day like it is a sprint, you also have to keep in mind that internship and residency are a marathon. We will talk about this later in one of our chapters, but we encourage you to remember to honor yourself, your personal relationships, and each other. Doing so will ensure that, when you need to be ready for your "surgical tightrope," during an overnight call when your patient's respiratory status is compromised and he needs a cricothyroidotomy, your hours of preparation will allow you to remain calm and focused as you remember your training and what you learned from *The Surgery Boot Camp Manual: A Multimedia Guide for Surgical Training* to help save the life of your patient.

Again, we welcome you to *The Surgery Boot Camp Manual: A Multimedia Guide for Surgical Training*, the first text and video resource of its kind in surgical education. It is our privilege to share our expertise with you as you make this difficult transition to your surgical residency. As alluded to above, this resource is intended to serve as both a practical and technical guide for the surgical novice. Likewise, the anticipated audience is primarily for newly minted surgical interns, but also includes medical students who are entering their surgical clerkships, as well as junior residents who are searching for a succinct resource to fine-tune and perfect their procedural skills. This is a high-yield curriculum that can either supplement the surgical boot camp experience offered by your medical school or it can be used exclusively on its own if you are unable to enroll in one.

1

INTRODUCTION TO THE SURGICAL SERVICES: THE WARDS

BLAINE T. PHILLIPS, MD, MPH | LUCY C. MARTINEK, MD

As a trainee, your first day working on the surgical services can be quite over-whelming. Your day starts early and everything moves at such a fast pace. To make matters worse, it is often initially unclear how one can be helpful. You will likely be confronted with numerous questions and insecurities: What is my role? Where do I fit in? What should I do and, even more importantly, what should I not do? The surgical services are inherently different from most other fields of medicine, and trainees are typically provided with only preliminary preparation (eg, proper scrubbing technique, knot tying, and suturing) before being sent to their teams on the surgical wards. Clearly, there will be a lot of on-site and hands-on learning.

The authors of this chapter were motivated to provide this content as we both come from families without anyone in the medical professions. In this sense, we both lacked a consistent figure who could provide us with guidance and we both coveted access to an introductory text, like this chapter, to help us prepare for our surgical training. Irrespective of your current level of training, it is our hope that you have already found a compatible and dedicated mentor who can help you through all the stages of your surgical career. However, whether you have secured consistent mentorship or are still seeking this, we hope this chapter provides perspective, answers some of the questions you must be asking yourself, and helps prepare you for your surgical training experience.

   BP and LM

OVERVIEW

As referenced in the Introduction, the primary audience for this resource is the surgical trainee. Since surgical training is a lengthy process, a variety of unique audiences who find themselves at different stages of training can benefit from the content provided through this multimedia guide. This includes fourth-year medical students who will soon become surgical interns, interns who just started their surgical residency, residents from other specialties who will rotate on a surgical service, junior residents who want to review their recently-acquired technical and procedural skill set, and even medical students who are about to begin their surgical clerkships. Additionally, a broad array of other healthcare professionals who work in the surgical subspecialties or other procedure-based fields can utilize this manual. With that said, this resource would be incomplete without a prelude dedicated to those who are completely new to and unfamiliar with the surgical services. Therefore, this chapter will serve to introduce the surgical services to novice surgical trainees and will specifically focus on topics pertinent to the surgical wards.

   This chapter will discuss team structure and dynamics, expectations, preparation, and troubleshooting for the surgical trainee as it relates to the wards to ensure that students and residents with varied surgical experiences have the same fundamental understanding of the basics for the surgical services. If you find this chapter to be on par with your present training experience, then we strongly encourage you to review this chapter prior to your work on the surgical services.

TEAM STRUCTURE AND DYNAMICS

The majority of surgical teams will have an attending, chief resident, and intern at the very minimum. However, there can also be variations to this composition, depending upon the institution or the specific service, in regard to who else makes up the team. This variation can manifest itself with the possible additions of a fellow, junior resident, and/or medical student. Furthermore, some hospitals may even have dedicated nurse practitioners or physician assistants who help with patient care on the floor or with procedures in the OR, especially for services that are typically high in volume or complexity of care.

The dynamic of any team in the hospital is one of hierarchy. The surgical team is a classic example of this. The overall scheme is one in which information is communicated from those of lower rank to those at the top, and then orders and directions are provided from the attending surgeon or chief resident back down to the intern. While this is certainly an oversimplification, as there are various degrees of autonomy at every level, this generally describes the team dynamic. This is not to say that those who find themselves at the "bottom of the totem pole" are not valued. In fact, the opposite is often the case as the intern, ultimately, is the individual who makes the service run smoothly. Moreover, a weak intern can break down the entire team dynamic and even endanger the lives of the team's patients. The medical student can also serve as a valuable member of the team. We will discuss the roles and expectations of medical students and other junior surgical trainees on the floor in the next section, but as with most other medical teams found within the hospital, the student can be of greatest use to the intern. The more a medical student is able to help the intern, the more efficient the service will run.

The intern will primarily be responsible for taking care of non-, pre-, and postoperative patients on the floor, writing discharge summaries, notifying the chief resident and/or attending when their expertise is required, and making sure that all tasks outside of the OR are completed each day. Meanwhile, more senior residents, such as the chief resident, will spend relatively more time in the OR than the intern but will also be responsible for taking care of patients on the floor.

Although the hierarchical structure of the surgical team on the wards manifests itself in essentially the same manner within the OR, there are other factors at play in this latter setting (eg, dedicated OR nursing staff and anesthesiology team) that make the overall dynamic here more complex. These subtle differences in team structure and dynamics in the OR will vary based on the preferences and practice style of the attending surgeon assigned to that case, and it will also vary based on the number of senior surgical trainees present in the room. Nevertheless, it is important for you as the surgical trainee to be familiar with what is generally expected of you while also exercising flexibility in your level of participation in the case.

Parts of the following three sections on Expectations, Preparation, and Troubleshooting were written specifically for the medical student starting his or her clerkship. Although this may seem rudimentary to readers who have already exceeded this level of training, there is still content provided that is pertinent to all surgical trainees, independent of their current level of training. The content that is specific to medical students, however, is still technically quite important to review for interns and junior residents. Our reasoning for this is that the life of a surgeon, or any physician for that matter, is one of both continuous learning and continuous teaching. We constantly need to learn, grow, and adapt in an ever-advancing field. Similarly, we always need to be prepared to help educate and train the next generation of surgeons. Furthermore, teaching is actually the most effective method of learning. In fact, we foster this idea to such an extent that the role of a resident as a teacher was actually dedicated as its very own chapter within this manual (see Resident as Teacher). In this light, interns and residents are, therefore, strongly encouraged to read these sections so that they can be best prepared to guide, teach, and properly assess the medical students who are assigned to their services as they rotate on their clerkships and subinternships. At the very least, this introductory chapter will serve as a succinct review of the basics when it comes to the surgical services.

EXPECTATIONS

The OR and surgical wards can be both exciting and intimidating places. As a junior surgical trainee, you are often eager to help but, at the same time, hesitant to offer assistance as you fear you will end up performing an action that either is beyond your scope or could ultimately harm the patient. Unfortunately, this fear is not unfounded. For example, medical students are often found to have a poor understanding of the indications for hand disinfection,[1] and patient mortality has been found to increase in hospitals because of academic year-end changeovers.[2] Therefore, as a surgical trainee in the early stages of training, if you find yourself in a situation where you are uncertain as to whether or not you should do something, trust your instincts and ask a superior before proceeding.

With that stated, where in this fast-paced and dynamic environment do you, the surgeon-in-training, fit? Although generalizations can certainly be made and will be described here, it is important to note that the trainee's role will depend on your specific level of training (ie, clerkship, subinternship, internship, or junior residency), the specific service to which you are assigned, and the individuals that make up your surgical team. Therefore, it is absolutely critical for the surgical trainee to approach the intern (if the trainee is a medical student), chief resident or fellow, *and* attending on the first day you join their service to clarify what their individual expectations are for you and how you can best help the team from *each* of their different perspectives. Although these expectations could very well overlap, they could also be quite different, and you will be required to deliver on each. Some questions that you should ask on your first day on your new service are:

MEDICAL STUDENTS:
How can I best help the intern prior to morning rounds?

ALL SURGICAL TRAINEES:
How many patients should I assume responsibility for at a given time?
How detailed should my presentations be on morning rounds and during sign-out?
How can I best help the team on the floor?
How can I best help the team in the perioperative holding area, OR, and postanes-
*   thesia care unit (PACU)?*

You should ask these questions and learn about your expectations on the first day you join a *new team* on any service (even if that *new team* is joining the specific service you have already been a part of for a few weeks).

You will eventually figure out your role, but the earlier you demonstrate this initiative and deliver on your team's expectations, the quicker your team will start to trust you and provide you with greater responsibility. As you are entrusted with greater responsibility, you will gain more from your time both on the wards and in the OR in terms of your education, enjoyment, and overall experience.

Just as we encourage surgical trainees to query their team's expectations when they first join a new service, we also urge you to regularly ask for feedback from your superiors. The career of a surgeon, or any healthcare professional for that matter, is one of constant feedback and evaluation. We can always improve. Even the most experienced and accomplished clinicians and surgeons can improve. Getting in the habit of asking for feedback early on in your medical career and, more importantly, implementing that feedback and constructive criticism into your daily practice and routine will only serve to improve you.

Although it is appropriate to ask your superiors for feedback relating to your performance in the OR on a more regular basis (eg, at the end of each procedure), you should ask for feedback on the wards with less frequency (eg, every 1-2 weeks depending on your specific service). The one exception to this pertains to asking your direct superior for feedback on your patient presentations during morning rounds and patient handoffs at the end of the day.

This feedback should be elicited on a daily basis or, at the very least, until improvement is noted by your superiors. On the wards, surgical trainees should ask their superiors if they can each schedule a time at the end of the week when they could informally discuss feedback with you. This accomplishes several things: it lets them know that you want to improve, it reminds them to observe you and make mental notes regarding your performance, and it lets them "pencil in" this feedback session into their busy schedules. All aspects of the feedback you receive are important. This includes both your strengths and your weaknesses. Although constructive criticisms can sometimes seem as though they are personal attacks, you should never view them as such.

Although the following may seem obvious and is discussed in its own chapter (see chapter on ACGME Professionalism), professionalism still deserves to be mentioned here regarding surgical trainee expectations. This means you should always be punctual (being "on time" means being "early" for medical students and interns), dressed in proper attire, and presentable in terms of your appearance and hygiene. You need to be courteous and respectful of all patients and colleagues, whether that be over the phone, via email, or in person. The surgical trainee also needs to be aware of his or her role on the team when talking to patients and their families and should not make promises that the team cannot keep.

We will organize the rest of this section based on the typical day of a junior surgical trainee on the surgical wards. As the medical student or intern, you should be the first one who arrives at the hospital in the morning. Once you get there, you should print up a list of all the patients on your service and record their most recent vital signs, including their ranges overnight; inputs and outputs ("ins and outs" or "I's and O's"); and pertinent lab values, if available. You should then make enough photocopies of these for all the members of your team. We suggest making a couple extra copies just in case extra students, residents, or attendings join rounds. If you are the team's medical student, this will significantly help make your intern more efficient each morning and will also help you learn about all the patients on your service. You should then *go see* your individual patients to ask them how they feel and if they have experienced any notable changes in function or pain (or with any other relevant sensory modalities). You should also conduct a *focused* physical examination (PE). For example, if your patient had an uncomplicated appendectomy the prior night, you may not need to perform a complete neurologic examination. You should also ask the nursing staff if they have any concerns or if there were any significant overnight events. Then, record a SOAP (subjective, objective, assessment, and plan) note of your findings for your patient presentations on morning rounds. For those who are unfamiliar with this process, we suggest allotting a generous amount of time for this initially until you get more accustomed with this ritualistic process and improve your efficiency.

On morning rounds, all patients will be discussed. You will be required to present your patients to the team and, as indicated earlier, should attempt to provide the level of detail your team desires to hear from someone at your designated level of training. You will learn over time what level of detail will be acceptable on the fast-paced rounds of the surgical services. Also, it is important to note that if you are a medical student and your intern starts presenting one of your patients (out of habit), you should politely interrupt him or her and ask if you can present your patient. Although this may seem obvious, if you are ever asked a question about one of your patients that you either do not know or are unprepared to answer, *do not* ever make up data or answer in the affirmative if you are uncertain. Communicating inaccurate information can be dangerous to patient care, so please do not be afraid to say that you do not know the answer. Data can be easily looked up during rounds. Likewise, you can always ask the patient additional questions or further examine him or her, if need be, when you go see the patient with your team.

For both your patients and all the patients on your service, you should catalog their respective daily action plans ("things to do" for each patient during the day) by using small boxes that denote the completion status of each task. As tasks are completed throughout the day, you can checkoff the associated box to help you keep track of your progress in delivering patient care At first, it will seem impossible and overwhelming to keep up with everything that is being communicated by your team. Becoming efficient at this takes time and experience. Everyone has a different method of taking these notes, whether that be color-coding information or using shorthand. We encourage you to ask your immediate superior what works for him or her before devising your own organizational system as you learn what works best for you.

In addition to taking notes on the tasks that need to be completed for each patient throughout the day while on morning rounds, you should also make sure that your white coat pockets are filled with all the necessary supplies that will help your team be more efficient on rounds. This is typically the role assigned to whoever is currently "lowest on the totem pole." If you are a medical student, your intern can generally help you regarding what supplies you should carry, but a variety of tape, scissors, bandages, gauze, gloves, saline flushes, suture removal kits, and a light source are a good place to start. If you find yourself on a service that requires a lot of supplies on morning rounds and your white coat pockets cannot accommodate the volume, we suggest carrying a pink plastic emesis bin filled with your supplies instead. As you round, you should attempt to think of what the next patient will require and be ready to assist your superiors. Being able to anticipate which supplies are needed will become easier as you learn the patients on your service and how the service functions. Also, make sure to sanitize your hands before and after each patient encounter, even if the next patient on your list is in the same room.

After morning rounds are completed, you will often head to the preoperative holding area to introduce yourself to your patient prior to heading to the OR if you were assigned cases for that day. However, your responsibilities in the preoperative holding area, OR, and PACU will not last the entire day. Once you have dropped your last patient off in the PACU, you should quickly make your way back to the floor to either return to your daily floor work if you are an intern or to check in with a member of your surgical team if you are a medical student.

While on the floor during the day, surgical trainees should ask their superiors how they can best help the team. Although this applies to both medical students and interns, it is more common with the former. Common tasks that a medical student can assist with include: checking in on the status of patients, writing discharge summaries and progress notes, communicating with nursing staff and floor managers, as well as calling consults, just to name a few. Outside of helping the team, medical students should always check in on their individual patients throughout the day and ask the nursing staff if they have any concerns. Medical students have more time than their interns to interact with and care for their patients. This extra time with their patients provides medical students with the opportunity to potentially learn valuable information (eg, by obtaining medical records from outside hospitals or calling family members if the patient is a poor historian) that could end up making a considerable difference in the outcome of the patient. At the end of the day, the trainee will be required to handoff their patients to the night team during sign-out (see chapter on Handoffs).

Surgical trainees will also be assigned to attend clinic. During clinic, surgical trainees will often be asked to see patients prior to their superiors. You should obtain a detailed history, perform a PE, and present the patient before he or she is seen by the attending surgeon. Trainees may even be asked to come up with a differential diagnosis and management plan and will typically be tasked with writing the outpatient note for each patient they see in clinic before having the attending sign off on this documentation.

Finally, our conversation on surgical trainee expectations would be incomplete if we did not emphasize that your *primary goal* is to learn and grow as a surgeon-in-training. If you are on the floor and one of your patients, or any patient on your service for that matter, is going for a procedure or test (eg, endoscopy, echocardiogram, or arteriogram), you should try to accompany that patient to learn about the procedure or test being carried out and what this specific experience is like for that surgical inpatient. Trainees should constantly be observing, always be reading, and never stop challenging themselves to become better. However, learning does not always strictly entail observation. Oftentimes, the best way to learn is to do something *yourself*. In fact, without incorporating yourself into all the various tasks that comprise the full spectrum of patient care, whether that be obtaining a guaiac stool sample, placing a nasogastric tube, or removing sutures, the trainee will be unprepared to move on to the next level of his or her training. Carrying out even the most menial tasks in patient care serves a role in advancing your education and experience. Therefore, the role of the medical student and resident is one of apprenticeship. We all have to "pay our dues," but it is a time-tested method to effectively and efficiently learn this wonderful craft as we ascend up the ladder of responsibility.

PREPARATION

Although we briefly mentioned how to prepare yourself for the wards in our section on Expectations, it deserves further emphasis and a succinct review in its own section. To recapitulate, the junior surgical trainee needs to be prepared with photocopies of the patient list with updated vitals, ins and outs, and lab values each morning for rounds; to give presentations on their patients each morning in the format desired by the team (eg, SOAP note or I-PASS format[3-5]); with supplies for morning rounds; for their surgical cases during the day; for handoff at the end of the day; and to troubleshoot unexpected complications, which will be described in our next section. Furthermore, surgical trainees can also improve their utility at the bedside on the wards and in the OR by continuously practicing their technical skill set (eg, knot tying and suturing) (see our chapter on Knot Tying and our chapter on Technical Skills).

Surgical trainees should prepare for each individual day and for the upcoming week. As previously indicated, what this preparation specifically entails should be determined on the first day of the surgery rotation when trainees ask their superiors what is expected of them and how they can best help the team during their time on the service. How surgical trainees can best prepare for *each day* on the surgical services was described in our section on Expectations and summarized above. However, surgical trainees can also prepare for the *week ahead* on the wards by reading about the patients they will see in clinic, reviewing the cases they will scrub in on in the OR, and by possibly getting an early start on any special conference presentations they might be asked to execute.

Of course, all this preparation can be completed on a daily basis the night before you return to the hospital. Nevertheless, we emphasize the importance of weekly preparation here because you will have little free time during your days on service and the best opportunity for you to prepare for your clinic, say on Thursday, may be the prior Saturday or Sunday when you are home or have less work. This will allow you to take advantage of whatever free time you may have during your busy week and weekend.

Finally, we think it is essential to highlight the value of review. In the Introduction to this multimedia guide, we mentioned the importance of being a motivated adult learner. If you do not review the key teaching points you learned each day and over the course of the week (eg, reading about interesting patients, cases, or pathology you saw, or practicing the procedures or techniques you attempted), you will not grow as a clinician and surgeon.

TROUBLESHOOTING

It is extremely fitting to include our section on Troubleshooting directly after our discussion on Preparation. No matter how exceptional the care is on the surgical services, foreseen and unforeseen complications are guaranteed to arise. Ironically, these expected and unexpected events always seem to occur when the vast majority of your team is either busy with other patients on the wards or in the OR. Therefore, these complications can provide *prepared* surgical trainees with unique opportunities to be of real help to both their surgical teams and to their patients. We place considerable emphasis on the preparedness of the trainee in this situation for obvious reasons and must acknowledge the foresight of the great Louis Pasteur when he stated, "…fortune favors the prepared mind." Although your preparation may not always coincide specifically with the complication at hand, especially those that are unexpected, the likelihood of experiencing a successful outcome when troubleshooting is undoubtedly enhanced if you are prepared. This principle not only applies to medical students and other junior surgical trainees but to all members of the surgical team and the team as a whole.

As a surgical trainee, how will you approach complications and unexpected events? Outside of adequate preparation, this comes down to attitude, communication, and perspective. The best surgeons-in-training are calm and collected during stressful situations, trusted by their superiors, independently resourceful, and efficient with task completion. They demonstrate initiative and a capacity to translate an impressive preclinical fund of knowledge to patient care. Finally, they are relentlessly helpful and always demonstrate a willingness to assist the team, no what matter the circumstances may be. However, depending on the situation, sometimes the most helpful act the surgical trainee can engage in is actually stepping aside, especially when the surgical trainee is still at the medical student level. What do we mean by this?

Despite the fact that the primary goal of the junior surgical trainee is to learn and, in the surgical context specifically, achieve proficiency in one's technical and procedural skill set through hands-on experiences, there are times when patient care supersedes the hands-on educational experience of the trainee. During these times, the impact of the surgical trainee should be minimized so as not to compromise the outcome of the patient. In other words, the trainee should not get involved in the intervention taking place, nor get in the way of those caring for the patient. However, the surgical trainee should *still* remain in the room to observe, as this is vital to his or her education. There are times when it is obvious that the surgical trainee should not get involved, but there are times when this decision is not as clear to the medical student or even to the novice intern. To make matters more challenging, knowing *when* and *how* to be helpful is a skill that is not always taught. Nevertheless, it is important to be able to recognize the occasional situation that requires the surgical trainee to step aside and become either the passive or active observer.[6] The common example of this occurs during a code in which a typical junior surgical trainee has little to no experience and should not insert himself or herself into the team trying to revive the patient. In situations like this, there is a code leader who will assign responsibilities and may either assign you no tasks or ask you to get in line to provide compressions. The former assignment designates you as a passive observer while the latter makes you an active observer. The key here is being able to recognize which role to assume if those around you are unaware of your preparedness. If your fund of knowledge and skill set is insufficient, then the role of passive observer is appropriate. If this is not the case, you can assume the role of an active observer and wait until you receive specific instructions to provide assistance. Alternately, there may be situations when you have to perform life-saving maneuvers if a more senior physician is not readily available. In these situations, it is important to know what maneuvers are included within a reasonable scope of practice for your level of training. An example of this may be providing cardiopulmonary resuscitation (CPR) until help arrives.

This ability to quickly assess one's surroundings and know how one is best suited to help or not help is a skill that is rarely addressed with surgical trainees in any formal manner and requires the development of situational and interpersonal awareness. Mastery of these salient but more subtle and less tangible skills is extremely beneficial to surgical trainees and will not only help you when navigating through the "culture" of surgery but will continue to serve you well throughout your entire medical career. Although it is challenging to succinctly explain situational and interpersonal awareness here, it is our hope that simply introducing these ideas to you will help you become more aware of both the environment around you, within you, and among those around you. Understanding these concepts will also help you appreciate the roles and contributions expected of certain team members in various situations, will bring you awareness to the interpersonal dynamics often at play, and help you better communicate with all actors in the field. This will help you, as the surgical trainee, adapt and succeed in the dynamic environment of surgery.

Any surgeon can attest to the fact that there are unspoken rules of etiquette that are only revealed during embarrassing moments of blunder. The goal of the surgical trainee is to learn, be actively engaged, and help the team but to also avoid putting themselves into situations where they *do* blunder, either by impeding patient care or, worse, hurting the patient.

SUMMARY

FOR MEDICAL STUDENTS

The second and third years of medical school are an exciting time for medical students. It is a time when you actually get to care for patients and a time when you get to apply all the knowledge you have learned from your preclinical years. We encourage you to make the most of your time on the wards. Some students enter their surgical rotation and cannot get enough of the OR. Other students are not as excited about surgery and prefer to stay on the floor with their intern and help out with the "medicine" component of their surgical clerkship. While this is a valid way to spend your time learning if you are certain you do not want to pursue a career as a surgeon, we still encourage you to completely dedicate yourself to your surgical rotations and try to spend a significant amount of time in the OR. We advocate this because your surgical clerkship will be the *only* time during your entire medical career that you will have the opportunity to learn and appreciate surgical medicine. Even if you decide that surgery is not the career for you, you will still have learned a great deal about how this will affect your future patients who will either have surgical histories of their own or need to undergo surgery as part of their care with you. It is also worth noting that only 20% to 45% of medical students ultimately pursue the specialty that they were interested in during their first year of medical school when compared to their fourth year.[7] Therefore, if you assume that surgery is not the field for you without giving it the chance it deserves, you truly might be missing out on the field of medicine that you were meant to join.

We encourage you to learn how and when to be helpful. Recognize opportunities to contribute and build a reputation as being invested and willing to help. Be mindful that the best way you can help in certain situations is to step aside and not get in the way. Strive to address your own weaknesses and continue to work on your strengths. Constantly ask for feedback and never take constructive criticism personally. Be professional. Demonstrate initiative and be a self-motivated adult learner.

Your job as a medical student on the floor is to help provide quality care for the patients your service is responsible for and to also make your superiors look good. Do not seek individual accolades for work you accomplish. This will be noticed and the moment you go out of your way to make sure people know it was *you* who accomplished something, it will rub your team the wrong way. Always be the first person on the floor each morning and, before you leave the wards each day, ask your superiors if there is anything else you can do to help them. Know your patients. Ask questions, but do not ask questions you could or already should have looked up yourself.

At the end of the day, residents want their students to succeed, learn, and appreciate their time on the surgical service. When you, as the medical student, are motivated and curious, it makes it more enjoyable and inspiring for your superiors to teach. Furthermore, when you demonstrate proficiency and understanding of techniques or concepts later in your rotation after they were taught to you earlier, this pleases your superiors as they can see you are listening and digesting their lessons and advice. And who knows? You may even end up loving surgery, just like the authors of this chapter did on their surgical clerkships.

FOR INTERNS AND JUNIOR RESIDENTS

We commend you for your years of sacrifice and studying that has allowed you to reach this point in your careers. We also applaud you for having read through the above sections. Undoubtedly, it was mostly review. However, as mentioned previously, this review is still pertinent to your role as a surgical educator. In this regard, the above sections will serve to reminder you of what you should expect from your medical students, how you recommend they prepare for your service, how best you can guide them and teach them to troubleshoot when you are not available, and how to properly assess them. You will find the remaining portion of this manual much more appropriate to your level of training.

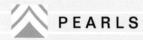

PEARLS

1. Understand your daily routine and what is expected of you early on in each rotation.
2. Do not hesitate to ask for support and be confident in voicing your opinion. Be sure to ask your seniors for feedback and avoid being defensive when receiving constructive criticism.
3. Development of situational and interpersonal awareness will help you navigate through the complex "culture" of surgery.

References

1. Graf K, Chaberny IF, Vonberg R-P. Beliefs about hand hygiene: a survey in medical students in their first clinical year. *Am J Infect Contr*. 2011;39(10):885-888.
2. Young JQ, Ranji SR, Wachter RM, Lee CM, Niehaus B, Auerbach AD. "July effect": impact of the academic year-end changeover on patient outcomes: a systematic review. *Ann Intern Med*. 2011;155(5):309-315.
3. Sectish TC, Starmer AJ, Landrigan CP, Spector ND; the I-PASS Study Group. Establishing a multisite education and research project requires leadership, expertise, collaboration, and an important aim. *Pediatrics*. 2010;126(4):619-622.
4. Starmer AJ, Sectish TC, Simon DW, et al. Rates of medical errors and preventable Adverse events among hospitalized children following implementation of a resident handoff bundle. *J Am Med Assoc*. 2013;310(21):2262-2270.
5. Starmer AJ, Spector ND, Srivastava R, et al. Changes in medical errors after implementation of a handoff program. *N Engl J Med*. 2014;371(19):1803-1812.
6. Miller DT, Norman SA. Actor-observer differences in perceptions of effective control. *J Personal Soc Psychol*. 1975;31(3):503-515.
7. Compton MT, Frank E, Elon L, Carrera J. Changes in U.S. medical students' specialty interests over the course of medical school. *J Gen Intern Med*. 2008;23(7):1095-1100.

2

HOW TO BE A SUCCESSFUL INTERN

ALESSANDRA STORINO, MD | WEI WEI ZHANG, MD

Surgery internship is both an exciting and difficult period for new physicians. Surgery is fast paced and dynamic and often can border on chaotic. Although this can be overwhelming at first, surgical interns have the opportunity to train in a stimulating field that few are ever exposed to. The following are a few guiding principles to ensure a productive and successful year.

BE PREPARED

Although it is impossible to be prepared for every challenge you will face, anticipating obstacles, being on time, and being ready for action will make you a valuable intern.

- **Be on time:** If the intern is late, the team is late. Being on time to work might seem an obvious, effortless task to accomplish for any motivated employee. However, when you are working 80 hours a week in 12- to

24-hour shifts, running up and down all day and often changing from days to nights, showing up on time demonstrates resilience. If you are late, you are putting a rough start on the day for everyone.

- Insider advice: Set up two independent alarms (night table and cellphone, for example) to minimize the risk that you sleep through your alarm. Eventually, you will figure out what works for you.
- **Write everything down:** Do not trust your memory. Instead, keep your list organized and have a pen and paper available at all times. You will be gathering information all day and it can easily get mixed up.
- **Know the jargon:** Learn abbreviations in advance. We use multiple abbreviations with the goal of keeping the census short. They might also be used verbally, for example, during sign out.
  - Insider advice: A few examples: AFVSS. ARBF. OOBx3. ADAT. HLIV or KOV.
- **Look the part:** Find out the dress code for meetings, lectures, and clinic and make sure you dress appropriately. It may seem trivial, but both your patients and your colleagues will make assumptions about you based on your appearance, so it is best to make the right impression. Do not let a dirty white coat or unkept hair take away from all that you have to offer.
- **Make transitions between services smooth:** Several times per year, you will be transitioning into a new service with a whole new dynamic. It is expected that you obtain sign out on all patients from your cointern coming off that service to ensure continuity of care.
  - Insider advice: It is useful to also ask how the service works, resources to study, most frequent surgeries performed, attending preferences, recovery protocols, etc.

DEVELOP YOUR OWN SYSTEM

Interns are a vital part of the surgical team and are sometimes referred to as the "floor general." They have the very important responsibility of executing daily plans discussed on morning rounds and handling new developments throughout the day. This is not an easy task, as workflow is frequently interrupted by attending rounds, clinic, consults, operating room (OR) cases, or other unplanned events. Regardless of all distractions, there is a set of tasks that must be invariably completed. Interns must be both organized and adaptable to get through the workday.

Although every surgical service workflow is unique, incorporating the following concepts into your day should improve efficiency:

- **Triage your day:** Your responsibilities are not all equally urgent. It is important to learn early on which tasks must be completed right away versus which can be saved for later. The goal is to complete time-sensitive tasks early so that everything is completed by the end of the day.
  - Insider advice: Always attend to sick or unstable patients first. Then work on coordinating procedures/consults and setting up discharges. If you are planning to have another team evaluate or perform a procedure on a patient, it is important to let them know early. Not only is this courteous to your colleagues but it also maximizes the chances of task completion by giving other services ample time to plan ahead.
  - Insider advice: Know which tasks may delay a patient's discharge. For example, advance a diet and remove a Foley early in the day on a patient who should be able to eat and void before being discharged, as compared with a dressing change that can happen anytime.
- **Follow up, follow up, follow up!** Timely review of pending workup is key. Allocate specific times to review pending results for *all patients*, so that interventions can be instituted in a timely manner. Carrying this out in a systematic way ensures that you do not miss *any* important results on *anyone*.
  - Insider advice: Be systematic. Review vital signs, urine output, laboratory work, pending cultures, imaging, and consultant recommendations for everyone, in the same order, every day. Highlight your "VIP players": on every service, there will always be patients who are sickest or at higher risk of complications. It is your responsibility to identify them and recognize any concerning signs early.
  - Insider advice: Check on these patients frequently. Find out who their nurse is and call them for updates if you are not immediately available to see them. Give advanced directives to nurses: I am worried about this patient, if he vomits, page me. If urine output is less than 25 mL in the next hour, page me. If they develop a fever, page me.

BECOME A PROBLEM SOLVER

It is natural for interns to take a more passive role in the beginning of the academic year, acting as "reporters of events" while they learn the dynamics of the team, work flow, and their new hospital. However, surgical interns often do not have their senior residents immediately available to them at all times. Thus, as interns gain more confidence and autonomy, they should be able to triage problems into those that they can solve on their own and those that need the attention of their seniors.

- **Just do it:** Get through your list to the best of your abilities so you can report them as resolved to your colleagues at sign out. Do not get used to leaving things pending for others to do. Your colleagues will appreciate it, and they will do the same for you.
  - Insider advice: If a dressing has to be changed, change it. If a patient needs consent for surgery, consent them. If a patient is out of surgery, do a postoperative check. If a family member requested an update, call them for an update.
  - Insider advice: At many institutions, the night team carries a large patient load and is only peripherally familiar with your patients. In addition, many elective subspecialty services are not available after hours. Because of this, many tasks are best completed during the day. Do not leave your night float colleagues to scramble for solutions with limited information and a skeleton crew.
- **Take ownership of your role as a doctor:** You have gone through many years of education to get to your internship and already have a robust fund of knowledge. Let go of your role as learner/observer as an MS4 and embrace your role as the patients' surgeon. The only way to becoming a sound clinician is through experience. When you identify an abnormal course, you should have a differential diagnosis, test your hypothesis, and make a plan for management before you report to your senior. This is the time to put all that theory into practice. And remember, your actions and decisions every day affect patient outcomes.
  - Insider advice: If a patient has low urine output, do not call your senior to report just that. Rather, take a minute to understand the problem, recall relevant events, and make recommendations accordingly. Is the urinary catheter clogged? Try flushing it. Do they need fluid resuscitation? Review the fluid balance. Do they have baseline kidney disease? Check baseline kidney function. You are often the person who knows the patient the best and are in the best position to troubleshoot the issue.

COMMUNICATE EFFICIENTLY

Effective communication is vital in the hospital environment. As an intern, you will be in constant communication with people of varying backgrounds, cultures, and educational attainments—from patients to floor nurses to other physicians. Each person you interact with has different perspectives regarding the patient's care. You must address their concerns as well as verbalize your own thoughts in a clear, concise, and nonjudgmental manner. Often times, your ability to communicate is just as important in determining your success as your technical performance and clinical accolades, so it is wise to invest time in developing your interpersonal skills early in your training.

Very few circumstances can be as stressful to an intern as is presenting patients to seniors or attendings, especially in the middle of the night. Similarly, rounds or sign-out can be stressful when you have many patients and events to report. Frequent flaws in communication include drowning in details of little relevance while overlooking important facts, not knowing critical information and failing to finalize the plan.

- **Know your patients well:** The more you know about your patients the more comfortable you will be talking about them. There is no shortcut in obtaining a good history, doing a focused but thorough examination and reviewing pertinent diagnostic studies. Similarly, round on patients frequently. Any team members can look up events recorded in the online medical record, but the bedside examination is irreplaceable. There are intangible data that cannot be obtained any other way, plus your patients appreciate the extra visit.
  - Insider advice: As you evaluate a patient, look around. Are there any drips going? What kind of vascular access do they have? Is there a Foley or a rectal tube?
  - Insider advice: A good intern has no surprises to disclose at sign out, including during overnight call. If you are concerned about a patient's status, let your senior know so that it can be addressed in a timely manner.
- **Keep it short:** A concise assessment is key. A good one-liner summarizes critical facts about a patient putting in context the information that will follow. They are often used to capture the attention of your senior/ attending when staffing a consult. However, the one liner is a good way to give a quick background before discussing a patient with any health care professional.
  - Insider advice: The one liner usually has four key components: Age, sex, distinguishing feature, and diagnosis. For example: "45M with atrial fibrillation on warfarin presents with an incarcerated umbilical hernia with bowel," "32F 15 weeks pregnant with uncomplicated appendicitis on MRI," "68M POD6 total knee replacement who now has an ileus."
  - Insider advice: When using a one liner to staff a consult, it is useful to predicate your statement with whether the consult is operative or not. For example: "Operative consult in ED, 45M with atrial fibrillation on

warfarin presents with an incarcerated umbilical hernia with bowel" or "Nonoperative consult on floor, 68M POD6 total knee replacement who now has an ileus."

- **Interpret clinical data:** When you are presenting a new patient, you should highlight the data points that provide the most information and that are more likely to change management. Indicate the severity of disease. Group data points together that are consistent with your clinical impression.
  - Insider advice: Do not read the whole computed tomography (CT) scan report or all laboratory results to your senior or attending. Rather, summarize the important results in a single sentence. Nevertheless, have all the information available in case it is requested.
  - Insider advice: Find out where the Radiology reading room is so that you can obtain preliminary results on images.
- **Key is in the follow-up:** Interventions have end points: a successful intervention is expected to have an effect over a lapse of time. Follow up with nurses and techs to make sure that the desired intervention is being carried out. Report to your seniors whether the end point has been met. Ask for the end point of interventions that you are not familiar with.
  - Insider advice: If a patient has a bowel obstruction, know whether they have had return of bowel function or not. If a patient has any type of drain (eg, nasogastric tube, abdominal drain, chest tube), know the output over time and quality of output. If a patient received diuretic therapy, know their change in weight or urine output.
  - Insider advice: Just because you place an order does not mean it will be completed. If it is a complicated or important task, make sure you communicate with the patient's care team so you are on the same page.

BECOME EFFICIENT

Per the Accreditation Council for Graduate Medical Education regulation, residents should work no more than 80 hours per week. If you use those 80 hours *efficiently*, you will be able to achieve your internship goals and keep a healthy rewarding life outside of the hospital.

- **Learn to multitask:** Although it might seem that we are frequently rushing to get things done in record time, we actually spend a lot of time just waiting for things to happen. The more prepared you are to make use of that time, the less likely you will be stuck at work after hours.

- Insider advice: Waiting for that CT to be completed, anesthesia to place an arterial line, a patient waking up after surgery, or your attending to show up for rounds? Work on your notes, return pages, or make some calls while you are waiting.
- **Anticipate delays during rounds:** Resident rounds tend to be very fast paced in comparison with attending rounds. Despite that, resident rounds are also thorough: wounds will be evaluated, pulses will be checked, nasogastric tubes will be flushed, and so on Anticipate what you can do to expedite rounds and assume an active role during them.
  - Insider advice: Make sure your list is prepped on time and is meticulously accurate.
  - Insider advice: Setting up a bucket with dressing supplies will expedite rounds and prevent you from running to the supply room repeatedly. Be sure to check which type of dressing will be needed for each patient and bring extra.
  - Insider advice: Have a Doppler available during Vascular Surgery rounds.
  - Insider advice: Premedicate for bedside procedures. If you are planning for a painful dressing change, coordinate for pain medication to be given in advance.
- **Keep the nurses in the loop:** There is no better way to ensure that tasks will be completed than personally discussing your plans with their nurse. Similarly, get used to asking nurses about events of the day. Remember that the only person who might know more about the patient than the intern is the nurse. Acknowledge their role and get them on board.
  - Insider advice: There is a lag time between writing an order online and nursing becoming aware of the order. You can overcome that delay by directly communicating your plans to the nurse.
- **Know your hospital system:** The hospital you rotated through during medical school may be very different from your training institution for residency. Hospital systems vary greatly in physical layout, patient population, culture, specialty strength, and services available. Familiarity with your local resources will make your life easier and your day run more smoothly.
  - Insider advice: Work smarter and not harder by maximizing the utility of your electronic medical records (EMR). Take the time to learn all the functions available in your system. Know how to find the information you need quickly. Save shortcuts and customize your home screen for easy access to commonly used functions. Use smart phrases and templates to make note writing easier and faster.
  - Insider advice: Get to know your work community. Meet the other doctors, nurses, administrators, and techs around you. Get to know their name and their role, engage in friendly banter, and exchange contact information if appropriate. You will find it easier to get things done if you are familiar with the people doing it.

WIN THE DISPOSITION GAME

In very brief terms, our goal as a surgical team is to identify patients' disease, treat the patients, and discharge them to continue their recovery elsewhere. Your role as an intern is to get them ready for that transition. Think daily about disposition for all patients. What is keeping this patient in the hospital today? Recognize barriers to discharge for your patients.

- Insider advice: Dig into their social history beyond drinking or smoking habits. Knowing where the patient lives, what kind of support they have, and their baseline performance status might help you recognize early who will benefit from social work, physical and occupational therapy, and case management consults to get them ready for discharge.
- Insider advice: Make sure you complete the medication reconciliation so that the appropriate home medications are started back for your patients. Failure to do so might cause complications and delays in discharge. Check with your team when is the right time to restart antihypertensives, diuretics, and anticoagulants postoperatively. Check if patients have chronic pain treated with analgesics at home and adjust accordingly in the postop setting.
- Insider advice: Work with social work and case management. Sending a patient to a rehabilitation facility involves assessing patient/family preference, bed availability, insurance authorization, and transport. Identify who the case manager is for your patients, and update them early on discharge plans.

PLAY NICE IN THE SANDBOX

For many new interns, residency may be their first experience in a professional environment. This shift of focus from learning to delivering patient care may be a difficult transition for some, as they must learn quickly how to work on a team, moderate conflict, and troubleshoot problems in a busy, high-stress environment. Success in residency is not just about clinical knowledge but depends heavily on how you interface with your workplace.

- **Be a team player:** Residency is hard enough, do not make it harder by making enemies. Throughout the 5 to 7 years of surgical training, you will spend countless hours with your coresidents and you will get to know them in nauseating detail. Help each other out and foster a collegial work environment. Residency is much easier when you have good people on your side.

- **Lies are the kiss of death:** You might think it is absurd that residents would make up information to please others, but it happens. This might be related to pressure from high expectations, fear to look like you are not prepared, and, most often, a sense that making an "educated guess" is better than admitting that you do not know. Regardless, do not do it. More often than not, you will be caught in the lie and your colleagues will stop trusting you. Over time, you will learn to anticipate what information is relevant. Meanwhile, when you are not sure about something, acknowledge that you do not know and rectify by obtaining the information that is needed.
  - Insider advice: Always check everything YOURSELF. Trust but verify. At the end of the day, you are accountable.
- **Treat EVERYONE with respect:** The hospital is a diverse work place, and you will interact with a multitude of people with different personalities and communications styles. There is guaranteed to be a difference of opinion at some point. When this occurs, you may feel the need to exert for authority as a physician, but this often leads to resentment. Instead, try to listen, develop mutual understanding, and diffuse the conflict tactfully. There is no substitution for a genuine appreciation for the people around you, what they do, and where they are coming from.
- **Be accountable:** As an intern, your daily work greatly affects the people around you, not just the patients who depend on you for their recovery but also your team and the entire hospital system. For example, if you forget to make someone NPO before surgery, the patient does not get his/her operation that day, your attending must rearrange his/her schedule, the OR reassigns staff and moves rooms, and the nurses' patient load changes. It is important to be responsible and have follow through. Stay organized and carry out your tasks to completion. It sounds simple, but if you were supposed to do something, do it in a timely fashion. This applies to clinical tasks as well as administrative duties.
- **Check your ego at the door:** New interns are often guarded when starting residency. They are eager to show off their knowledge and often look at being wrong as a sign of failure. However, in medicine, information is imprecise and the variables are ill defined and unpredictable. As a result, patients will frequently surprise you and you are going to be wrong often. It is best to embrace the unpredictability and stay humble.
  - Insider advice: You can learn something from everyone. When you are starting out, it is not just your senior residents and attendings who are teaching you. The people around you all have different perspectives and skill sets and are filled with useful information. Take the time to hear what they have to say and learn what they know. Similarly, you do not have to

100% agree with someone to learn from them. Just hear them out, process it, and decide whether the information is useful to you.

KNOW HOW TO RECEIVE FEEDBACK

As an intern, everyone is expecting to train you and feedback is an essential part of getting you to your potential. Although criticism is good for you, it may be difficult to take in and process at times. Regardless of how much effort you have dedicated to your job and how you think you performed, you should always be prepared for criticism. Receiving criticism is to your advantage, regardless of whether you think it is good or bad, fair or unfair.

- Insider advice: Ask your seniors and attendings for feedback halfway into your rotation so that you can actually act on their suggestions before you come off service.
- Insider advice: Do not compare yourself with others. During residency, it is very hard to gauge your performance relative to others because unlike college or medical school, everyone's experience is different. Furthermore, in residency there are no hard facts about your performance other than your ABSITE scores, which are important but might not fully reflect your surgical and clinical ability. Focus on your own progress.
- Insider advice: Your chief resident is instrumental to your education. You will learn how to manage the floor and function as an intern from your chief resident. Your chief resident has a lot of insight into your performance because you work so closely together, so take the time to process and internalize the feedback you receive from her/him.

YOU NEED TO STUDY

It may seem impossible to squeeze in study time into your routine as a new intern. However, becoming a surgeon requires a broad scope of knowledge, and self-directed learning is an integral part of your education. As you get settled into your intern year, you should develop a learning regimen that works for you.

- **Identify resources early:** There are so many studying resources available that it might be difficult to choose where to start. Ask other residents about their choices and try them before you spend a lot of money on a book that you might not like and will not use.

- **Study every day:** Developing the habit makes a lot of sense if you recognize that 30 minutes daily translate into 182 hours of studying over a year.
  - Insider advice: Consider videos, podcasts, and question banks as study resources for those days in which you do not have the energy or focus to read a whole book chapter.
- **Preparing for cases pays off:** Doing cases is a very effective way to solidify previous knowledge. If you study for your cases in advance, you will be learning a lot more than what you would if you did not have that first-hand exposure. Get in the habit of reading for every case, including both the disease process and the surgical technique.
  - Insider advice: Summarize your surgery in five essential, easy-to-remember steps. Over time, you will be able to add more details such as different type of incisions, instrument names, type of staplers, and suture material.
- **Take the time to learn at work:** Although it is extremely important to be efficient as an intern, do not forget to take a minute to take things in. When someone stops to give you a teaching point, focus on it and learn from it. When there is an interesting case, take a few minutes and read about it. When you get the opportunity to do something in the OR, take a deep breath, take your time, and try your best to absorb the experience.
  - Insider advice: Efficiency and learning are tied together. The quicker you can get through your daily tasks the more time you will have to focus on educational activities such as reading, attending lectures, or scrubbing cases in the OR.

LEARN TO SELF-CARE

Intern year is filled with transitions and obstacles. During this year, interns face long work hours, steep learning curves, a constant demand for efficiency, and lack of sleep. New interns face a big change in their lifestyle as they transition from a fostered learning atmosphere to the rigid structure of surgical residency. They have much less flexibility and control of their time than they did in medical school. In addition, new interns often fixate on living up to expectations, which may or may not be realistic. As a result, many interns have difficulties adjusting to their new life, which can range from insomnia to burn out to major depression. Finding a healthy way to adjust to the hardships of intern year is one of the most important things you can do for yourself. After all, your ability to take care of others will be impaired if you cannot manage to keep yourself together.

- **Know your limits:** The first step to self-care is self-awareness. Surgical residents are some of the strongest, most level-headed and hard-working people, but everyone has their limits. At some point during your residency, you *will* feel overwhelmed, either physically, emotionally, or intellectually. This is normal; residency is something that is meant to push you so that you grow. However, it is important to recognize when you have had too much.
- **Set boundaries and get some rest:** Few people realize that the adage "eat when you can, sleep when you can, and don't mess with the pancreas" is all about self-care. Residency is a stimulating experience filled with both opportunities and obligations. Although you want to maximize your experience during this time, it is also important to rest up while you can. You may want to always stay post call to cover cases and agree to every research opportunity that comes up, but you should be strategic about what you sign up for. Do not spread yourself too thin or you will be in danger of getting nothing done or burning out quickly. Try your best to spend some time outside of work and maintain a healthy lifestyle amid the chaos.
- **Avoid dehumanization:** Dehumanization is endemic in health care. The surreal and overwhelming experience of internship may lead some to view their patients and colleagues as tasks and obstacles. They may also be so consumed in their training that they lose a sense of themselves and what makes them a person. Although dehumanization can be viewed as a necessary defense mechanism, it can lead to a lack of empathy and cruelty toward oneself and others. Throughout your residency, try your best to treat those around you as individuals, and do not lose sight of the things that make you who you are.
- **Find social support:** Residency is difficult, and you will need people to support you through it. Whether it is family, friends, or colleagues, it is important to develop a social network during residency to keep you balanced and grounded.
- **Get help if you need it:** Just like urine output, your well-being is a dynamic variable that changes based on your current circumstance. It is important to periodically check in with yourself to make sure you are doing okay, especially if you are on a particularly difficult rotation or experiencing stressors outside of work. Many residents experience issues coping at one point or another during their residency. Just as you would not leave a patient oliguric on the floor, you should not leave your mental health unaddressed.
  - Insider advice: You should seek help if you experience insomnia, depression, anxiety, or substance abuse. Most residencies offer confidential counseling for trainees for situations like these.

CONCLUSION

Internship can be stressful and overwhelming, as well as a period of tremendous personal and professional growth. It will be an unparalleled learning experience, give you long-lasting friendships, and prepare you for the next stage in your career. It is impossible to anticipate every challenge you will encounter during internship. Perhaps, the best advice is to give the best of you every day: to your patients by taking excellent care of them, to your colleagues by being a helpful and reliable team player, and to yourself by taking ownership of your education.

 PEARLS

1. Know your patients well; learn to communicate efficiently. Develop your own system to increase efficiency.
2. Interpersonal relationships are important. Remain polite and respectful with your colleagues. If you feel burnt out, seek out assistance and support from available resources.
3. Read, read, read. Get in the habit of studying daily; this is your career not just an examination you need to pass anymore.

3

COMMON MEDICATIONS RESIDENTS USE

NISHA NARULA, MD | MADHU SIDDESWARAPPA, MD, MRCS (GLASGOW)

There are a host of medications that residents commonly use. These are categorized by organ system.

NEUROLOGIC/PSYCHIATRIC

A common call is one about a patient's agitation or delirium. The first step is to evaluate the patient and determine the severity, with a key part being determining if the patient is a danger to himself/herself or the staff. If yes, an antipsychotic is the best choice—a medication such as haloperidol that can be rapidly administered via the intramuscular route. If the agitation or delirium is mild, you have time to think of a thoughtful approach of how to address this both in the short and long term. Common medications for this are still antipsychotics and benzodiazepines, but do not forget nonpharmacologic means. Nonpharmacologic measures include reorienting the patient, encouraging family members to be at the bedside, maintaining a night/day sleep cycle, limiting tubes/lines/drains if medically possible, and not waking up the patient in the middle of the night: making the hospital room as close to home as feasible. However, these are not always effective. Restraints can be employed especially if the patient's agitation is either interfering with care, eg, due to pulling out lines (like intravenous lines), or harmful to others. Benzodiazepines are sometimes used, but these, although effective for sedative effects in the short term, can end up worsening delirium.

Benzodiazepines do have a use, however. Their strongest indications are for anxiety or panic disorders, as well as for insomnia. Nighttime pages for sleep medication are common and benzodiazepines are one option. Their main side effects include respiratory depression, somnolence, and delirium, so avoid in an already sleepy patient or one who will have trouble protecting their airway. Commonly used ones are midazolam (very short acting), alprazolam (by mouth only), lorazepam (short to medium length), diazepam (long acting), and clonazepam (long acting). Typically, for insomnia or acute anxiety, give lorazepam. Be wary of using these in patients with liver problems as they get metabolized slowly. Also include holding parameters. Although nurses will usually not administer these to sedated patients, the safest order would be to write holding parameters for a low respiratory rate (eg, lower than 10 breaths per minute) or sedation. Also avoid benzodiazepines in the elderly.

Another big category of medications is analgesic medication. Surgeons commonly prescribe opioids. When assessing what to give and how much, first see if patients are taking these long term, as they can develop tolerance. If they have never had adverse reactions to any opioids, you can start with any. Hydromorphone, morphine, and fentanyl are the commonly used intravenously; oxycodone, hydromorphone, morphine, or any of these medications in combination with acetaminophen orally; morphine or hydromorphone intramuscularly; morphine sublingually; and fentanyl as a transdermal patch. There are multiple conversions used for opioid equivalence to switch from one medication to another, but you quickly learn approximately how much each one is equivalent to. For instance, oxycodone usually starts at 5 mg by mouth (PO), morphine at 15 mg immediate release PO, or hydromorphone at 2 mg PO, and these are roughly equivalent. You can also give as a PCA (patient-controlled analgesia) or an epidural. Acetaminophen, nonsteroidal anti-inflammatory drugs (ibuprofen, Toradol), muscle relaxants, and others are good adjunctive measures. When writing a prescription make sure to include patient information, medication, instructions, and number to dispense. Include your Drug Enforcement Administration number and national provider identifier number to avoid getting phone calls from the pharmacy about these.

CARDIAC

Beta blockers (such as metoprolol, atenolol) should be continued on the day of surgery and postoperatively. If the patient is NPO (nothing by mouth), they can be converted to intravenous (IV) form (conversions available to be looked up). Angiotensin-converting enzyme inhibitors should be held on the day of surgery and restarted if low concern for kidney injury. Usually these are restarted when the patient can take oral medications. Hydrochlorothiazide is held postoperatively and restarted when the fluid balance is established. For all antihypertensives, holding parameters should be written for blood pressure, and for beta blockers and other medication affecting the heart rate, holding heart rate parameters should be written.

For hypertensive urgency or emergency, beta blockers or vasodilators can be used. Labetalol is best to bring down the blood pressure, metoprolol is best for heart rate, and with hydralazine the patient can get reflex tachycardia. Choosing between these depends not only on the patient's blood pressure and heart rate and what they can tolerate but also on what the floor is allowed to give IV because there are different policies. If in the intensive care unit (ICU), nicardipine, nitroprusside, and labetalol drips are other options.

For atrial fibrillation and flutter, if the patient is stable, choices of medications are metoprolol (three attempts), diltiazem, amiodarone, and finally digoxin. If unstable, will need to cardiovert, but at this point an ICU team or cardiology consult team should be involved in an urgent fashion.

Statins (eg, atorvastatin) are continued during the perioperative time unless the patient is strict NPO, as it has been shown to reduce postoperative adverse cardiac events.

PULMONARY

Albuterol is a beta-2 agonist and should be continued in the perioperative setting unless the patient has tachycardia. Ipratropium is an anticholinergic and similarly should be continued. Fluticasone is an inhaled steroid and can be continued. These can all be given as an inhaler or nebulizer. Encouraging the patient to get out of bed to a chair, ambulate, and use an incentive spirometer are also important for pulmonary rehabilitation.

GASTROINTESTINAL

A bowel regimen should be given (although first the patient should be passing flatus if he/she has undergone gastrointestinal [GI] surgery). Be careful about a per rectal regimen if the patient had an anorectal procedure or low colon/rectal anastomosis. Colace is a stool softener, whereas Senna, metoclopramide, and others are prokinetics. MiraLAX, magnesium citrate, and lactulose are osmotic agents. Fleet enemas can also be given. Methylnaltrexone is a mu receptor antagonist that can be given for ileus, although it is expensive. Disimpaction can be required for severe constipation at times.

For diarrhea, first infection needs to be ruled out, at minimum consisting of a *Clostridium difficile* workup. Once this is negative, fiber and loperamide are common agents to help with diarrhea.

Stress ulcer prophylaxis is needed for those who are critically ill. Sucralfate is typically given if it is a home medication or a patient has a known ulcer. An H2 blocker such as famotidine is best for general prophylaxis. A proton pump inhibitor such as omeprazole is associated with higher risks of *C. difficile* but can be continued if the patient already takes it at home. Lansoprazole comes in a sublingual formulation, which is useful. If a GI bleed is in the differential, a proton pump inhibitor should be used and given IV.

Antiemetics are commonly prescribed after surgery. Sometimes if a patient is distended or vomiting, a nasogastric tube is the best option. Medications to treat nausea, common after anesthesia and especially GI surgery, include ondansetron, prochlorperazine, promethazine, scopolamine patch, metoclopramide, steroids (although use with caution given risk of wound infection), and benzodiazepines. Erythromycin given IV is useful for gastric emptying.

GENITOURINARY

Patients frequently get urinary retention in the hospital. A bladder scan is frequently done to approximate the amount of urine in the bladder. It is often the only choice to get a sense of how much the patient is retaining or how much he/she has remaining after voiding, but it can be inaccurate, especially in patients who just had an abdominal operation or patients with cirrhosis. Straight catheterization is usually the best option and has a lower risk of urinary tract infection than replacing a Foley catheter, even if multiple straight catheterizations need to be done. Tamsulosin has long-term effects in men to reduce the risk of further retention.

In the early postoperative fluid, be judicious about restarting furosemide. If administering these newly for diuresis, PO and IV furosemide are converted in a 2:1 ratio. Other diuretics, such as hydrochlorothiazide and spironolactone should also be restarted judiciously.

Of note, for renally dosed medications, these need to be adjusted for those who develop kidney injury.

HEMATOLOGY

For DVT prophylaxis, either heparin subcutaneously or enoxaparin is used and continued in the perioperative period, sometimes even after discharge.

Therapeutic anticoagulation is administered in surgical patients either because they develop deep vein thrombosis (DVT)/pulmonary embolism (PE) postoperatively or because they come in already on it. Heparin drips are usually started at a stable dose (rather than a weight-based protocol), but in the case of an acute PE or lower extremity embolus, these can be administered as a weight-based bolus followed by a drip. It is quick on and quick off. Enoxaparin can also be administered and continued as an outpatient for high-risk patients. Warfarin for long-term anticoagulation sometimes needs a bridge with heparin depending on the indication. Many medications interact with it, and so choices should be made accordingly. It can be reversed with KCentra, fresh frozen plasma, and vitamin K (which takes longer). There are other new oral anticoagulants. In preoperative patients, these need to be held at various time frames most of the time. Make sure to look up half-lives and hold these accordingly. It is common to hold anticoagulants for four half-lives before surgery, and perhaps less if the consequences of a thrombotic complication would be devastating, for example, mechanical cardiac valve.

Antiplatelet agents include aspirin, which needs 7 days to wash out, but for most operations these do not need to be stopped preoperatively, and clopidogrel, which take 5 to 7 days to wash out.

Heparin-induced thrombocytopenia should be suspected with a drop in platelet count after heparin is administered. It can result in severe thrombosis. If suspected, stop heparin, get a PF4 antibody as a screening test and serotonin release assay to confirm, and start argatroban or bivalirudin in the meantime.

ENDOCRINE

Insulin sliding scales should be given to patients with diabetes or those on total parenteral nutrition. Those who are NPO should have finger stick blood glucose checked q6 hours and those who are on a diet QACHS (before each meal and before bedtime). Start administering insulin at a glucose of 150 and give 2 units subcutaneously, increasing by 2 for every 50. Always include orders for hypoglycemia. If a patient is NPO, give long acting at 50% to 80% of the dose. An insulin drip can be used on certain floors and in the ICU.

Steroids should be continued for those who were taking them preoperatively and given on the day of surgery. Stress dose steroids were commonly administered in the past, but for many operations, even if the patient is taking them long term, these are not always necessary. Discuss with an attending and the anesthesia team to clarify. Look up PO to IV conversions.

Levothyroxine can be given PO or IV (2:1 conversion) and continued in the perioperative period, although missing a few doses is okay because it has a long half-life.

MISCELLANEOUS

Contrast can be given PO (barium, which is not water soluble, or gastrografin, which is water soluble) and/or IV (iodinated for a computed tomography scan or gadolinium for magnetic resonance imaging). For certain instances, it can be given per rectum or through a tube or ostomy. Be careful in those with acute kidney injury or chronic kidney disease; some patients need prehydration with IV contrast. Consider allergies, as some may need desensitization with steroids and diphenhydramine if they need contrast.

In pediatrics, remember to use weight-based dosing for medications. In pregnant or lactating patients, look up medications to ensure they are safe. For patients who get enteral medications through a nasogastric tube, make sure to use crushed or liquid medications. Nasojejunal tubes (such as a Dobhoff) easily get clogged and medications are required to be given in liquid form.

Resources to ask for questions on medications include senior residents, nurses, pharmacists, Epocrates, and UpToDate.

LIST OF COMMON MEDICATIONS

ANALGESICS

Tylenol 325 to 650 mg PO/PR q6
Tylenol #3 (codeine/APAP 30/300) 1 to 2 tabs PO q4-6
Percocet (oxycodone/APAP 5/325) 1 to 2 tabs PO q4-6
Oxycodone 5 mg PO q4-6
Vicodin (hydrocodone/APAP 5/500) 1 to 2 PO q4-6
Ketorolac 15 to 30 mg IV q6-8 (avoid in kidney insufficiency)
Morphine 1 mg IV q2 (dose can be increased if needed)
Fentanyl 25µg IV q2 (dose can be increased if needed)

Dilaudid 1 mg IV q4 (dose can be increased if needed)
Fentanyl patch 25 to 100 µg transdermal q3 days
PCAs (starting doses):
    Morphine 1 mg q8 minutes, 32 mg lockout
    Fentanyl 10 µg q10 minutes, 240 µg lockout
    Dilaudid 0.1 mg q8, 3.2 mg lockout

ANTIEMETICS

Zofran 4 mg IV q6
Phenergan 12.5 to 25 mg IV/PO/PR q6 (be cautious in the elderly)

ANTIBIOTICS

Ampicillin/sulbactam 3 g IV q6
Cefazolin 1 g IV q8
Clindamycin 600 mg IV/PO q8
Fluconazole 200 to 400 mg IV/PO q24
Ertaenem 1000 mg IV q6
Levaquin 500 mg IV/PO q24
Linezolid 600 mg IV/PO q12 (usually needs ID approval)
Metronidazole 500 mg IV/PO q8
Piperacillin/tazobactam 3.375 mg IV q6
Vancomycin 1 g IV q12

PROPHYLAXIS

Heparin 5000 units SQ q8
Enoxaparin 30 mg SQ BID
Famotidine 20 mg IV/PO q12
Esomeprazole 40 mg IV/PO q24

CARDIOVASCULAR

Metoprolol 5 mg IV q6 converts to 12.5 mg PO BID, 5 mg IV ×1 is a good start
    for AF
Diltiazem 10 mg IV ×1 for AF with RVR, SVT, also used as a drip in the ICU
Hydralazine 10 mg IV q20 minutes (only to bring down hypertension acutely)
Furosemide 10 to 80 mg IV/PO, PO dose = 2× IV dose

ELECTROLYTE REPLACEMENT

Potassium 10 mEq for every 0.1 below 4.0. Ex. K = 3.6, give 40 mEq (PO better than IV)

Magnesium 1 g for every 0.1 below 2.0. Ex. Mg = 1.8, give 2 g IV. Mg oxide PO can cause diarrhea but is 400 to 800 mg. Phosphate is given either as K-Phos or Na-Phos. Dose is usually in the range of 15 to 21 mMol IV

OTHERS

Diphenhydramine 12.5 to 25 mg IV/PO q6 (be cautious in the elderly)

Hydroxyzine 25 to 100 mg PO q6-8

Zolpidem 5 to 10 mg PO qHS

Colace 100 mg PO BID

Dulcolax 10 mg PR

Lovenox 1 mg/kg SQ BID (treatment dose for DVT)

 PEARLS

1. Place patients on their home medication regimen whenever permitted.
2. Approach your patients systematically; be sure to take note of all relevant comorbidities and conditions to select the most appropriate medications to prescribe.
3. Switch from IV to oral preparations when possible. If using IV preparations, be sure to adjust the dose accordingly. The pharmacy can help with this step if necessary until you get a strong grasp over the conversion rates.

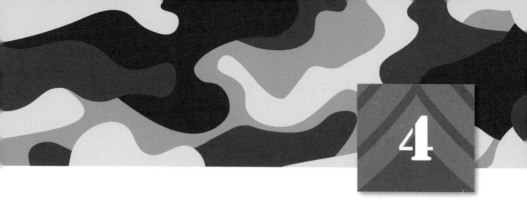

FLUID RESUSCITATION AND MANAGEMENT

CARLY D. COMER, MD | CHARLES S. PARSONS, MD

Fluid resuscitation and management is a main component of preoperative and postoperative care for the operative patient. As surgeons, we are often making patients NPO (nothing by mouth), decompressing the stomach or gastrointestinal tract, leaving drains, or otherwise altering a patient's innate ability to maintain their fluid status. The same holds true during a trauma situation. A patient with a traumatic injury that requires operative intervention must first be stabilized via fluid resuscitation before heading to the operating room. Thus, it is important that, as surgeons, we understand the clinical implications for fluid resuscitation and management alongside electrolyte needs.

ASSESSING A PATIENT'S FLUID STATUS

In the immediate postoperative period, a patient will have fluid deficits resulting from preoperative and intraoperative fluid losses. Surgery induces an inflammatory state in the body, resulting in cytokine release and consequential vascular permeability and low intravascular volume (even if their overall fluid balance is positive). Therefore, it is important to properly assess a patient's fluid status (ie, are they euvolemic, hypovolemic, or hypervolemic) through physical examination and review of their "in's and out's" and laboratory tests. Common signs and symptoms to look out for are tachycardia, hypotension, dry mucous membranes, poor skin turgor, altered mentation, and oliguria. Urine output is also a reliable way to monitor a patient's volume status. The average adult should be producing at a minimum of 0.5 mL/kg/h, which for most adults, is an hourly urine output of 30 to 50 mL/h.

When looking a patient's fluid status, it is important to think if the patient is volume depleted, requiring resuscitative fluid, or if the patient is adequately hydrated but needs assistance maintaining the volume status with maintenance fluid.

RESUSCITATIVE FLUIDS

Resuscitative fluids share the common characteristic of isotonic volume expansion. The two main types of volume expander solutions are crystalloids and colloids. Crystalloids are aqueous solutions of mineral salts or other water-soluble molecules. Colloids contain larger insoluble molecules. Colloid solutions, such as 5% albumin, assists with volume resuscitation by increasing and preserving intravascular oncotic pressure, which consequently increases intravascular volume. Although it takes a lesser amount of colloid than crystalloid to fully resuscitate a patient, liberal use of colloid fluid has not demonstrated improved patient outcomes or survival in comparison with crystalloid fluid use, and it is much more expensive. One liter of normal saline (NS) can be <$1, whereas an equivalent dose of albumin is $100.

Two common isotonic crystalloid solutions to choose from are lactated Ringer (LR) solution or NS (0.9% NaCl). LR is more similar to extracellular fluid composition, as it not only includes more comparable physiologic concentrations of sodium (Na^+) and chloride (Cl^-) but also includes potassium (K^+), bicarbonate (HCO_3^-) and calcium (Ca^{2+}). NS includes only Na^+ and Cl^- and at a higher concentration than extracellular fluid. Normosol and PlasmaLyte are two other types of crystalloid fluids utilized. Like LR, these fluid solutions have a more alkalized pH and are more closely equivalent to that of extracellular fluid (ie, plasma). For a complete look at the electrolyte composition (mEq) of crystalloid fluids, refer to Table 4.1.

Crystalloid fluid boluses can be given at volumes of 10 to 20 mL/kg until adequate resuscitation (as measured by clinical end points such as urine

TABLE 4-1 Electrolyte Composition (mEq) of Crystalloid Fluids

Fluid	Na⁺	K⁺	Cl⁻	Ca²⁺	Buffer	Dextrose (g)	pH	Osmolality
Extracellular fluid	142	4	103	5	27 (HCO_3^-)	0	7.4	280
Lactated Ringer	130	4	109	2.7	28 (lactate)	0	6.5	275
Normal saline (0.9% NaCl)	154	0	154	0	0	0	4.5	308
½ Normal saline (0.45% NaCl)	77	0	77	0	0	0	4.5	154
5% Dextrose in water	0	0	0	0	0	50	5.0	278
Normosol	140	5	98	0	27 (acetate) 23 (gluconate)	0	6.6	294
Plasma-Lyte	140	5	98	0	27 (acetate) 23 (gluconate)	0	7.4	294

output). In the hospital you will see 500 mL or 1 L fluid boluses given, which does roughly correspond to the resuscitation volume of 10 to 20 mL/kg for the vast majority of adult patients. When deciding between LR and NS, typically either can be chosen, although surgeons are partial to LR because of it being closer to physiological concentrations. There are some patient types, however, where surgeons would prefer NS to be used for resuscitation. The first is a neurosurgery patient or a patient who comes in with head trauma or a traumatic brain injury. In these patients NS is preferred in an attempt to drive up their intravascular sodium concentration to draw fluid out of the parenchyma in the brain and reduce intracranial pressure. A second patient type where the use of NS is preferred is with transplant patients. It is better for these patients to not receive the additional K+ or lactate (when discussing kidney or liver, respectively) that is found in LR.

Colloid solutions are solutions that contain large insoluble molecules, generally proteins or complex polysaccharides, which are dispersed evenly throughout the solution. Albumin, packed red blood cells, platelets, and fresh frozen plasma are all colloid solutions, and each is utilized when clinically indicated. Albumin comes as 5% and 25%, differing only in the dilution of the protein within NS. One unit of 5% albumin is approximately 250 mL of fluid and 1 unit

TABLE 4-2 Electrolyte Composition (mEq) of Albumin Versus Plasma

Fluid	Na+	K+	Cl−	Ca²⁺	HCO₃−	Dextrose	pH	Osmolality
Plasma	142	4	103	5	27	0	7.4	280
5% Albumin	145	0	0	0	0	0	7.4	290

of 25% albumin is 50 mL of fluid. For a complete look at the composition of 5% albumin in comparison with plasma, refer to Table 4.2. It is important to note that the best colloid solution, if clinically indicated, is packed red blood cells.

MAINTENANCE FLUIDS

Maintenance fluids replace a patient's sensible (ie, quantifiable losses, such as urine) and insensible fluid losses (ie, unquantifiable losses, such as cutaneous losses from the skin and upper respiratory tract if on mechanical ventilation). The average daily amount of insensible losses is 8 to 12 mL/kg. The daily maintenance fluid rate for a patient can be calculated utilizing the hourly "4-2-1 rule" or the 24-hour "100-50-20 rule," also known as the Holliday-Segar method. Both are weight-based rules. According to the 4-2-1 rule, for the first 10 kg of the patient's body weight 4 mL/kg/h of fluid is administered, for the second 10 kg of the patient's body weight 2 mL/kg/h of fluid is administered, and for each kilogram >20 kg 1 mL/kg/h is administered. As an example, according to the 4-2-1 rule, a 70-kg patient would receive a maintenance fluid rate of 110 mL/h (ie, 40 + 20 + 50). According to the Holliday-Segar Method, for the first 10 kg of the patient's body weight 100 mL/kg/d is to be given, for the second 10 kg of the patient's body weight 50 mL/kg/d is to be given, and for each kilogram >20 kg 20 mL/kg/d is to be given. Referring back to our 70-kg patient example, per the Holliday-Segar Method, this patient should receive a total of 2500 mL/d (ie, 1000 + 500 + 1000) of maintenance fluids, which comes to 104 mL/h. A common maintenance fluid rate written for both surgical and nonsurgical patients in the hospital is 100 mL/h. This again is open to variation depending on the patient's weight and clinical situation.

Postoperative patients get maintenance fluid if they cannot eat or drink. The standard maintenance fluid is half normal saline (½NS; 0.45% NaCl) with 5% dextrose (a glucose source), with the shorthand form written as D5 ½NS. It is important to remember to never bolus a postoperative patient with maintenance fluid. If you are giving a patient a bolus, it is because he/she is showing signs or symptoms of underresuscitation and requires resuscitative fluid, ie LR or NS. Furthermore, if a patient is diabetic, it is appropriate to write him/her for maintenance fluids without dextrose, ie ½NS. This will help mitigate the pages you get regarding their increasing serum glucose levels and increasing insulin requirements.

CONCLUSION

Fluid resuscitation and management creates its own set of clinical challenges and should be reassessed for each patient regularly, with increasing frequency for critically ill or quickly evolving patients. For stable postoperative patients, you will be providing them with fluid and monitoring their electrolytes until they are properly tolerating a diet of some kind, at which time their body usually will no longer require assistance to maintain proper fluid status. However, until they are normalized, each patient deserves regular assessment to develop an appropriate fluid repletion and maintenance plan.

 PEARLS

1. It is important to assess a patient's fluid status. The clinical picture helps in assisting if the patient requires more or less fluid. For the majority of adult patients, an hourly urine output of 30 to 50 mL/h is appropriate and expected.
2. Common fluid bolus amount given in the hospital is 500 mL or 1 L of NS or LR.
3. D5 ½NS is the usual maintenance fluid provided. The hourly 4-2-1 rule or 24-hour Holliday-Segar Method can assist you in determining the rate to run a patient's maintenance fluid.

Suggested Reading

1. Kuglar N, Paul JS. Fluid and electrolyte therapy. Cameron JL, Cameron AM, eds. *Current Surgical Therapy.* 12th ed. Philadelphia, PA: Elsevier; 2017.

5

COMMON INFECTIONS AND ANTIBIOTICS

AMMARA WATKINS, MD | MOLLY J. DOUGLAS, MD

Becoming familiar with common infections and antibiotics is important. This chapter does not delve into the details of antibiotic mechanism of action. Rather it provides a quick, pragmatic reference for common infections and antibiotic regimens in the hopes to familiarize the reader with these everyday scenarios. Depending on institutional hospital antibiograms and prescribing practices, there may be some differences in regimens noted here. As always, when starting antibiotics, it is important to consider appropriate indications. Starting antibiotics early, specifically within 1 hour of suspicion of a severe infection/sepsis, may be life saving. At the same time, it is important to de-escalate antibiotics as cultures become available and plan a tentative stop date when initiating antibiotic therapy. Source control must also be achieved, as antibiotics are minimally effective if there is an ongoing source for infection such as undrained abscess, infected foreign body, or perforated bowel.

HOW TO THINK ABOUT INFECTIONS

Managing infections can be boiled down into three basic steps:

1. Diagnosing that infection is present (done with clinical examination, imaging, and cultures)
2. Source control (eg, drainage, operation and washout, removal of infected foreign bodies)
3. Match up the bugs and drugs (treat with appropriate antimicrobial therapy. This should include discontinuing antibiotics when no longer needed)

KEEPING UP TO DATE

Microbes and their response to antibiotics are constantly changing, and the recommendations in this guide may quickly become out of date (last updated August 2018).

Please consult your local/institutional antibiogram to choose regimens appropriate for your local resistance patterns. For general guides to antimicrobial sensitivities, apps such as the Johns Hopkins ABX app or Sanford Guide may be useful.

The Infectious Disease Society of America (IDSA, www.idsociety.org) is an excellent resource for updated evidence-based guidelines on infection diagnosis and treatment and is the source for the majority of the therapy regimens included in this chapter.

URINARY TRACT INFECTIONS

Urinary tract infections (UTIs) are common among hospitalized patients, particularly when there has been an indwelling Foley catheter in place (ie, CAUTI, catheter-associated urinary tract infection).

DIAGNOSIS

- SUSPECT based on symptoms (dysuria, frequency), laboratory tests (leukocytosis without alternate source), or global changes such as altered mental status (particularly in the elderly) or sepsis.
- TEST with urinalysis and culture—positive findings include nitrites, leukocyte esterase, and bacteria on urinalysis and >100,000 colony forming units (cfu)/mL of a particular bacteria on culture.

- If coexisting sepsis or back pain, consider computed tomography (CT) for pyelonephritis or obstructing ureteral stone.

SOURCE CONTROL

- Remove any urinary tract foreign bodies if permissible, eg. Foley catheters. (Also, reduce risk by avoiding unnecessary urinary catheters.)
- Upper urinary tract infections may require urology consultation for removal of obstructing stone.

BUGS AND DRUGS

- Mostly gastrointestinal (GI) tract organisms due to anatomy.
- *E. coli* accounts for the majority of UTIs. Other organisms include other Enterobacteriaceae (*Proteus mirabilis, Klebsiella pneumonia*), *Staphylococcus saprophyticus*. Organisms such as lactobacilli, enterococci, group B streptococci, and coagulase-negative staphylococci (except *S. saprophyticus*) are usually contaminants.
- Do not treat asymptomatic bacteriuria (except in pregnancy).
- Recommended regimens (in order of preference):
  - Nitrofurantoin 100 mg by mouth (PO) twice a day (BID) for 5 days (uncomplicated, non-CAUTI UTI only)
  - Bactrim DS 160/800 PO BID for 3 days
  - Ciprofloxacin 500 mg or Levofloxacin 750 mg PO BID daily for 3 days
  - Fosfomycin 3 g single dose
  - *Increase regimen duration to 7 days if catheter-associated UTI*
  - Augmentin, cefdinir, cefpodoxime-proxetil for 3 to 7 days are appropriate if above cannot be used; beta-lactams usually less effective than the above-mentioned alternatives.
  (Resistance to ampicillin/amoxicillin is common—do not use for UTI.)

HOSPITAL-ACQUIRED PNEUMONIA AND VENTILATOR-ASSOCIATED PNEUMONIA

DIAGNOSIS

- SUSPECT based on fever, cough, increased sputum, and often leukocytosis.
- TEST usually with chest x-ray—positive is infiltrate/consolidation in conjunction with above-mentioned symptoms. (Do not treat an x-ray finding on an asymptomatic patient.)

- In intubated patients, endotracheal aspirate (rather than directed or blind bronchoalveolar lavage) is recommended by the IDSA to obtain sample for culture. Positive culture is >100,000 cfu/mL of a single organism.
- In nonintubated patients, attempts at culture via expectorated sputum, induced sputum, or nasotracheal suctioning are recommended by the IDSA to guide therapy. However, samples are often inadequate and grow multiple contaminants, and strength of this recommendation is low.

SOURCE CONTROL

- Usually nothing to drain in early pneumonia
- In more advanced infections, parapneumonic effusions may develop and progress to empyema, which would require chest tube drainage. Loculated/fibrotic empyemas may require video-assisted thoracic surgery (VATS) decortication for full source control and lung re-expansion.

BUGS AND DRUGS

- Hospital-acquired pneumonia (HAP) treatment should be influenced by recent antibiotic use, known hospital flora, and underlying/preexisting conditions. Once culture and sensitivity are available, narrow antibiotics accordingly.
- Generally, empiric therapy should cover methicillin-resistant *Staphylococcus aureus* (MRSA) (gram-positive coccus), *Pseudomonas aeruginosa* (gram-negative rod), and gram-negative bacilli.
- Regimens are broadly divided into those with coverage of multidrug-resistant organisms (MRSA, multidrug resistant (MDR) *Pseudomonas*) and those without.
  - How do you know which to use?
  - Factors that contribute to MDR pneumonia include previous intravenous (IV) antibiotics within 90 days, hospitalization >5 days, high frequency (>10%) of MDR pneumonia at the hospital or intensive care unit, septic shock at the time of HAP, and immunosuppression.
- HAP with no risk factors for MDR may be treated with one of the following:
  - Fluoroquinolone: Levofloxacin 750 mg PO/IV daily or Ciprofloxacin 400 mg IV q6h
  - Cephalosporin: Cefepime or ceftazidime 2 g IV q8h

- Zosyn (piperacillin-tazobactam) 4.5 g IV q6h
- Carbapenem: Imipenem 500 mg IV q6h or Meropenem 1 g IV daily.
- If risk factors for MRSA, ADD to above:
  - Vancomycin 15 mg/kg IV q8-12h (adjust for vancomycin trough of 15-20 mg/mL)
    or
- Linezolid 600 mg IV q12h
- If there is concern for gram-negative (GNR) bacilli resistance (*Enterobacter, Serratia, Pseudomonas*), use *two* anti-GNR antibiotics together, usually a beta-lactam (Zosyn, cephalosporin, or carbapenems as listed earlier) and a non-beta-lactam agent such as:
  - Fluoroquinolones: Levofloxacin or ciprofloxacin as earlier
  - Aminoglycosides: Amikacin 15 to 20 m/kg IV daily, gentamicin 5 to 7 mg/ kg IV q24h
  - Polymixins: Colistin or polymyxin B
- Seven days of treatment is adequate for most patients with ventilator-associated pneumonia. Longer durations may be indicated depending on the improvement of clinical, radiological, and laboratory parameters (be aware the chest x-ray appearance will lag behind clinical improvement).

CLOSTRIDIUM DIFFICILE INFECTION

Clostridium difficile (C. diff) is a gram-positive anaerobic rod that mainly infects the colon. It most commonly occurs in people with altered GI flora due to recent antibiotic use and is more common in those who have spent time in institutions (eg, nursing home, hospital). Disease can cover a spectrum from mild with diarrhea and abdominal pain to fulminant colitis with life-threatening sepsis.

DIAGNOSIS

- SUSPECT in patients with new otherwise-unexplained diarrhea, abdominal pain, and/or rising WBC (very high white blood cell counts, eg, 30 to 40k cells/mL can be associated with C. diff).
- TEST for C. diff toxin in stool sample (usually polymerase chain reaction, but varies by laboratory). Do not test asymptomatic patients, as asymptomatic carriage is possible.

SOURCE CONTROL

- Generally achieved with antibiotics alone (see later text)
- Fulminant colitis with life-threatening infection may require total abdominal colectomy for source control
- Stool microbiota transplant is useful for multiply-recurrent disease

BUGS AND DRUGS

- First, stop the inciting antibiotic if possible. (Commonly implicated medications are clindamycin, penicillin, fluoroquinolones, and cephalosporins. If antibiotics are indicated, use those that are less implicated in C. diff infections (vancomycin, macrolides, and tetracyclines).
- Next, start anti-C. diff antibiotics.
  - First line: Oral Vancomycin 125 mg PO q6h *or* Fidaxomicin 200 mg BID for 10 days
  - Severe disease: Oral Vancomycin 500 mg q6h *plus* Metronidazole 500 mg IV q6h; *add* rectal Vancomycin enemas (500 mg in 100 mL NS q6h) if ileus
  - If vancomycin not available: metronidazole 500 mg PO/IV TID for 10 days (previously considered first line)
  - Recurrent disease: options included tapered/pulsed dosing of oral vancomycin, use of fidaxomicin if vancomycin previously used
  - Multiple recurrences: Stool microbiota transplant improves cure rate
- Be aware—Vancomycin works on C. diff in the **lumen** of the colon, thus enteral therapy is required. IV vancomycin will not treat C. diff. Also, enteral vancomycin is not systemically absorbed and will not treat infections elsewhere in the body. Enteral vancomycin also has no effect on renal function and can be used at the same dose in patients with renal failure.

SURGICAL SITE INFECTIONS

Wound classification strongly predicts the incidence of surgical site infections (SSIs).

- Clean wound (no breaks in sterility, eg, hernia): <2%
- Clean-contaminated (contact of the field with a nonsterile body compartment, with minimal contamination/spillage, eg, elective colon resection with prepped bowel): <5%
- Contaminated (spillage of infectious material, followed by rapid source control, eg, gunshot wound to colon): 13% to 20%

- Dirty (established infection, generally delayed source control compared with contaminated wounds. eg, abscess, perforated diverticulitis with fecal contamination): 30% to 40%

SSIs may be **superficial** (in the skin, subcutaneous tissue) or **organ space** infections.

DIAGNOSIS

- SUSPECT based on wound redness, swelling, or purulent/turbid drainage for superficial SSI or based on increased surgical site pain, fevers, leukocytosis, functional problems (ie, ileus) for deep/organ space infections.
- TESTING rarely required beyond clinical examination for superficial infections. Consider CT or ultrasound depending on site for concern for deeper infections.

SOURCE CONTROL: THIS IS THE MAINSTAY OF TREATMENT

- Superficial SSI: Open the wound (can usually be done at bedside) and drain any purulence. Continue local wound care (packing or vac dressing, until healed)
- Deep space SSI: Depends on location; may require image-guided drain or operative washout
- Explant of prosthetics (eg, hardware, hernia mesh) may be needed if infected

BUGS AND DRUGS

- Antibiotics rarely required for superficial SSIs as long as adequately drained. Consider a short course (3-5 days) if there is significant surrounding cellulitis
- Deep space: Often 4 to 14 days of antibiotics in addition to source control; target drugs to likely pathogen by site and narrow when cultures available

CENTRAL VENOUS LINE INFECTION

Central venous catheters are infamous for creating an entry site for bacteria and may precipitate systemic infection with bacteremia or local insertion site infection with cellulitis or abscess. The femoral site carries the highest risk of catheter infection, followed by internal jugular then subclavian. Total parenteral nutrition (TPN) administration increases the infection risk. The most common species isolated include *Staphylococcus epidermidis*, *S. aureus* and yeast. Infection prevention is best achieved through adhering to "bundles" to ensure sterility during placement and each time the catheter is accessed, placing catheters only when needed and removing them as soon as no longer indicated.

DIAGNOSIS

- SUSPECT in patients with indwelling central venous catheters with new fevers, sepsis, leukocytosis, or signs of insertion site infection (redness, swelling, purulent drainage).
- TEST with blood cultures (one peripheral and one from the catheter); consider culture of catheter tip after removal. Culture any purulence at insertion site.
- Check surveillance cultures q48h to determine when bacteremia clears.
- Further reading: CLABSI and CRBSI (central line–associated versus central line–related blood stream infections) have different definitions based on the rigor with which the catheter is implicated as the source of infection, using differential time to positivity and quantitative culture results. This is beyond the scope of this chapter, but a good overview is found at lifeinthefastlane. com/ccc/central-line-infections.

SOURCE CONTROL

- Consists of removing the infected line and draining any local abscess at the insertion site (if present).
- Give a 24- to 48-hour "line holiday" if possible after line removal before inserting a new line.
- Negative blood cultures are preferred before inserting a new line, particularly if it will be a long-term line (eg, tunneled dialysis catheter, Hickman for long-term TPN).

BUGS AND DRUGS

- Will almost always be able to target to culture data
- Potential etiologies and drugs include:
  - Gram-positive cocci (GPCs) (non-MRSA): oxacillin, cefazolin
  - MRSA: vancomycin, linezolid, daptomycin

- GNR: Zosyn, cefepime, carbapenems
- Yeast (cover empirically in immunosuppressed patients and those with hematologic malignancy or who have already been on broad-spectrum antibiotics): fluconazole, amphotericin (preferred in neutropenic patients)
- Duration of treatment is 7 to 14 days from the time of the first negative blood culture and longer in cases of immunosuppression
- If blood cultures fail to clear, look for other uncontrolled sources (eg, endocarditis, osteomyelitis, prosthetic infections)

GASTROINTESTINAL INFECTIONS (APPENDICITIS, CHOLECYSTITIS, DIVERTICULITIS)

These infections often require surgery for definitive treatment. A complete discussion of their workup and operative management is beyond the scope of this chapter. However, antibiotics will frequently be needed as the patient awaits surgery or if nonoperative management is chosen. GI infections require broad-spectrum coverage against gram-negative rods and anaerobes.

Duration of treatment depends on clinical situation and may include stopping antibiotics after surgery (as for uncomplicated appendicitis or cholecystitis), a short course (eg, 4 days) after adequate source control/washout (eg, diverticulitis managed with sigmoidectomy), or a longer course (7-14 days or more) if source control is suboptimal or there is ongoing illness. Common regimens include:

- Ciprofloxacin 400 mg IV q12 (gram negatives) and Flagyl 500 mg IV q8h (anaerobes)
- Ceftriaxone 1 g IV (gram negatives) and Flagyl 500 mg IV q8 (anaerobes)
- Unasyn (ampicillin-sulbactam) 3 g IV q6
- Zosyn (piperacillin-tazobactam) 4.25 IV q6
- Ertapenem 1 g IV daily
- Exception to the rule: perirectal abscesses are well managed with drainage alone; no antibiotics

WHAT COUNTS AS "BROAD-SPECTRUM" COVERAGE?

This includes antibiotics that cover many gram-positive (often including MRSA), gram-negative (including *Pseudomonas*), and anaerobic organisms.

1. Vancomycin (MRSA) + cefepime (gram positives and negatives) + metronidazole (anaerobes)—main weakness is weak *Enterococcus* coverage

2. Vancomycin (MRSA) + Zosyn—broader owing to excellent anaerobe coverage, some non–vancomycin-resistant enterococcus (VRE) strains also covered
3. Vancomycin (MRSA) + carbapenem—broadest anaerobic coverage

> Alternatives for MRSA include linezolid and daptomycin.
> VRE may require addition of linezolid.

- What does IV Vanc/Zosyn cover?

This is a common go-to regimen and is a good starting point until more culture data are available. It covers gram positives (including MRSA), gram negatives (including *Pseudomonas*), and anaerobes.

- What does IV Vanc/Zosyn not cover?
  - Atypical infections (ie, community-acquired pneumonia)
  - Extended-spectrum beta-lactamase-producing organisms (often in patients with prolonged hospitalizations; primarily gram negative: *Klebsiella*, *E. coli*, *Pseudomonas*)
  - Vancomycin-resistant enterococcus
  - Fungal infections
  - *Clostridium difficile*
  - Mycobacterial infections
  - Viral infections
  - Parasites
  - *Stenotrophomonas maltophilia*
  - Source control

 PEARLS

1. Learn the bacterial coverage of various antibiotics and the organisms that cause common infections.
2. Be aware of your institute's unique antibiotic regimens and common strains of infections. Refer to resources such as the Johns Hopkins ABX app for fast reference or call your hospital pharmacist when in doubt.
3. Begin empiric antibiotics early when infection is suspected. De-escalate as soon as culture data allow.
4. For SSIs, make sure to mark out the initial erythema with a marking pen so you can monitor for progression/regression

6

SURGICAL PAIN MANAGEMENT— PERSPECTIVE 1

KORTNEY ROBINSON, MD, MPH | GABRIEL BRAT, MD, MPH

INTRODUCTION

Patients experience pain in multiple physiologic and personal ways. Each form should be treated with medications that target appropriate receptors and have different mechanisms of action. Multimodal therapy, expectation management, and personalization encompass this philosophy. Each surgical patient can have acute surgical pain that requires surgeons to be equipped with the proper knowledge and tools.

BACKGROUND

In the late 1990s, it became common to describe pain as the "fifth vital sign" to underline the need to explicitly reduce pain as part of medical management. In parallel, prescriptions for opioids increased exponentially. As the number of opioids prescribed grew, there was an equivalent increase in opioid-related overdose deaths.[1] By 2014, overdoses surpassed motor vehicle collisions as the most common cause of accidental death among adults.[2] However, as opioid abuse became a major public health crisis, a new lens was focused on the prescribing of opioids for pain. With the rise in deaths from opioids, prescribers, government agencies, insurers, and pharmacies began to regulate the dose and length of prescriptions. Many states developed or are in the process of enacting legislation regulating opioid prescribing to patients.

The recent literature has reported that 5.9% to 6.5% percent of opioid-naive patients who undergo surgery continue to use opioids 6 months after discharge.[3] Drug diversion, where unused prescriptions are acquired by someone other than the intended patient or used for an unintended purpose, is known to be a source of exposure to opioids and a gateway to opioid addiction and abuse. This is particularly a potential problem in surgery, where studies have shown that only ~30% of opioid-containing pills are used by general surgery patients and >70% of opiates are left unlocked at home.[4,5] Because more than 50% of surgical patients receive postdischarge opioids, surgeons have a responsibility to be careful and conservative in their prescribing habits. Most states have now adopted online prescription monitoring programs to display total opioid exposure from recent prescriptions for a given patient. This tool should be used before prescribing opioids.

Most surgical patients will experience acute pain from surgery. Therefore, managing acute pain is a necessary skill set for surgeons. These key concepts will help to improve patient care and pain control[6]:

- Set expectations.
- Use validated tools for pain assessments.
- Use multimodal therapy for the treatment of pain.
- Minimize or avoid opioids when possible.
- Patients with acute uncontrolled pain need prompt action and require adjustment of their pain regimen.
- Identify patients at increased risk of opioid misuse.
- Patients with chronic pain may require multidisciplinary care.
- Naloxone is used to treat opioid overdose.
- Discharge prescriptions should be customized to the patient.

SET EXPECTATIONS

Patients should hear explicitly—ideally while in the preoperative period—that they will have significant pain after surgery. Patients need to know that the provider will not be able to rid them of **all** pain and the goal is to achieve a manageable pain level. It builds rapport and trust when care teams engage patients in the management and setting of expectations clearly and before surgery. In the postoperative period, emphasizing the natural progression of pain—from more acute to reduced levels over time—allows for setting thresholds for use of opioids. It is now commonly accepted that opioids should be reserved for moderate to severe uncontrolled pain.

Furthermore, some patients adamantly refuse any type of opioids; narcotic contracts are growing in popularity as an increasing number of patients are recovering from addiction and overdose. Providers need to respect patient preferences and devise a plan for pain management that incorporates appropriate adjuncts.

USE VALIDATED TOOLS FOR PAIN ASSESSMENTS

The most common tool for pain assessment is the visual analog scale. This scale represents faces with pain ratings from 1 to 10, 1 being no pain and 10 being the worst pain. In surgery, it is virtually impossible to have a patient with a "0" pain score.

USE MULTIMODAL THERAPY FOR THE TREATMENT OF PAIN

Multimodal therapy is extremely important. Providers should always apply multiple types of medications and approaches to managing pain (Figure 6.1).

Adjunct medications: Adjunct medications include acetaminophen, nonsteroidal anti-inflammatory drugs (NSAIDs), and neuropathic agents such as gabapentin.

- Tylenol
  - Generally, there should be a standing order for every 6 to 8 hours immediately after surgery. A standing order often better controls a patient's pain.
    - Typical doses: 650 mg Q6 hours or 1000 mg Q8 hours to remain in the range of 3000 mg per 24-hour period.
    - Acetaminophen is hepatotoxic at doses greater than 4000 mg per 24 hours and is contraindicated in hepatic failure.
- NSAIDs
  - Two common NSAIDs are ibuprofen and ketorolac. Ketorolac can be given by intravenous, intramuscular or oral route, whereas ibuprofen is most commonly given orally.
    - Contraindications include renal failure, gastrointestinal bleeding, and peptic ulcer disease, as NSAIDs can precipitate or worsen these pathologies. NSAIDs are also often withheld in renal transplant patients.

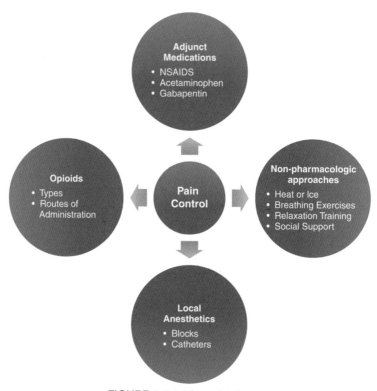

FIGURE 6.1 Multimodal therapy.

- Gabapentin
  - Use in low doses (100-300 mg) when prescribing to a patient who has not been taking gabapentin long term.
    - Caution in elderly patients and in patients with renal impairment as it is associated with significant sedation.
    - High-dose coprescription of this medication with opioids has been reported to increase mortality from overdoses.[7]

Nonpharmacologic approaches: Local pain can often be treated with heat or ice to ease muscular pain or swelling. The psychological state of the patient can also play a role in the perception of pain. Relaxation training and breathing exercises can be useful. Furthermore, the patient's social support system can either inhibit or promote the healing process.

Local anesthetics: Local anesthetics can be used in the preoperative, intra-operative, and postoperative setting. Depending on the type of procedure performed, blocks or catheters may be placed in the perioperative setting. These can substantially reduce patient's pain. For smaller or localized procedures and incisions, the area can be infiltrated with local anesthetics to reduce pain.

- Common types of blocks: spinal, transversus abdominus plane, extremity (eg, femoral, adductor canal), paraspinal
- Common locations of catheters: epidural, preperitoneal, extremity (eg, supraclavicular, femoral)

Opioids: The term opioid is used to describe substances that bind to the opiate receptors in the brain. There are multiple types and routes of opioids. We will discuss the most common opioids prescribed, contraindications, patients at higher risk for misuse, and the reversal agent.

- Routes of administration
  - Oral: optimal route of administration and best when patients can take oral medications.
  - Intravenous or intramuscular: reserved for patients who have uncontrolled severe pain or those who are NPO (taking nothing by mouth). Intravenous (IV) opioids are also used in patient-controlled analgesia (PCA), whereby the patient has the ability to administer a set dose over time with a button. There is a lockout mechanism to prevent multiple doses. In general, a basal rate **should not** be written in the order. If available, an acute pain service or anesthesia team is often involved or can be consulted when writing for PCAs.
  - Transdermal: do not use in an opioid-naive patient. Patients with chronic pain may use patches (most commonly composed of fentanyl) to deliver a constant dose.
- Common opioids (Table 6.1)
  Dose adjustments are necessary with:
  - Hepatic insufficiency or failure
  - Respiratory compromise or obstructive sleep apnea
  - Elderly patients
  - Concurrent use of benzodiazepines, sleep medications, or antiepileptics

MINIMIZE OR AVOID OPIOIDS WHEN POSSIBLE

Opioids are effective medications to treat acute pain. However, they have significant side effects (Figure 6.2) and can be addicting. Risk of misuse increases with the duration of prescriptions and number of refills. Efforts should be focused on weaning patients off opioids as quickly as possible.[8]

TABLE 6-1 Information on Commonly Prescribed Opioids

Drug	Common Starting Dose	Caution/Contraindications
Morphine	2-4 mg IV 7.5-15 mg PO	Metabolites accumulate in renal failure
Oxycodone	5-10 mg PO	
Hydrocodone	5-10 mg PO	
Hydromorphone	0.25-0.5 mg IV 2-4 mg PO	
Tramadol	25-50 mg PO	Contraindicated in patients with seizure history Maximum daily dose of 400 mg

IV, intravenous; PO, by mouth.

PATIENTS WITH ACUTE UNCONTROLLED PAIN NEED PROMPT ACTION AND REQUIRE ADJUSTMENT OF THEIR PAIN REGIMEN

Uncontrolled acute pain can lead to chronic pain in surgical patients.[9] When necessary, patients may require a breakthrough dose of an IV opioid to control pain. As discussed previously, local anesthetics, including postoperative blocks and catheters, can also be used.

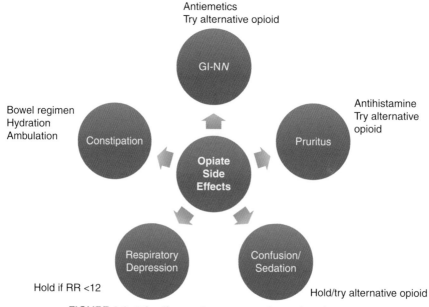

FIGURE 6.2 Side effects and treatments of opioid medications.

When a patient has uncontrolled pain, immediate breakthrough treatment should be combined with an analysis of the existing regimen. The provider should ask themselves the following questions:

- Does the pain regimen contain all possible adjuncts? Is it missing key components?
- Are doses appropriate for the patient and type of surgery?
- Is there another source of pain? Is there a possible complication that should be investigated?

IDENTIFYING PATIENTS AT INCREASED RISK OF OPIOID MISUSE

A subset of patients is at increased risk of opioid misuse, abuse, or overdose. Prescribers should be aware of the factors that increase the risk of misuse[10]:

- Age 16 to 45 years
- Psychosocial factors
  - Depression
  - Bipolar
  - Schizophrenia
  - Obsessive-compulsive disorder
  - Posttraumatic stress disorder
  - Attention deficit disorder and attention-deficit/hyperactivity disorder
  - History of drug or alcohol abuse
  - History of preadolescent sexual abuse
- Family history
  - Drug or alcohol abuse

PATIENTS WITH CHRONIC PAIN MAY REQUIRE MULTIDISCIPLINARY CARE

The US Food and Drug Administration defines opioid tolerance as daily consumption of 60 or more morphine milliequivalents for a week or longer. Patients taking long-term opioids may have tolerance to opioids or reduced response and a narrowed therapeutic window. These patients will often benefit from perioperative evaluation by a pain specialist to develop an appropriate management plan. There are basic steps to aid in the treatment of opioid-tolerant patients.

- Identify doses of preoperative opioids. Call the provider or pharmacy or use the state physician monitoring program.
- Use home dose as "baseline" and add typical coverage of operative pain.
- Ensure multimodal therapy is being utilized.
- Consult outpatient providers about management of the postoperative prescription, and investigate if there is a narcotics agreement in place.

NALOXONE IS USED TO TREAT OPIOID OVERDOSE

- Signs and symptoms of opioid overdose are confusion, altered mental status, meiotic pupils, and respiratory depression.
- Goal of reversal is adequate ventilation.
- The half-life of naloxone is much shorter than that of the opioid it is reversing, so it may need to be redosed. These patients should be on continuous oxygen monitoring.
- A provider should also rule out alternative reasons for altered mental status: stroke, sepsis, and metabolic derangements.

DISCHARGE PRESCRIPTIONS SHOULD BE CUSTOMIZED TO THE PATIENT

Unfortunately, research has shown that inpatient postoperative opioid use does not correlate with discharge prescriptions.[11] When discharging a patient, discuss pain control expectations with the patient, prescribe adjuncts, and write the prescription with reference to the surgery. Prescriptions should meet state and federal guidelines and be based on expected need over the next week and opioid requirement in the last 24 hours before discharge. Encourage patients to lock up their opioids and dispose of them as soon as they are no longer needed, either at drop boxes or through their garbage by mixing the pills with coffee grounds, dirt, or cat litter in a plastic bag.

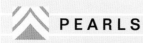

PEARLS

1. Set patient expectations, and use a multimodal approach to pain management.
2. Limit and discontinue opioid use as soon as possible to avoid dependence and related side effects.
3. Approach each patient individually; observe for high-risk indicators of dependence, address acute pain and chronic pain appropriately, and employ a multimodal approach as appropriate.

References

1. CDC. *Vital Signs: Overdoses of Prescription Opioid Pain Relievers – United States, 1999-2008.* 2011. Retrieved from https://www.cdc.gov/mmwr/preview/mmwrhtml/mm6043a4.htm.
2. CDC. *Increases in Drug and Opioid Overdose Deaths – United States, 2000-2014.* 2016. Retrieved from https://www.cdc.gov/mmwr/preview/mmwrhtml/mm6450a3.htm.
3. Brummett CM, Waljee JF, Goesling J, et al. New persistent opioid use after minor and major surgical procedures in US adults. *JAMA Surgery.* 2017;48109:e170504. doi:10.1001/jamasurg.2017.0504.
4. Bicket MC, Long JJ, Pronovost PJ, Alexander GC, Wu CL. Prescription opioid analgesics commonly unused after surgery. *JAMA Surgery.* 2017:1-6. doi:10.1001/jamasurg.2017.0831.
5. Hill MV, Mcmahon ML, Stucke RS, Barth RJ. Wide variation and excessive dosage of opioid prescriptions for common general surgical procedures. *Ann Surg.* 2016;265(4):1-6. doi:10.1097/SLA.0000000000001993.
6. CDC. *Guideline for Prescribing Opioids for Chronic Pain Improving Practice Through Recommendations.* 2017. doi:10.15585/mmwr.rr6501e1.
7. Gomes T, Juurlink DN, Antoniou T, Mamdani MM, Paterson JM, van den Brink W. Gabapentin, opioids, and the risk of opioid-related death: a population-based nested case–control study. *PLoS Med.* 2017;14(10):1-13. doi:10.1371/journal.pmed.1002396.
8. Brat GA, Agniel D, Beam A, et al. (2018). Postsurgical prescriptions for opioid naive patients and – association with overdose and misuse: retrospective cohort study. *BMJ.* 2018;360:j5790. doi.org/10.1136/bmj.j5790.
9. Lovich-Sapola J, Smith CE, Brandt CP. Postoperative pain control. *Surg Clin.* 2015;95(2):301-318. doi:10.1016/j.suc.2014.10.002.
10. Webster LR, Webster RM. Predicting aberrant behaviors in opioid-treated patients: preliminary validation of the opioid risk tool. *Pain Med.* 2005;6(6):432-442. doi:10.1111/j.1526-4637.2005.00072.x.
11. Chen EY, Marcantonio A, Tornetta P. Correlation between 24-hour predischarge opioid use and amount of opioids prescribed at hospital discharge. *JAMA Surg.* 2017;e174859. doi:10.1001/jamasurg.2017.4859.

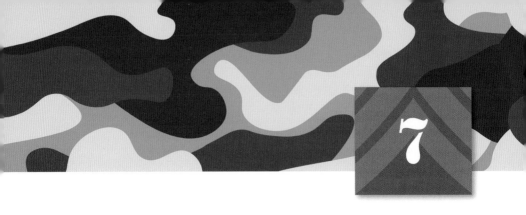

SURGICAL PAIN MANAGEMENT— PERSPECTIVE 2

BIJAN J. TEJA, MD, MBA | CINDY M. KU, MD | STEPHANIE B JONES, MD

INTRODUCTION

As a surgery intern and resident, pain will be one of the issues you are most frequently asked to manage. Pain and nausea are two of the things patients fear most when undergoing surgery.

The first thing to think about when a patient has pain is whether there is an underlying cause that needs to be addressed. In many cases, patients complaining of severe pain before discharge out of proportion to what would be expected end up returning to the hospital with missed complications such as pseudoaneurysms from vascular procedures, anastomotic leaks, wound infections, compartment syndrome, or intraabdominal abscesses. Be sure to take severe pain seriously before treating it with pain medications. There have been numerous cases of missed complications such as dead gut when bowel obstructions and other conditions have been treated reflexively with escalating doses of narcotics rather than careful assessment.

Pain from surgery can be particularly difficult to manage in patients with chronic pain, long-term opioid users, and patients who have a history of heroin or other opiate abuse. Using a multimodal approach described later and involving your acute or chronic pain service colleagues early for these challenging patients can make a substantial difference in the overall quality of pain control they receive.

ORAL AND INTRAVENOUS NONOPIOID ANALGESICS

Multimodal analgesia (ie, treatment with multiple classes of analgesics) is the gold standard for pain control. Using modalities other than opiates can reduce opioid requirements significantly and reduce opioid side effects such as nausea and vomiting, constipation, and delirium.

Commonly used agents include[1]:

Acetaminophen: Reversible COX inhibitor (predominantly COX-3). Can reduce opioid requirements by as much as 40%. The intravenous (IV) form is ~$20 per dose but is often appropriate for patients with severe pain not able to take the oral form. Some hospitals use rectal Tylenol routinely as a replacement for IV Tylenol in patients who cannot take oral medications.

Ibuprofen: Reversible COX-1 and 2 inhibitor. Effective in controlling pain. Contraindicated in patients with active bleeding, peptic ulcers, and history of bariatric surgery and in those with hyperkalemia or severe renal impairment.

Ketorolac: Reversible COX-1 and 2 inhibitor. This medication can be extremely effective and provides a higher level of analgesia than acetaminophen or ibuprofen. In fact, every 30-mg dose of IV ketorolac is approximately equivalent to 10 mg of morphine in pain reduction/opioid-sparing ability.[2] The IV form is less expensive than IV acetaminophen; roughly $2 per dose. Contraindications are the same as for ibuprofen. Ask the chief or the attending before administering owing to concern for increased bleeding risk (although meta-analyses show no increased risk). Do not administer for procedures where bleeding could be rapidly fatal (ie, neurosurgery). Reduce dose in the elderly and in patients with mildly increased creatinine.

Gabapentin/pregabalin: These have a structure similar to that of gamma-aminobutyric acid (GABA) but do not bind GABA receptors; exact mechanism unknown. Helpful as an adjunct to decrease narcotic use. Can cause dizziness and sedation. Pregabalin is more expensive but has a quicker onset (1 versus 3-4 hours), similar half-life, and more reliable absorption/pharmacokinetics.

Tizanidine/baclofen/cyclobenzaprine: Antispasmodics are helpful for pain associated with sprains, muscle spasms, or contractures. Tizanidine is a centrally acting α2 agonist, baclofen is a GABA agonist, and cyclobenzaprine has an unknown mechanism. Do not discontinue baclofen abruptly, as doing so can cause delirium and even rhabdomyolysis.

OPIOIDS

Whenever you start administering opioids, make sure you pay close attention to bowel function. Do not discharge patients given oral opioids without advising them to take stool softeners to ensure they are having bowel movements every day. Even though the stool softeners are available over the counter, many residents give prescriptions for Miralax (polyethylene glycol), senna, or other agents to make sure patients remember to buy them. You will likely see at least a few patients in your residency who require a partial or total colectomy for colitis caused by opioid-induced constipation, a completely preventable complication. Be sure to help patients avoid this as best you can.

Opioids are often effective but are associated with adverse effects including respiratory depression, reduced bowel motility/constipation, and tolerance.

- Morphine/hydromorphone/oxycodone: Long half-lives of these medications facilitate pain control in the postoperative period. Hydromorphone is more lipophilic and has a much faster time to peak effect than morphine (IV form/patient controlled analgesia doses take ~15 minutes to peak for hydromorphone versus 30-60 minutes for morphine). Morphine lasts slightly longer. All three can be used as oral agents. Which one works better tends to be very patient specific, and it can be helpful to ask a patient if one has worked well or not worked well for them in the past.
- Tramadol: Combined opiate receptor agonist and serotonin–norepinephrine reuptake inhibitor. Some elderly/frail patients find that they tolerate tramadol slightly better than other opioids.
- Fentanyl: Much shorter half-life with single dose because of rapid distribution into fat. Infusion, patch, or high number of repeated doses causes drug accumulation and prolonged elimination time (can take days to eliminate after long infusions). Note that infusions or large doses of fentanyl or fentanyl analogues can cause opioid-induced hyperalgesia, in which the patient becomes more sensitive to painful stimuli and can require much larger doses of opioids for postoperative pain control.

TABLE 7-1 Opioid Conversions

	IV	IV to PO Conversion	PO
Morphine	5 mg	×2-3	10-15 mg
Hydromorphone	0.75 mg	×5	4 mg
Tramadol	50 mg	×1.5-2	75-100 mg
Oxycodone	N/A		7.5-10 mg
Codeine	N/A		100 mg
Hydrocodone	N/A		15 mg

- Meperidine: Used primarily for the treatment of perioperative shivering. Unique because it has minor local anesthetic properties in addition to narcotic properties. Its metabolite, normeperidine, is excreted by the kidneys and can cause seizures in patients with chronic kidney disease.
- Methadone: Used primarily for the treatment of chronic pain or opiate addiction. Has N-methyl-D-aspartate antagonist properties as well (similar to ketamine), which help with pain control in patients with opioid tolerance. Interns and residents usually obtain a chronic pain service consult and/or assistance from a pharmacist to help with dosing and close follow-up after discharge.

Conversions between opioids are provided in Table 7.1.

LOCAL ANESTHETICS

Subcutaneous injection of lidocaine or bupivacaine (Marcaine) for port sites has been shown to improve perioperative pain and decrease hospital costs after laparoscopic surgery.[3,4]

Epinephrine 5 µg/mL prolongs effect and reduces systemic absorption/toxicity, allowing higher doses to be administered (most effect with lidocaine). This tiny subcutaneous dose rarely, if ever, has any hemodynamic effect.

Maximum dosages for common local anesthetics are provided in Table 7.2.

SPECIAL SITUATIONS

Large abdominal or thoracic incision/multiple rib fractures: Strongly consider getting an epidural for your patient. Large abdominal and thoracic cases are usually booked with an epidural, and the anesthesia team will typically discuss

TABLE 7-2 Maximum Local Anesthetic Doses

	Plain (mg/kg)	With Epi (mg/kg)	Duration of Effect (minutes)	Maximum Volume With Common Formulations
Lidocaine	3-5 (max 300 mg)	7 (max 500 mg)	30-60 plain 120-360 w/epi	1% plain: 3-5 mL/kg (max 30 mL) 1% with epi: 7 mL/kg (max 50 mL)
Bupivacaine (Marcaine)	2.5 (max 175 mg)	2.5 (max 200 mg)	120-240 plain 180-240 w/epi	0.25%: 1 mL/kg 0.5%: 0.5 mL/kg

epi, epinephrine.

this with the attending surgeon beforehand at most hospitals. For laparoscopic procedures converted to open procedures or for patients with multiple rib fractures, you will need to request placement of an epidural from the acute pain service. Many surgical services routinely perform transverse abdominis plane (TAP) blocks for large abdominal incisions or intercostal nerve blocks for large thoracic incisions. These blocks can also be done by the anesthesia pain service under ultrasound after the case (either in the operating room or in the postanesthesia care unit).

Contraindication to epidurals include international normalized ratio ≥1.5, therapeutic anticoagulation (eg, for deep vein thrombosis/pulmonary embolism), and cellulitis at the planned epidural site.

For patients with large incisions and narcotic tolerance, ketamine infusions (usually ordered by the acute pain service) can be extremely effective. At low doses, ketamine provides effective analgesia without the dysphoria seen at high doses and without the respiratory depression and constipation associated with narcotics (ketamine preserves respiratory drive, unlike narcotics).

Long-term IV narcotic abusers presenting with injection site abscesses: Long-term opioid use causes hyperalgesia (excessive pain sensation with minimally painful stimuli) and tolerance to narcotics, which makes pain in patients with narcotic use history very difficult to control. Injection site abscesses sometimes require large/multiple incisions and multiple dressing changes, and these patients require large narcotic doses and other agents that most physicians do not have experience titrating. Nerve catheters (continuous injection nerve blocks) can be especially effective for these patients and allow for frequent dressing changes over 4 to 5 days. Strongly consider consulting the acute pain service at your hospital early when these patients are admitted to your service.

PEARLS

1. If a patient is complaining of pain out of proportion to what you would expect, make sure you have thought about and ruled out potentially serious complications, including pseudoaneurysms from vascular procedures, anastomotic leaks, wound infections, and bowel ischemia.
2. Consider talking to a more senior physician early in your training if you are unable to find an explanation for the pain severity.
3. If possible, when patients with long-term opioid use or large incisions are admitted to your service, it is helpful to page the acute pain service early on during daytime hours. Otherwise, the patient may not get their epidural, TAP block, or continuous nerve catheter until the next day when the acute pain service attending is back in the hospital and able to perform or supervise the procedure.

References

1. Jones D. *Pocket Surgery.* 2nd ed. Philadelphia: Lippincott Williams & Wilkins; October 2017.
2. Buckley MM, Brogden RN. Ketorolac. A review of its pharmacodynamic and pharmacokinetic properties, and therapeutic potential. *Drugs.* 1990;39(1):86-109.
3. Protic M, Veljkovic R, Bilchik AJ, et al. Prospective randomized controlled trial comparing standard analgesia with combined intra-operative cystic plate and port-site local anesthesia for post-operative pain management in elective laparoscopic cholecystectomy. *Surg Endosc.* 2017;31(2):704-713.
4. Hasaniya NW, Zayed FF, Faiz H, Severino R. Preinsertion local anesthesia at the trocar site improves perioperative pain and decreases costs of laparoscopic cholecystectomy. *Surg Endosc.* 2001;15(9):962-964.

8

WHEN TO CALL THE CHIEF RESIDENT

NAKUL RAYKAR, MD, MPH | MARK P. CALLERY, MD

Common advice to new surgical interns often includes that chief residents must be informed of... "everything." Although the chief resident *should* be informed of all relevant clinical updates that impact patient care on the service, this advice is rarely useful to the beginning surgical resident as what constitutes "relevant" is rarely defined. Obviously, the chief resident should be alerted if a recent postoperative patient is having respiratory distress and is facing likely reintubation, but does he or she need to be alerted when placing an order for a higher dose of acetaminophen? Similarly, although it is fairly obvious that morning rounds are a good time to update and to ask questions, what about in middle of the night?

A growing body of research demonstrates a link between patient safety and effective health care team communication.[1] With aging populations, growing team censuses, and surgical intern patient loads ever increasing,[2] the room for error further decreases. Questions will arise even among competent and confident residents and must be communicated to senior oversight. In the first year, it can be hard to discern what is and is not important. Seemingly benign interventions can have outsized impact. Acetaminophen, for example, although generally considered harmless by many physicians and the general public, may not be harmless for a patient with liver insufficiency on the transplant waitlist. Hence, titrating a pain regimen on such a patient may, in fact, warrant inclusion of the chief resident.

So why not err on the side of caution and ask for help when uncertain? A common impediment is a surgical culture that may suggest that those who ask for help may lack competence, confidence, or both.[3] Resident trainees continue to report belittlement and unprofessional behavior from senior house staff and faculty in the context of clinical care.[2]

This chapter aims to provide a general framework for when to let the chief resident know of evolving clinical circumstances while balancing the desire for autonomy, the desire to not be viewed as lacking confidence or competence, and the desire not to spark belittlement from a chief resident for "bothering" them on "trivial" concerns.

THE ROLE OF CHIEF RESIDENT

Before delving into a framework for when to engage the chief resident, we may benefit from an understanding of the chief resident's role on a surgical service. Unlike in many specialties where interns command a fair amount of autonomy in managing daily patient care, the chief resident on a surgical service continues to serve as the primary point person for all matters related to patient care on the service. As such, very few things (should) happen on a surgical service without the knowledge of the chief resident. In many ways, this structure can be immensely protective of junior residents and interns. The chief resident will shoulder responsibility for patient care decisions even if the intern put in the order. If a nasogastric tube was inserted on a patient overnight without the chief resident's knowledge, though, he or she may be unable to defend any negative consequences of that action to the attending surgeon.

In congruence with the chief resident serving as the "quarterback" of the service comes the recognition that the chief resident, too, has anxieties, concerns, and uncertainties about the ultimate course of patients and must report to their own set of demanding bosses (attending surgeons). As such, the hesitation involved in calling a chief resident is often unnecessary; most conscientious chief residents are just as anxious about not being called and not knowing what is happening in the hospital as the intern who is uncertain as to when to dial.

FRAMEWORK FOR WHEN TO INVOLVE THE CHIEF RESIDENT

In the attempt to provide a practical guide for when to pull the figurative "trigger" in calling a chief resident, we differentiate scenarios into categories of "must" call, "should" call, and "can" call, each with decreasing levels of urgency (Table 8.1).

TABLE 8-1 When You Can, Should, and Must Call the Chief Resident

Contact Emergently ("Must Call")	Contact Urgently ("Should Call")	Contact Per Discretion ("Can Call")
Active clinical scenario beyond the expected scope of the surgical intern that may benefit from senior-resident expertise Examples: ■ Active clinical deterioration (eg, active MI, respiratory failure, pulmonary embolism, hemodynamic instability, worsening abdominal examination) ■ Need for ICU transfer ■ Marked nursing concern These situations mandate emergent communication with the chief resident, regardless of whether in the middle of a surgical case or overnight	Subacute clinical scenario within the scope of practice of the surgical intern that may benefit from reassurance or direction from chief resident Subacute clinical scenario well within the scope of practice of the surgical intern but that is key information for the scope of responsibility for a chief resident *Example may include NGT placement (or this might be in the above section)* Examples: ■ New fever ■ Abnormal and unexpected laboratory values including, eg, a rise in WBC or subacute drop in Hct ■ Medication error ■ Issue with surgical consent ■ Persistent emesis and abdominal distention requiring NGT These situations benefit from communication with chief resident on urgent basis. If in the middle of an active surgical case, one may wait for a pause in intense focused activity. If overnight, resident should still be alerted	Nonacute clinical scenarios that rest comfortably within the scope of practice of the surgical intern but are necessary updates for the chief resident. If there is any uncertainty as to clinical significance of any of these situations, they should be treated with urgency and a chief resident should be called Examples: ■ Pathology report results ■ Radiology report results ■ Self-limited musculoskeletal chest discomfort ■ IV access ■ Urinary frequency ■ Renewal of delirium treatment ■ Heparin drip adjustments

Hct, haematocrit; ICU, intensive care unit; IV, intravenous; MI, myocardial infarction; NGT, nasogastric tube; WBC, white blood cell.

Must call scenarios consist of deteriorations in patient condition and any scenario that requires senior-level expertise outside of the scope of a surgical intern. These situations include obviously serious conditions in which a patient is in respiratory distress and may require intubation and/or transfer to the intensive care unit. Must call scenarios also include clinical puzzles that are simply unclear to the treating intern. For example, "Mrs. X is complaining of a lot of pain at the surgical site, and I'm not sure if I should treat her with pain medications or further interrogate the surgical site?" Finally, must call scenarios also include logistical issues that may interfere with timely clinical care and require a higher level of intervention. If a consulting service, for example, refuses to see a patient that the team is expecting them to see for critical input, the issue should be elevated through the chief resident. If a patient is expected to be on the schedule for a procedure the next day but is not actually on the operating room schedule, this should be reconciled and the chief resident informed.

Should call scenarios rest within the scope of practice of the surgical intern; however, the residual uncertainty of the situation would benefit from reassurance from a more seasoned clinician. These situations may include, for example, a patient who is stable but "doesn't look right" to the intern. The patient admitted with diverticulitis, for example, who was started on antibiotics but has spiked a new fever and is visibly diaphoretic and potentially a worse abdominal examination should warrant a phone call to a chief resident. In fact, we suggest the surgical intern should contact the chief resident to report any deviation from the expected clinical course as was discussed previously with the chief resident and even if the intern has already sent the routine laboratory and clinical workup for a new fever. To this end, it is critical that the surgical intern takes it upon himself or herself to establish a mental "what is expected" for every patient on the list that they are covering either during the day or overnight. Although it is nice when coresidents signing out patients to you provide you with this background, the ultimate onus is on you to specifically request this information if you are unclear of the expected clinical course for the patient during the day or overnight.

A second category of should call scenarios includes those in which the phone call serves mostly as a critical update. These scenarios may rest well within comfort level of the surgical intern, but the chief resident needs to be updated nonetheless in order for them to effectively serve as the leader of the service. Imagine, for example, that the intern astutely asked if the team was expecting a particular intensive care unit patient to deteriorate clinically and require vasopressor support overnight. She received an answer in the affirmative. When the patient *is* started on vasopressors, it may be important to let the chief resident know so that he or she can update the attending surgeons as appropriate. Again, these situations benefit from prediscussion between the surgical intern and the chief resident.

Finally, we define situations in which a surgical resident can update the chief resident, at his or her discretion. These involve scenarios that rest comfortably within the scope of practice of the surgical intern, are unlikely to benefit from higher-level expertise, and of questionable utility for the chief resident to know on an emergent basis. For example, the finalization of pathology results on the patient recovering from pancreatic resection. Scenarios that fit this situation should also be presettled between the surgical intern and chief resident.

ADDITIONAL CONSIDERATIONS

TEXT MESSAGE VERSUS PHONE CALLS

Text messaging has quickly become a preferred mode of communication for a large number of patient issues over the course of the day. It affords many benefits, including being a rapid means of communication, and is often less disruptive to those being "called." Many of the can call issues and some of the should call issues are well suited for communication over text message. Often times a text message giving a senior resident or attending physician a "heads up" about a must call issue can be very helpful to set the tone of the conversation. Use of text message requires a few important considerations. First, never assume that a text message sent is equivalent to a text message read. Use of messaging in this context requires careful attention on the part of the sender and a follow-up phone call or page for critical matters. Second, institutions have varying policies on the use of text message for communication. A US federal requirement, however, is the need to protect patient data and to avoid using patient identifiers over a potentially insecure medium.[4] Review relevant institutional guidelines!

EXPECTED SCOPE OF PRACTICE FOR SURGICAL INTERN

Many surgical trainees of all levels, particularly interns, are afraid that asking for help exposes weaknesses in their own fund of knowledge or ability to manage a situation. The successful surgical intern should never give in to this falsehood. Good chief residents and faculty understand that all trainees enter with varied clinical experiences and, as such, should expect very little at baseline. And although it is true that expectations will evolve over the course of the year, good chief residents will keep in mind that the intern who has spent the first 3 months of the year in the off-service or nonclinical activities will not have the same clinical exposure of the resident who spent the first 3 months taking care of critically ill patients on a busy inpatient surgical service. If you think they do not remember, a gentle reminder is always appreciated.

THERE IS NO GOLD STANDARD FOR WHEN TO CALL: PATIENT SAFETY ABOVE ALL!

Although the individual intern may be poring over the "appropriateness" of a particular clinical situation to demand waking a chief resident at 3 AM, he or she must keep in mind that there is no clear right or wrong. A study at the University of Pittsburgh examining resident-attending communication showed that, although as groups residents and attending physicians had a high rate of agreement on what events require in person communication (eg, cardiac arrest, respiratory failure), individual pairs of residents and attending physicians had noticeable discordance on the same specific scenarios.[5] In other words, a specific pairing of a resident with a specific attending often disagreed on the need to notify or be notified about a specific clinical situation. These results can be extrapolated to the relationship between a surgical intern and chief resident to provide the intern with reassurance that there is no "gold standard" or firm rules.

As such, try your best to establish the rules with your particular chief resident early in the rotation, early in the day, or before night falls. *"What types of issues do you want me to call you for?"* Anticipate issues or potentially unstable patients and ask early. *"Mrs. R had an elevated temperature this morning and her WBC increased this morning, if she spikes another temperature overnight do you want me to send the standard workup or would you like a phone call?"*

Finally, ask for feedback, early and often. Ultimately, your relationship with your chief resident is a critical dynamic that you can work to improve throughout your time together. Ask for feedback the morning after on the chief resident's perception of the "appropriateness" of your handling of these situations overnight.

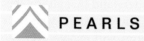

PEARLS

1. Be sure to communicate efficiently with your chief resident. Ask and have a firm understanding of what your role is and what level of communication the chief resident requires of you.
2. Communicate important messages promptly and clearly to ensure there are no misunderstandings.
3. Should you feel your chief resident takes an important concern of yours without much urgency, be sure to emphasize you are worried and ask why your chief resident is not as concerned. At times, this can clarify a misunderstanding that would otherwise be disastrous.

References

1. Greenberg CC, Regenbogen SE, Studdert DM, et al. Patterns of communication breakdowns resulting in injury to surgical patients. *J Am Coll Surg.* 2007;204(4):533-540.
2. Patel SP, Lee JS, Ranney DN, et al. Resident workload, pager communications, and quality of care. *World J Surg.* 2010;34(11):2524-2529.
3. Novick RJ, Lingard L, Cristancho SM. The call, the save, and the threat: understanding expert help-seeking behavior during nonroutine operative scenarios. *J Surg Educ.* 2015;72(2):302-309.
4. U.S. Center for Medicare & Medicaid Services. Texting of patient information among healthcare providers. Memorandum S&C 18-10-ALL. 2017. Available at https://www.cms.gov/Medicare/ Provider-Enrollment-and-Certification/SurveyCertificationGenInfo/Downloads/Survey-and-Cert-Letter-18-10.pdf.
5. Gary T, Rubin F, Hanusa BH, Roberts MS. Expectations of groups versus pairs of attendings and residents about phone communications and bedside evaluation of hospitalized patients. *Teach Learn Med.* 2005;17(3):217-227.

9

HANDS-OFF AND SIGN OUT

LORENZO ANEZ-BUSTILLOS, MD, MPH | MICHAEL N. COCCHI, MD

INTRODUCTION

Developing the skills to transfer a patient's care and responsibility from one team to another is of utmost importance. As key members of the health care team, patient safety is one of our top priorities. Our commitment to patients must preserve the continuity of care through effective communication. Every day of your residency you will deal with hand-offs, a process that can put you either in a position of giving or receiving important information. You may find yourself on the receiving end when signing in during the start of a shift or as you get called by other teams for a surgical consult. On the other hand, you will be the one giving information when transferring a postoperative patient to the intensive care unit or to your fellow residents after a shift. Regardless of your role in the process, active participation is paramount to ensure a quality hand-off; this will ensure the patient's safety and continuity of care, and your colleagues will appreciate the proper sharing of information.

Whatever you do, do not take hand-offs lightly. There is a reason why accreditation agencies in the United States have raised concern about failed hand-offs and how these can compromise patient safety. Inadequate hand-offs are one of the main reasons behind in-hospital adverse events. An added concern is the increasing number of hand-offs required given current residency work-hour restrictions. As your experience builds, you will become better and more efficient in the hand-off process. However, we will provide you with a few tips and tools that have proven to work for being an effective communicator in both verbal and written hand-offs. For the process of verbal hand-offs, the key is to be succinct yet include the essential information. Although it may seem normal to assume that more information is better, this is not always the case, especially in a field where more often than not time is of the essence.

I-PASS

As you build experience in doing appropriate hand-offs, we recommend you build a framework in your mind with a series of steps to follow as you relay patient information to others. The I-PASS mnemonic was developed by experts in effective communication in the hospital setting and has proven to work well in many specialties.[1] This standardized process follows 5 steps, 4 of which are to be taken by the sender of information, whereas the remaining one is the responsibility of the receiver.

   You should start hand-offs by stating the illness severity of the patient (I) and letting the receiver know whether the patient is stable or unstable or if the patient is someone who needs close monitoring. In surgery, when calling in consults to a chief or attending, a good habit is to start your presentation by stating whether this patient will require an emergent or urgent surgical intervention. This step can prime the listener and set the tone for the rest of the process. The next step is to provide the patient's summary (P). This includes a brief statement of the events that led to the admission, hospital course, ongoing assessment, and plan. The action list (A) follows, during which time you specify the things that need to be done pertaining to the patient's care, with a specific timeline and ownership. After this, you should make sure that you build the situational awareness (S) and let the receiver know of the things that could happen and how to deal with them if they happen (contingency plan). The last step in the process is performed by the receiver and aims to close the loop to ensure effective communication. The receiver should summarize the information that was given (S), emphasizing the things that need to be done and asking pertinent questions.

WRITTEN HAND-OFFS

Written hand-offs in surgery are often summarized in the form of patient lists. If done well, this tool can streamline the hand-off process and improve efficiency. As with verbal hand-offs, be succinct and do not add more than what is actually needed. Numbers to be added include vital signs (maximum and latest temperature, heart rate, blood pressure, respiratory rate), breathing source (room air, nasal cannula, or ventilator settings), input (oral or intravenous fluid intake), and output (urine, stool, nasogastric/chest tubes, or drains). You should also add information regarding the patients current diet status (NPO, regular, soft, or clear liquids diet), intravenous fluids (type and rate of infusion), and medication drips (drug and rate of infusion).

CONCLUSION

Time permitting, you may be able to spend more time doing hand-offs (usually with coresidents). In such cases, avoid getting lost in superfluous information. When losing focus, go back to I-PASS. More time, however, can provide you with the opportunity of giving useful details about the patient's preferences and bedside care. For example, you could add details on previous conflicts with the patient or family members that can be avoided in future encounters. You can also include tips and tricks on dealing with drains, vacuum-assisted closure devices, tubes, or any other special care that the patient may need. A good rule of thumb to follow is to share the information that you wish would have been given to you. Avoid adding personal opinions about patients that would not improve the quality of care that they receive.

HAND-OFF ETIQUETTE RULES

- Know your audience. Intern-to-intern hand-offs are different from intern-to-chief or intern-to-attending hand-offs. As you move up in the chain of command, you should aim to be more succinct and efficient with the amount of information being relayed.
- Know your patient. A quality hand-off starts with complete understanding and knowledge of what is happening and what has happened to the patient. You should be aware of the rationale behind everything that has been done.

- Avoid distractions during hand-offs. Find a place where you can minimize interruptions during the transfer of information. However, if urgent, do not delay the hand-off process regardless of the location. You will often need to give hand-offs to a chief or attending while they are operating; remember in this case to be succinct.
- Do not assume. Remember that your role on the receiving end of the hand-off process is that of an active participant. Make sure you listen carefully and voice any concerns or point out those things that seem off.
- Request hand-offs at the appropriate time. Similarly, do not expect hand-offs when either member in the process is dealing with an urgent situation.
- Avoid informal hand-offs. Refrain from requesting or accepting "curbside" consultations from other teams. Adequate patient care will be ensured if a formal request and a full, proper hand-off is requested.
- Be honest. If you do not know something being asked by the recipient, admit to that fact. Offer to find out this information and follow up as soon as possible.
- Provide information for written hand-offs by ensuring that the patient list is complete and accurate. Make sure vital signs, inputs and outputs, diet, medication drips, and any other relevant information is summarized in handouts.
- Do not hand off tasks to your fellow residents that should and could have been done by you. Follow the action plan and take ownership of what needs to be done.

 PEARLS

1. Hand-offs are one of the most important aspects of improving patient care. They should not be taken lightly and are appreciated by incoming staff.
2. Develop and hone your style and system for hand-offs. This will ensure that the most pertinent information is successfully handed off. I-PASS is an extremely valuable tool.
3. Do not assume, be as detailed as possible without overburdening your colleague. That said, take as much time as necessary.

Reference

1. Starmer AJ, Spector ND, Srivastava R, et al. I-PASS, a mnemonic to standardize verbal handoffs. *Pediatrics*. 2012;129(2):201-204.

10

BLOOD PRODUCT TRANSFUSION

BLAINE T. PHILLIPS, MD, MPH | JULIA LARSON, BS | KERRY L. O'BRIEN, MD | BRIAN O'GARA, MD, MPH

It is essential for the surgical team to appreciate the nuances and overall concepts of transfusion medicine. This chapter will highlight some of the obstacles that the surgical intern or resident may encounter, and it will describe the steps required for safe and appropriate blood product administration. The topics presented in this chapter include types of blood products and their indications, transfusion preparation, transfusion complications, and informed consent.

BLOOD PRODUCTS AND THEIR INDICATIONS

Component therapy, as opposed to whole blood transfusion, is currently the standard of care in the United States. You should be aware that research on whole blood transfusion is rapidly evolving and it is a promising new frontier in surgical resuscitation but is beyond the scope of this chapter. You will likely use component therapy most of the time. The most commonly used blood products are packed red blood cells (pRBCs), platelets, fresh frozen plasma (FFP), and cryoprecipitate (Table 10.1). Blood components are either processed from whole blood collections or collected via apheresis technology.

PACKED RED BLOOD CELLS

A single unit of pRBCs (product volume: ~350 mL) contains approximately 200 to 250 mL of red cells and 100 to 150 mL of plasma. To reduce the risk of febrile nonhemolytic transfusion reactions (FNHTRs) and cytomegalovirus transmission, the final product is often filtered at the donor center to remove white blood cells (a process known as leukoreduction).[1] pRBC transfusion is indicated in the settings of hemorrhage or symptomatic anemia. The decision to transfuse is typically based on clinical status, but certain thresholds are sometimes used to direct transfusion timing for conditions in which slow or chronic blood loss is common. Historically, strategies targeting a hemoglobin of 10 g/dL (hematocrit of 30%) were implemented. However, two recent major randomized, controlled clinical trials in the setting of gastrointestinal bleeding and critical care revealed that, for most patients, a hemoglobin transfusion threshold of 7 g/dL (hematocrit of 21%) is sufficient to maintain adequate hemodynamics and prevent organ failure.[5,6] Therefore, restrictive transfusion strategies are now frequently utilized to ensure adequate oxygen-carrying capacity while simultaneously decreasing the risk of fluid overload and direct transfusion-related complications. Often, a hemoglobin transfusion threshold of 8 to 10 g/dL (hematocrit of 24%-30%) may be indicated for those patients with active cardiac ischemia,[7] but data for this population are mixed and ongoing. Transfusion of a single RBC unit is expected to increase a patient's hemoglobin by 1 g/dL (hematocrit by 3%).

It is important to remember that the hemoglobin and hematocrit of actively bleeding patients may appear normal if insufficient time has elapsed for blood component levels to equilibrate after initial fluid resuscitation. Do not allow "normal-appearing" laboratory values to prevent you from considering transfusion in actively bleeding patients.

PLATELETS

A single unit of platelets is either collected through apheresis of blood from a single donor (product volume: ~300 mL) or pooled from the whole blood of six donors (product volume: ~50 mL; commonly referred to as a "six pack"). Platelets are typically leukoreduced at the donor center. Platelet transfusion is indicated to both prevent *and* treat bleeding in thrombocytopenic patients. In

TABLE 10.1 Commonly Used Blood Products[1-4]

Blood Product	Primary Indications	Quantitative Change in Laboratory Values	Duration of Effect	Volume	Shelf Life
pRBCs	Clinical status (eg, sickle cell crisis, acute hemorrhage, or symptomatic anemia) Hemoglobin of 7-8 g/dL Hematocrit of 21%-24%	1 unit of pRBCs: Hemoglobin ↑ 1 g/dL Hematocrit ↑ 3%	≤2 wk	~350 mL	42 d
Platelets	Thrombocytopenia (≤10,000/μL for bleeding prophylaxis but thresholds for administration vary depending on clinical situation) Platelet function defects *Contraindicated in TTP and HIT unless there is life-threatening bleeding*	1 apheresis unit (most common) or 1 six pack of platelets: Platelet count ↑ 30,000-60,000/μL	3-4 d	Apheresis platelets: ~300 mL Pooled platelets: ~50 mL per each concentrate (ie, ~300 mL per six pack)	5 d
FFP	Coagulopathy (eg, INR≥1.7, factor deficiencies, emergent reversal of anticoagulation effects, or DIC)	4-6 units of FFP (10-20 mL/kg): Factor concentration ↑ 20%	6-8 h	~225 mL	365 d when frozen 24 h after thaw
Cryoprecipitate	Hypofibrinogenemia (<100 mg/dL and often in the setting of hemorrhage or consumptive coagulopathy)	1 unit of cryoprecipitate: Fibrinogen ↑ 5-10 mg/dL	Varies based on each factor[a]	~12.5 mL	365 d when frozen 6 h after thaw

Cryoprecipitate contains fibrinogen, factor VIII, factor XIII, von Willebrand factor, and fibronectin.

DIC, disseminated intravascular coagulation.; FFP, fresh frozen plasma; HIT, heparin-induced thrombocytopenia; INR, international normalized ratio; pRBCs, packed red blood cells; TTP, thrombotic thrombocytopenic purpura.

general, spontaneous bleeding does not occur until a patient's platelet count falls below 5000 to 10,000/μL. Consequently, the threshold for prophylactic platelet transfusion in most medical centers is ≤10,000/μL. There are no studies showing that preprocedural platelet transfusion prevents bleeding. However, the risks of microvascular bleeding-related complications may vary by procedure type. Common thresholds for platelet transfusion are summarized in Table 10.2. Transfusion of a single unit of apheresis platelets (>80% of the platelets utilized in the United States are apheresis derived) can be expected to increase a patient's platelet count by 30,000 to 60,000/μL.

Owing to an increased risk of arterial thrombosis and mortality, platelet transfusion is contraindicated in patients with thrombotic thrombocytopenic purpura and heparin-induced thrombocytopenia, unless they have life-threatening bleeding.[10] Platelet transfusions are relatively contraindicated in patients with immune thrombocytopenic purpura as there is no evidence that they are clinically beneficial in this setting. Furthermore, platelet transfusions are of no value in uremic patients. Instead, management options for these patients include dialysis, desmopressin acetate (DDAVP), and cryoprecipitate.

TABLE 10.2 Common Threshold Values for Platelet Transfusion[8,9]

Indication	Examples	Platelet Transfusion Threshold
Nonbleeding patients	Hematopoietic stem cell transplantation Chemotherapy	≤10,000/μL
Low-risk invasive procedures	Elective central line placement	<20,000/μL
	Paracentesis Thoracentesis Nonelective central line placement	≤30,000/μL
High-risk invasive procedures	Elective lumbar puncture Transbronchial biopsy	≤50,000/μL
Actively bleeding patients	Esophageal varices	≤50,000/μL
Neurosurgical bleeding risk	Spinal anesthesia	≤50,000/μL
	Epidural anesthesia	≤80,000/μL
	Elective neurosurgery	≤100,000/μL
Invasive cardiac surgery	Coronary artery bypass grafting	<50,000/μL

TABLE 10.2 Common Threshold Values for Platelet Transfusion[8,9] (Continued)

Indication	Examples	Platelet Transfusion Threshold
Invasive orthopedic surgery	Hip replacement	≤50,000/μL
Acute intracerebral bleeding	Spontaneous intracerebral hemorrhage	Platelet transfusion is indicated if the patient is thrombocytopenic *Contraindicated for patients with spontaneous intracranial hemorrhage who are on antiplatelet therapy*
	Traumatic intracerebral hemorrhage	≤100,000/μL
Congenital platelet disorders	Bernard-Soulier syndrome Glanzmann thrombasthenia Wiskott-Aldrich syndrome	Platelet transfusion threshold is independent of platelet count in high-risk patients with platelet function defects and thrombocytopenia who either have significant bleeding or are undergoing an invasive procedure

FRESH FROZEN PLASMA

A single unit of FFP (product volume: ~225 mL) is derived either from whole blood or through apheresis. FFP may be used to correct coagulopathy resulting from clotting factor deficiencies and disorders, which most frequently manifest themselves as bleeding or abnormal coagulation studies (international normalized ratio [INR] and prothrombin time/partial thromboplastin time). Common scenarios include warfarin use; liver failure with decreased hepatic synthetic function; consumptive coagulopathy in the setting of trauma or hemorrhage; vitamin K deficiency through prolonged antibiotic use, malabsorption syndromes, or malnutrition; disseminated intravascular coagulation (DIC); massive transfusion with subsequent dilutional coagulopathy; or multiple factor deficiencies in patients who are either bleeding or at risk for spontaneous or procedural hemorrhage. Although there is no evidence that preprocedural prophylactic transfusion of FFP prevents bleeding complications, observational studies suggest that an INR of 2.0 is safe for procedures with a low bleeding risk and 1.5 is safe for those procedures with high risk. A dose of 10 to 20 mL/kg of FFP (~4-6 units) should increase circulating factor concentrations by 20% immediately after transfusion.

FFP should *not* be solely used for volume expansion owing to concerns over proper resource utilization and avoiding unnecessary infectious and non-infectious risks associated with blood products. For a life-threatening bleed in a patient given warfarin (INR >1.5), a four-factor (II, VII, IX, and X) prothrombin complex concentrate may be a superior choice to plasma as it is fast and corrects factor levels with a much smaller volume.

CRYOPRECIPITATE

Cryoprecipitate is indicated in hypofibrinogenemic patients (<100 mg/dL) who are bleeding and is often used in the settings of major surgery or DIC. A single unit of cryoprecipitate (product volume: ~12.5 mL) will increase the fibrinogen level by 5 to 10 mg/dL.[1,2,4] A typical adult dose is 10 single units given in two pools of 5 units for an increase in fibrinogen of 75 to 100 mg/dL.

TRANSFUSION PREPARATION

TYPE AND SCREEN

A type and screen determines the patient's ABO and RhD type and screens for clinically significant red cell alloantibodies. If the antibody screen is negative (ie, the patient has no history of clinically significant red cell antibodies) and there have been at least two ABO types performed (including a current sample), no other tests are required and the patient is eligible for electronic cross-match. Electronic cross-matching is conducted by a computer that matches an RBC unit with the known type of the patient. It typically is performed much faster than traditional cross-matching, which is carried out by laboratory personnel. If the antibody screen is positive, then those specific antibodies need to be identified before a safely matched product can be transfused (see following section Type and Cross). During an inpatient stay on the surgical wards, blood samples need to be sent frequently (every 3 days) for type and screen testing because minor antibodies can change with various disease states, pregnancy, and recent RBC transfusions.

If an inpatient is scheduled for a complicated surgery, a type and screen should be ordered the day before surgery if an up-to-date sample is unavailable. This also applies to inpatients undergoing uncomplicated surgeries (eg, hernia repair) who have a high risk of bleeding. Similarly, an outpatient preoperative type and screen should be ordered only if the procedure is complicated or long

TABLE 10.3 Type and Screen Results and Their Risk of a Major Transfusion Reaction

Type and Screen Results	Risk of a Major Transfusion Reaction (%)
ABO compatible	0.6
ABO and RhD compatible *(type)*	0.2
ABO and RhD compatible with negative antibody screen *(type and screen)*	0.06
ABO and RhD compatible with negative antibody screen and indirect Coomb test *(type and cross-match)*	0.05

in duration or if there is a reason why blood may be required for that specific patient. Permutations of type and screen results and their corresponding risks of a major transfusion reaction due to incompatibility are provided in Table 10.3.

TYPE AND CROSS

A type and cross involves performing a type and screen and then identifying a compatible match of the patient's blood type and antibody profile to a donor unit within the available supply to ensure a compatible transfusion. This is typically done in preparation for an imminent blood transfusion (eg, in the setting of hemorrhage or anticipated blood loss). A cross-match may take minutes to hours depending on the type of cross-match (eg, electronic, immediate spin, or full serologic) and the relative rarity of the patient's antibody profile within the donor population. A laboratory cross-match is an indirect Coombs test, in which the patient's serum is tested by mixing it with a sample from the donor unit and observed for agglutination. If no agglutination occurs, the unit is deemed a match.

RBCs and plasma must be ABO compatible, but whole blood (where available) must be ABO identical as it contains both RBCS *and* significant amounts of plasma. Platelets and cryoprecipitate do not require ABO matching.

EMERGENCY TRANSFUSION

In the setting of acute hemodynamic instability requiring blood product transfusion before the results of a type and screen or cross-match, emergency blood product release with O+ or O(−) blood is necessary. Group O blood is a precious resource that requires appropriate stewardship and should not be given unless there is reasonable certainty that the patient cannot wait for the results of blood bank testing. In most hospitals, O+ RBCs are given to males and women outside of child-bearing years. O(−) RBCs are reserved for women in their child-bearing years to prevent anti-D formation that could lead to hemolytic disease of the fetus and newborn in RhD-negative women. As an intermediate solution, if the blood type of the patient is known, "type-specific" blood can be transfused with a high degree of safety (ie, avoiding a major hemolytic reaction due to ABO incompatibility).[11]

MASSIVE TRANSFUSION PROTOCOL

Massive transfusion protocols (MTPs) are activated by a clinician in response to massive bleeding and are usually considered after transfusion of 4 to 10 units within a 24-hour period or in the setting of an acute and life-threatening large-volume hemorrhage. MTPs have a predefined ratio of pRBCs, FFP/cryoprecipitate, and platelet units (random donor platelets) in each pack (eg, 1:1:1 or 2:1:1) for transfusion. Ratios will vary in each hospital but, in general, are between 2:1:1 and 1:1:1 to balance the needs of sustaining life, preventing transfusion-related coagulopathy and DIC, and preserving blood bank resources.

TRANSFUSION COMPLICATIONS

There are numerous risks associated with blood product transfusion. They are often classified as acute or delayed. Acute complications from blood product administration are rare and include, but are not limited to, transfusion-transmitted bacterial infections and parasitic infections, allergic reactions, febrile reactions, anaphylaxis, acute hemolytic transfusion reactions, FNHTRs, transfusion-related acute lung injury (TRALI), transfusion-associated circulatory overload (TACO), and metabolic derangements such as hyperkalemia (Table 10.4).[12,13] Timely identification and intervention of acute complications can be potentially life saving. If an acute transfusion reaction is suspected, the transfusion should always be immediately stopped and the patient should be evaluated. Meanwhile, delayed complications of blood product transfusion include, but are not limited to, transfusion-transmitted viral infections (TTVIs; eg, hepatitis B virus [HBV], hepatitis C virus [HCV], and human immunodeficiency virus [HIV]), secondary hemochromatosis, delayed hemolytic transfusion reactions, transfusion-associated graft-versus-host disease, posttransfusion

TABLE 10.4 Acute Transfusion Reactions[12]

Risk	Incidence	Etiology	Signs/Symptoms	Management
Allergic (urticarial) reactions	1:33-1:100	Antibody in recipient to donor plasma protein	Urticaria Flushing Itching	SUSPEND transfusion Administer antihistamines Report to blood bank
Anaphylactic reactions	1:20,000-1:50,000	Antibody to donor plasma proteins	Hypotension Urticaria Bronchospasm Local edema	STOP transfusion Maintain blood pressure Report to blood bank
Febrile reactions	1:100	Antibody to donor white blood cells or presence of cytokines in blood product	Fever Chills	STOP transfusion Administer antipyretics Report to blood bank
Acute hemolytic reactions	1:76,000	Red cell incompatibility (often ABO incompatibility)	Fever Chills/rigors Hypotension Back/flank pain Pain at injection site Hemoglobinemia Hemoglobinuria Renal failure/oliguria DIC	STOP transfusion Manage hypotension Maintain renal perfusion Report to blood bank
TRALI	1:5000	Donor HLA or white cell antibodies	Respiratory distress Fever Tachycardia Hypotension Chest x-ray with bilateral infiltrates	STOP transfusion Provide respiratory support *Mechanical ventilation* Report to blood bank
TACO	1:100	Excess volume	Respiratory distress Orthopnea Cough Hypertension	STOP transfusion Diuretic therapy Respiratory support

(Continued)

TABLE 10.4 Acute Transfusion Reactions[12]   (Continued)

Risk	Incidence	Etiology	Signs/Symptoms	Management
Bacterial contamination	RBCs: 2.6:100,000 Platelets: 1:75,000	Bacterial contamination of blood product	Fever Chills/rigors Hypotension Nausea/vomiting	STOP transfusion Maintain blood pressure Administer antibiotics Obtain blood cultures Report to blood bank

Republished with permission of McGraw-Hill Education, from McKean SC, Ross JJ, Dressler DD, Scheurer DB. Principles and Practice of Hospital Medicine, 2nd edition. 2017; permission conveyed through Copyright Clearance Center, Inc.

DIC, disseminated intravascular coagulation; HLA, human leukocyte antigen; RBC, red blood cell; TACO, transfusion-associated circulatory overload; TRALI, transfusion-related acute lung injury.

purpura, changes to patient antibody profiles, and transfusion-related immunomodulation (TRIM), which can be especially detrimental for patients with cancer undergoing surgery.[13]

Although rare, some transfusion reactions can be acutely fatal. The most common cause of transfusion-associated mortality from allogenic blood product administration in the United States is TRALI, and the second leading cause of death is TACO (Figure 10.1).[14] Hemolytic transfusion reactions, which may be fatal when they occur, can be due to ABO and non-ABO incompatibility. Reactions due to ABO incompatibility are usually from clerical or identification error.

It is important to keep in mind that each RBC and plasma unit contains ~350 and ~225 mL of volume, respectively. Multiple transfusions over a short amount of time in a patient who is elderly, of small body habitus, or with a history of congestive heart failure can quickly cause TACO. Rapid administration of blood products during MTPs can also cause numerous complications that require monitoring. These include, but are not limited to, dilutional effects, coagulopathy due to factor depletion in the setting of trauma (eg, DIC), and metabolic derangements (eg, alkalosis and hypocalcemia due to an increase in serum citrate). Hypocalcemia may result from multiple transfusions given that citrate, which actively binds calcium as a chelating agent, is added to units to prevent coagulation.

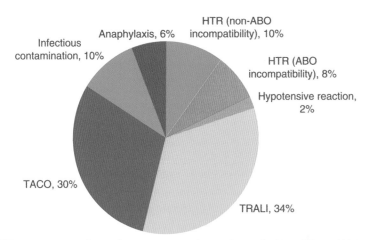

FIGURE 10.1 Causes of Transfusion-Associated Mortality in the United States.[14] (Data from the 2012-2016 fiscal year.) HTR, hemolytic transfusion reaction. (Data from Food and Drug Administration. Fatalities Reported to FDA Blood Collection and Transfusion – Annual Summary for FY2016. Center for Biologics Evaluation and Research.)

FNHTRs are the most common type of transfusion reaction, with allergic reactions occurring with the second greatest frequency. Anaphylaxis is rare but can be fatal. Platelet transfusion carries an increased risk of bacterial sepsis because platelets must be stored at room temperature. The risk of bacterial sepsis from RBC and plasma transfusion is much lower as these components are stored at lower temperatures (RBCs are stored at 1-6°C, and plasma is frozen and then stored at 1-6°C after being thawed).

Although some of these acute risks are most worrisome to the intern and surgical team, patients are most often concerned with TTVI. Among the TTVIs, viral hepatitis and HIV provide the greatest health risk and can lead to significant disease. In the United States, the risk of TTVI with HBV and HCV is 1/205,000 and 1/2,000,000, respectively.[13] For HIV, the risk of TTVI is also 1/2,000,000.[13] The highest risk of transmitting any type of infectious agent occurs acutely with platelets via bacterial sepsis. The development of hemochromatosis is also chronic in nature and results from serial blood transfusions without adequate phlebotomy or chelation therapy in patients with thalassemia, sickle cell disease, or other forms of anemia. Lastly, there has been recent active investigation into the potential for TRIM, which can weaken a patient's immune system for weeks to months after receiving a plasma-containing transfusion and may alter susceptibility to infection and the recurrence of cancer.[15] Ongoing research in this important field is needed to establish the long-term risk of transfusion in patients with immunosuppression or cancer.

INFORMED CONSENT AND REFUSAL OF BLOOD PRODUCT TRANSFUSION

In the elective or semielective setting, informed consent for blood product transfusion should be obtained, and the patient should be informed of the aforementioned risks. Consent is not required in emergent, life-threatening clinical scenarios.

Jehovah's Witnesses may refuse transfusion of human-derived blood products because of their religious beliefs, even in the setting of life-threatening hemorrhage. However, they may accept non-human-derived replacement fluids, including crystalloids (eg, Ringer lactate and normal saline) and some colloid solutions (eg, albumin, dextran, and hetastarch).[16,17] It is important to have an individual conversation with each patient about which products he or she will accept. Never assume that every Jehovah's Witness will hold the same values and belief system. Some Jehovah's Witnesses will accept autologous blood donation, depending on the manner and timeframe in which it returns to the body, and some may be comfortable with component therapy.[16,17] Other options include preoperative erythropoietin, preoperative iron supplementation, or cell salvage machines during surgery.[17] If a patient is a Jehovah's Witness, it is still considered best practice to offer him or her the standard of care, to explain the risks and benefits of accepting and refusing transfusion, and to document this conversation. Neither Jehovah's Witnesses who are minors nor their parents or guardians may be able to refuse blood product administration in some states and jurisdictions. Consult your hospital legal counsel for further assistance.

SUMMARY

As we conclude this chapter, we want to emphasize the importance of communication within the surgical team before blood product administration. In particular, medical students, interns, and junior residents should always inform their chief resident or attending when they are considering blood product transfusion owing to its status as a vital resource that can be associated with significant harm. When a patient is being considered for transfusion, this likely indicates that the patient is unstable and your superiors should be made aware of this change in clinical status. Also, blood product administration can be accompanied by severe, albeit rare, complications, and your superiors need to consider these complications before intervention.

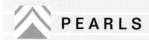

PEARLS

1. The decision to transfuse pRBCs is typically based on clinical status, but restrictive strategies (eg, hemoglobin transfusion threshold of 7 g/dL) are frequently utilized.
2. If an acute transfusion reaction is suspected, immediately stop the transfusion and evaluate the patient.
3. Always inform your chief resident or attending when considering blood product transfusion.

References

1. King KE, Bandarenko N. *Blood Transfusion Therapy: A Physician's Handbook.* 9th ed. Bethesda, MD: American Association of Blood Banks; 2008:236.
2. Sharma S, Sharma P, Tyler LN. Transfusion of blood and blood products: indications and complications. *Am Fam Physician.* 2011;83(6):719-724.
3. Klein HG, Spahn DR, Carson JL. Red blood cell transfusion in clinical practice. *Lancet.* 2007;370(9585):415-426.
4. Callum JL, Karkouti K, Lin Y. Cryoprecipitate: the current state of knowledge. *Transfus Med Rev.* 2009;23(3):177-188.
5. Hebert PC, Wells G, Blajchman MA, et al. A multicenter, randomized, controlled clinical trial of transfusion requirements in critical care. *N Engl J Med.* 1999;340(13):409-417.
6. Villanueva C, Colomo A, Bosch A, et al. Transfusion strategies for acute upper gastrointestinal bleeding. *N Engl J Med.* 2013;368(1):11-21.
7. Carson JL, Stanworth SJ, Roubinian N, et al. Transfusion thresholds and other strategies for guiding allogeneic red blood cell transfusion. *Cochrane Database Syst Rev.* 2016;10:CD002042.
8. Kaufman RM, Djulbegovic B, Gernsheimer T, et al. Platelet transfusion: a clinical practice guideline from the AABB. *Ann Intern Med.* 2015;162(3):205-213.
9. Al-Shahi Salman R, Law ZK, Bath PM, Steiner T, Sprigg N. Haemostatic therapies for acute spontaneous intracerebral haemorrhage. *Cochrane Database Syst Rev.* 2018;(4):CD005951. doi:10.1002/14651858.CD005951.pub4.
10. Goel R, Ness PM, Takemoto CM, Krishnamurti L, King KE, Tobian AA. Platelet transfusions in platelet consumptive disorders are associated with arterial thrombosis and in-hospital mortality. *Blood.* 2015;125(9):1470-1476.
11. Yazer MH, Waters JH, Spinella PC, et al. Use of uncrossmatched erythrocytes in emergency bleeding situations. *Anesthesiology.* 2018;128(3):650-656.
12. Chajewski OS, Squires JR. Postoperative blood transfusion. In: McKean SC, Ross JJ, Dressler DD, Scheurer DB, eds. *Principles and Practice of Hospital Medicine.* 2nd ed. New York, New York: McGraw-Hill Education; 2017. https://accessmedicine.mhmedical.com/content.aspx?bookid=1872&sectionid=138891186. Accessed September 4, 2018.
13. U.S. Department of Health and Human Services. *Blood Transfusion: What are the Risks of a Blood Transfusion?* National Heart, Lung, and Blood Institute; 2018. https://www.nhlbi.nih.gov/node/3593. Accessed July 27, 2018.

14. Food and Drug Administration. Fatalities Reported to FDA Blood Collection and Transfusion – Annual Summary for FY2016. Center for Biologics Evaluation and Research. https://www.fda.gov/downloads/BiologicsBloodVaccines/SafetyAvailability/ReportaProblem/TransfusionDonationFatalities/UCM598243.pdf. Accessed August 12, 2018.
15. Vamvakas EC, Blajchman MA. Transfusion-related immunomodulation (TRIM): an update. *Blood Rev.* 2007;21(6):327-348.
16. Dixon JL, Smalley MG. Jehovah's Witnesses: the surgical/ethical challenge. *J Am Med Assoc.* 1981;246(21):2471-2472.
17. El-Hamamy E, Newman DS. Jehovah's Witnesses and those who refuse blood transfusion. In: Arulkumaran S, Karoshi M, Keith LG, Lalonde AB, B-Lynch C, eds. *A Comprehensive Textbook of Postpartum Hemorrhage: An Essential Clinical Reference for Effective Management.* 2nd ed. London, England: Sapiens Publishing; 2012:587-601. https://www.glowm.com/pdf/PPH_2nd_edn_Chap-72.pdf. Accessed August 12, 2018.

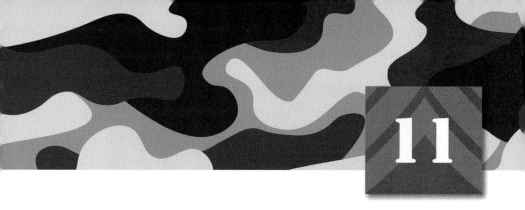

RADIOLOGY FOR THE SURGICAL RESIDENT

ANDREW D. CHUNG, MD, FRCPC | ROBIN B. LEVENSON, MD

INTRODUCTION TO DIAGNOSTIC IMAGING MODALITIES

The past few decades have seen a vast increase in the breadth of imaging options available to clinicians as well as the fidelity of data that is obtained from that imaging. However, like any other diagnostic test, from a complete blood count to a colonoscopy, effective utilization of medical imaging requires consideration of appropriateness. This begins with a clear clinical question to which an answer is being sought and then considers the strengths and weaknesses of the available imaging modalities to select a test that will advance the available clinical information.

PLAIN RADIOGRAPHY AND FLUOROSCOPY

Plain radiographs (CR) are formed through the transmission of X-rays in one direction through the patient. The resultant image is a 2-dimensional amalgamation of all the tissue densities that the transmitted X-rays passed through en route to the film (or digital detector). Five basic radiographic densities can

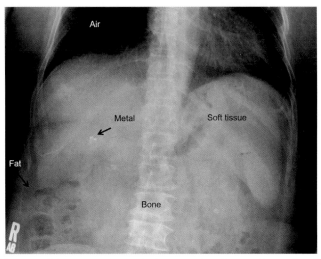

FIGURE 11.1 Abdominal radiograph depicting the 5 basic radiographic densities.

be discerned, and these are, from darkest to lightest: air, fat, water (soft tissue), bone, and metal (Figure 11.1). Tissues with low optical density, such as air in the lungs, allow for greater exposure of the detector and appear dark. Tissues with high optical density, such as metal, block the majority of X-rays and appear white.

The advantages of plain radiography lie predominantly in its availability, speed of acquisition, portability, and low cost. It is commonly used to assess for line placement or foreign body, evaluate for gross chest pathology (eg, pneumonia, pneumothorax, pulmonary edema, or effusion) or abdominal free air, or screen for mechanical bowel obstruction. However, their 2-dimensional nature lacks the anatomic localization and diagnostic fidelity of cross-sectional counterparts.

Fluoroscopy is the application of low-dose X-ray in real time. It further sacrifices spatial and contrast resolution in favor of temporal information. This is often used for procedural guidance by interventional radiology or intraoperatively by vascular surgeons, orthopedic surgeons, and trauma surgeons. It may also be combined with oral or injected contrast to give dynamic information, such as in the case of upper gastrointestinal studies for dysphagia or to rule out perforation/leak or in the case of hysterosalpingography to evaluate for tubal patency. Attention must be paid to study duration, as despite the low-dose technique, dose accumulated over long procedure times can accumulate sufficiently to cause burns and other patient morbidity.

COMPUTED TOMOGRAPHY

Computed tomography (CT) is generated through the transmission of X-rays through the patient over 360° and provides 3-dimensional spatial information at the cost of higher radiation dose. The same basic radiographic densities applicable CR apply to CT; on unenhanced CT, most soft tissues will demonstrate a similar homogeneous soft tissue density (~40 Hounsfield units [HU]). However, unlike in CR, tissue contrast can be augmented through the use of intravenous contrast material. The tissue contrast that is obtained depends on 2 major factors: organ vascularity/perfusion and timing of study acquisition (Figure 11.2). Viscera or tumors that are highly vascular will enhance faster and thus should be imaged earlier. Similarly, interrogation of the arterial versus venous anatomy will require different study timing. The portal venous phase, which is obtained approximately 70 seconds after contrast injection, is the workhorse of abdominal imaging, providing excellent tissue contrast for most organs and opacification of both the arteries and veins. However, clarity of the diagnostic question is of critical importance when requesting a CT, so that the study can be most appropriately protocoled to answer the clinical question.

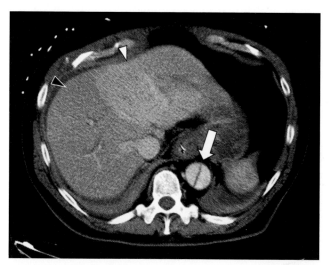

FIGURE 11.2 Contrast-enhanced axial CT image in late arterial phase demonstrates an aortic dissection (arrow) with resultant occlusion of the right hepatic artery (not shown). The left lobe of the liver demonstrates homogenous enhancement (white arrowhead); however, the right lobe of the liver demonstrates diminished enhancement (black arrowhead) due to decreased arterial supply. Tissue contrast after injection of intravenous contrast depends both on the time of scan acquisition and vascular supply.

Common applications of CT include investigation for a source of acute abdominal pain, trauma evaluation, source of bleeding (including active extravasation), evaluation of vascular anatomy and patency, and staging assessment for suspected or known malignancy. However, CT can lack sensitivity for biliary and gynecologic pathologies, which may be better evaluated at ultrasound (US) or magnetic resonance imaging (MRI). Evaluation for pathology within the bowel lumen is also limited and is better achieved at endoscopy, although specialized CT and MR enterography protocols, which involve meticulous bowel preparation before scanning, may be used for evaluation of the small bowel lumen.

ULTRASOUND

US relies on the transmission of sound waves through the body, with images assembled from the reflection of sound waves at tissue interfaces. US is also useful for the evaluation of moving tissues, such as flowing blood, with Doppler US providing information about both the velocity and direction of flow. US is inexpensive, readily available, portable (can be performed bedside), and lacks ionizing radiation. Thus, it is often a first-line examination for abdominal pain, such as suspected appendicitis or renal colic, as well as for biliary and gynecologic pathology, which may be suboptimally evaluated at CT (Figure 11.3). However, examinations are time intensive and operator dependent, with only selected images of the live examination captured and sent to workstations for review. Furthermore, study quality may be severely limited by body habitus, owing to poor acoustic penetration, or by gas or bone. For this reason, US is not suitable for evaluation of the bowel and may be quite limited in the evaluation of central abdominal structures, which may be obscured by gas-filled bowel loops.

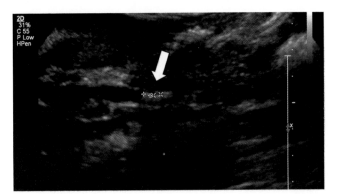

FIGURE 11.3 Grayscale ultrasound image demonstrating multiple echogenic filling defects within the common bile duct (arrow) consistent with choledocholithiasis. Ultrasound is an excellent first-line imaging modality for evaluation of suspected biliary pathology.

MAGNETIC RESONANCE IMAGING

MRI relies on the alignment of protons (H$^+$) in a strong magnetic field, typically 1.5 or 3.0 T for modern clinical scanners. The protons in the patient's body are then deflected by a radiofrequency pulse, and tissue properties will determine the rate at which protons realign in the x- and y-planes. Complex mathematical algorithms are then used to generate images from these properties, and imaging parameters may be tweaked to give different types of tissue contrast.

MRI provides excellent tissue contrast, even on unenhanced studies, which provides an advantage over CT. However, spatial resolution is lower than that of CT. Furthermore, unlike CT examinations, which may be completed in a matter of seconds, MRI examinations are often long and laborious, with some studies taking up to an hour and requiring extensive patient cooperation in the form of breath holding and motionlessness. Study quality can be markedly compromised by motion, susceptibility artifact from metal or gas, or ascites. As such, MRI more than any other modality, is best used as a problem-solving tool to answer a very specific clinical question. This may include further characterization of an indeterminate lesion identified at CT/US, better evaluation of biliary or pelvic/gynecologic pathology, or for local staging of pelvic tumors. However, attempts to use MRI as a screening modality for a nonspecific clinical complaint will likely result in a suboptimal and lengthy study, which would likely be better served by another imaging modality, particularly CT. There are also some circumstances (eg, pregnancy) when MRI is the preferred cross-sectional imaging modality over a CT scan with radiation.

NUCLEAR MEDICINE

Nuclear medicine consists of imaging tests whereby a particular molecule or cell type is radiolabeled and introduced into the patient. The radiolabeled molecule or cell will then localize to a particular organ, cell type, or excretion pathway, which provides information about the localization and/or function of certain organ systems or pathologies. Because radiation is being emitted from the patient in all directions, rather than transmitted in a known direction through the patient, spatial resolution is low. However, in exchange, functional information is obtained. Nuclear medicine may be used to highlight a source or location of pathology that is occult on other anatomic forms of imaging. For example, nuclear medicine red blood cell scans may detect gastrointestinal bleeding at rates of 0.1 mL/min, which is approximately 5 times more sensitive than angiography.[1,2] Nuclear medicine studies may be used as a problem-solving tool when other modalities are inconclusive. This includes assessment for acute cholecystitis (hepatobiliary iminodiacetic acid [HIDA] scan), determination of presence and site of a bile leak, and distinguishing infection from other pathologies.

BASICS OF CHEST PLAIN FILM

CENTRAL LINE PLACEMENT

Central lines are most commonly placed from an internal jugular or subclavian approach. The appropriate tip position is at the cavoatrial junction, which can often be discerned by the bulging contour of the right atrium from the relatively straight superior vena cava. When not discernible, placement approximately 4 cm below the level of the carina may be used as an estimate for the location of the cavoatrial junction.[3] Any kinking or deviation from the expected course of the central line should raise the suspicion of abnormal position (Figure 11.4), either within a venous collateral or artery, and should prompt further evaluation with a lateral radiograph or, if necessary, CT.

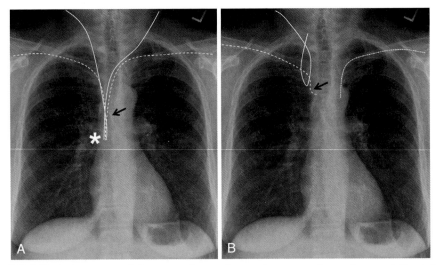

FIGURE 11.4 A, Pictorial depiction of normal central venous catheter placement. Frontal chest radiograph with the expected courses of bilateral internal jugular (solid lines) and subclavian (dashed lines) central venous catheters is depicted. The tip of the catheter should terminate at the cavoatrial junction (asterisk), where the straight contour of the superior vena cava meets the convex border of the right atrium. This is approximately 4 cm below the level of the carina (arrow). B, Pictorial depiction of abnormal central venous catheter placement. Frontal chest radiograph with right internal jugular line (solid arrow) coiled within the right internal jugular vein, with tip directed retrograde. Right subclavian line (dashed line) shows an abnormal angulation (arrow) suggestive of deviation into the azygos vein. Left subclavian line (dotted line) dives inferiorly to the left of the expected course of the left brachiocephalic vein, suggestive of intra-arterial placement.

ENDOTRACHEAL TUBE PLACEMENT

The ideal position of an endotracheal tube tip is 5 ± 2 cm above the level of the carina (Figure 11.5A).[4] Placement too close to the carina may risk bronchial intubation, because the position of the endotracheal tube will change with neck position. The principle "hose goes with the nose" is a reminder that the tip of the endotracheal tube will ascend when the neck is in extension and descend when the neck is in flexion. A low endotracheal tube that is deviated to one side, most commonly the right (right mainstem), should raise the suspicion of bronchial intubation. Unilateral intubation will often result in collapse of the contralateral lung (Figure 11.5B).

ENTERIC TUBE PLACEMENT

Appropriate enteric tube placement should demonstrate a near-vertical course through the thorax with tip distal to the diaphragm (Figure 11.5A). If deviation to either side is seen in the thorax, attention should then be drawn to the carina to identify whether the tube follows the course of one of the mainstem bronchi.

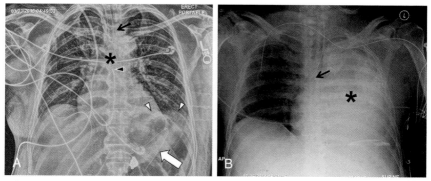

FIGURE 11.5 A, Normal placement of endotracheal and enteric tubes. Frontal chest radiograph shows the tip of the endotracheal tube (black arrow) is approximately 5 cm above the level of the carina (asterisk). The tip of the enteric tube (white arrow) is below the level of the left hemidiaphragm (white arrowheads). Note also the Swan Ganz catheter coursing through the right-sided heart chambers with tip in the main pulmonary trunk (black arrowhead). B, Right mainstem bronchial intubation. Frontal chest radiograph showing deviation of the endotracheal tube toward the right (black arrow) and below the level of the carina is consistent with right mainstem bronchial intubation. There is complete white out of the left lung consistent with collapse of the contralateral lung (asterisk).

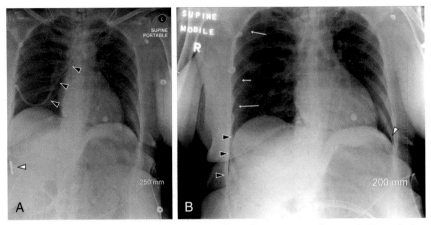

FIGURE 11.6 Malpositioned enteric tube and resultant pneumothorax. A, Frontal chest radiograph shows a weighted feeding tube following the course of the right mainstem bronchus (black arrowheads). The tip appears below the level of the diaphragm owing to its position within the deep posterior costophrenic sulcus (white arrowhead). B, Frontal supine chest radiograph after removal of the feeding tube demonstrates a pleural line within the right hemithorax, consistent with a pneumothorax (arrows). Note the lack of lung markings peripheral to the pleural line. There is prominence of the costophrenic sulcus (deep sulcus sign) on the right (black arrowheads), which is a sign of pneumothorax on supine radiographs due to accumulation of air anteriorly. The normal left costophrenic angle (white arrowhead) is available for comparison.

This is critical, as the tip may appear below the diaphragm on a frontal radiograph even if inappropriately placed through the bronchus given the depth of the posterior costophrenic sulcus (Figure 11.6A).

PNEUMOTHORAX

A pneumothorax is best identified on upright chest radiograph and should appear as a well-defined thin white pleural line, beyond which lung markings are typically not seen. When the patient is upright, the apex is the most common location of small pneumothoraces, as air rises to the nondependent portion of the chest. These diagnostic criteria are helpful in identifying pneumothorax mimics, such as skin folds or artifactual "Mach bands." When the patient is in the supine position (common in trauma or intensive care unit patients) pleural air tends to collect anterior and basal (nondependent), leading to the "deep sulcus sign." The costophrenic sulcus looks deeper and more lucent (Figure 11.6B).

Pneumothorax with deviation of the mediastinum to the contralateral side should raise the suspicion of tension (Figure 11.7). Other findings in tension

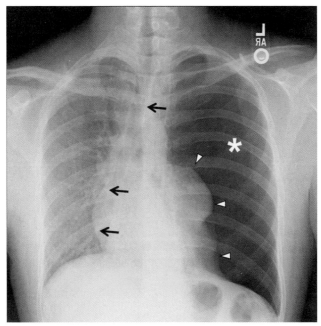

FIGURE 11.7 Tension pneumothorax. Frontal chest radiograph shows that the left lung is collapsed and retracted toward the mediastinum. Note the well-defined pleural line at the lung-pneumothorax interface (arrowheads). The left hemithorax is abnormally lucent and demonstrates a complete absence of lung markings (asterisk), confirming the diagnosis of pneumothorax. Deviation of the trachea and mediastinum to the contralateral side (arrows) is indicative of a tension pneumothorax.

pneumothorax may include ipsilateral expansion of the rib interspaces and ipsilateral flattening of the hemidiaphragm. The ipsilateral lung may also be compressed.

ATELECTASIS/PNEUMONIA

Atelectasis refers to partial collapse of the lung parenchyma, whereas pneumonia is space occupying and refers to consolidation filling the lung parenchyma due to infection/pus. On CR, the 2 may be difficult to distinguish. Atelectasis is characterized by volume loss (including ipsilateral shift of the mediastinum, hemidiaphragm elevation), but in reality, these findings may be quite subtle and this is a concept with which even Radiology trainees may struggle. Both may appear as dense opacification (increased "white") over a segmental or lobar distribution of the lung. Silhouetting (loss of definition) of the hemidiaphragm or

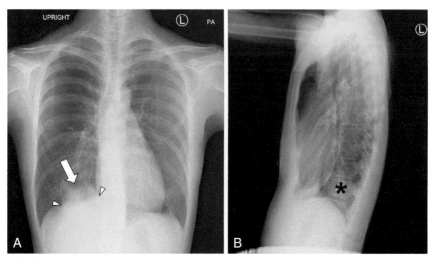

FIGURE 11.8 Right lower lobe pneumonia. A, Frontal radiograph demonstrates a dense opacity over the right lower lung (arrow) with silhouetting of the right hemidiaphragm (arrowheads). B, Lateral radiograph in the same patient demonstrates increased density over the lower vertebral bodies (spine sign) confirming right lower lobe consolidation.

increased density over the vertebral bodies (spine sign) may be seen in lower lobe atelectasis or pneumonia (Figure 11.8). Air bronchograms (dark branching airways visible through the area of consolidation) favor infection. Associated pleural effusions may be seen.

PLEURAL EFFUSION

Pleural effusions are characterized by menisci seen at the costophrenic angles and are best identified on lateral decubitus or lateral chest radiographs (Figure 11.9). When large, they may cast a veillike opacity over the affected lung, which may be difficult to distinguish from and may mask underlying consolidation. Chronic pleural thickening may mimic a small effusion.

WIDENED MEDIASTINUM

Mediastinal widening may be seen in the context of various pathologic conditions, the most acute of which is traumatic aortic injury. Other causes of mediastinal widening include but are not limited to tumors, lymphadenopathy, mediastinal collections, and vascular enlargement or anomalies. However, given variability, the best indicator of a truly widened mediastinum is comparison

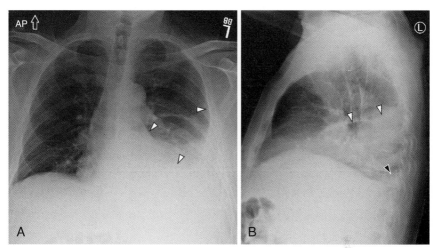

FIGURE 11.9 Pleural effusions. A, Frontal chest radiograph demonstrates a veillike opacity over the left lower lung with silhouetting of the left hemidiaphragm. There is a curvilinear meniscus at the interface of this opacity with the lung (white arrowheads) consistent with a pleural effusion. B, Lateral chest radiograph in the same patient again demonstrates a moderate left pleural effusion (white arrowheads). There is a small meniscus at the posterior costophrenic angle on the right (black arrowhead) consistent with a small effusion. Lateral chest radiographs are more sensitive for small effusions than frontal radiographs.

with previous. Even then, a wide array of technical factors may simulate the appearance of a widened mediastinum, including degree of inspiration/presence of atelectasis, patient positioning, and whether the film was acquired portably in the anteroposterior (AP) direction rather than posteroanterior (PA). As such, one should be cautious in interpreting a widened mediastinum, particularly in patients with low clinical suspicion of aortic injury, as apparent widening due to technical factors is far more common.[5]

INTRODUCTION TO ABDOMINAL IMAGING CONCEPTS AND COMMON PATHOLOGIES

PNEUMOPERITONEUM

In the absence of recent surgical history, pneumoperitoneum is worrisome for hollow viscus perforation. On CR, pneumoperitoneum is best detected with the patient in the upright position; gas in the nondependent portions of the abdomen will be contrasted against the soft tissue density of the liver and diaphragm (Figure 11.10A).

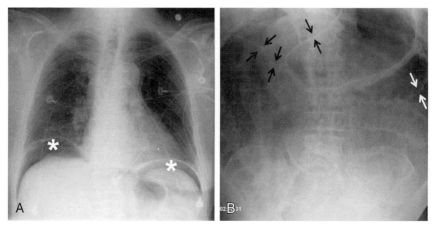

FIGURE 11.10 Pneumoperitoneum. A, Upright frontal chest radiograph demonstrates lucency between the diaphragm and the liver/spleen (asterisks). B, Supine abdominal radiograph demonstrates lucency outlining both sides of the bowel wall (arrows), which is referred to as Rigler sign. It is important to look where there is no other bowel loop adjacent to the outer surface of the bowel, as 2 gas-filled bowel loops in close proximity may simulate Rigler sign.

Detection of pneumoperitoneum on supine films is difficult, although it can be suggested when both sides of the bowel wall appear well defined (Rigler sign, Figure 11.10B) or by increased central lucency (football sign) due to gas collecting along the protuberant portion of the anterior abdomen.

ILEUS VERSUS OBSTRUCTION

Ileus can be difficult to distinguish from obstruction on CR (Figure 11.11). Findings that may be suggestive of ileus include gaseous distention of the entire gastrointestinal tract, including the rectum. Mechanical obstruction more commonly presents with a greater degree of bowel dilatation, with more focal distribution of dilated bowel loops (due to distal collapse), lack of gas in the rectum, and multiple differential air-fluid levels on upright or decubitus films. In general, normal small bowel loops should not exceed 3 cm in diameter, large bowel loops 6 cm, and the cecum 9 cm.

FREE FLUID VERSUS ABSCESS

Free fluid is a nonspecific intra-abdominal finding and may be related to inflammation with or without infection, trauma, fluid overload, or malignancy. Abscesses are organized intra-abdominal fluid collections, typically secondary

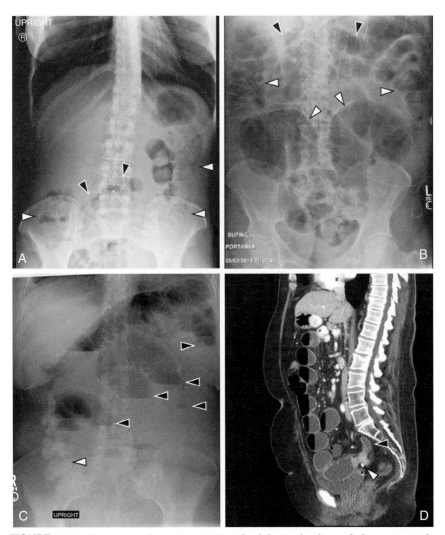

FIGURE 11.11 Ileus versus obstruction. A, Upright abdominal radiograph demonstrates the normal bowel gas pattern with relative paucity of gas within nondilated loops of small bowel (black arrowheads) and mottled stool within nondilated large bowel (white arrowheads). B, Supine abdominal radiograph shows diffuse distention of the small bowel (black arrowheads) and large bowel (white arrowheads), suggestive of generalized ileus. C, Upright abdominal radiograph shows diffuse dilation of the small bowel, concentrated in the upper abdomen, with multiple differential air-fluid levels (black arrowheads) and nondistended ascending colon (white arrowhead), in keeping with mechanical small bowel obstruction. D, Sagittal contrast-enhanced CT image in the same patient as in (C) demonstrates an abrupt transition point in the pelvis (white arrowhead) with collapsed distal small bowel loops (black arrowhead).

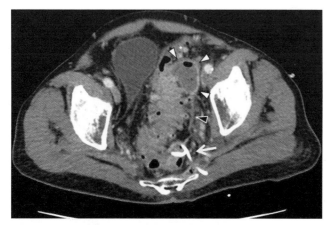

FIGURE 11.12 Diverticular abscess. Axial contrast-enhanced CT image shows a gas- and fluid-containing collection adjacent to the sigmoid colon. Note the thick hyperdense enhancing wall (white arrowheads), which is the characteristic feature of an organized collection/abscess. There is adjacent peritoneal thickening (black arrowhead) consistent with inflammation. A pigtail drainage catheter (white arrow) had previously been placed in a second collection.

to infection. The hallmark feature of an abscess is a circumscribed, enhancing wall at cross-sectional imaging with central hypodensity/fluid (Figure 11.12). Fluid density may be slightly higher than that of simple fluid because of purulent contents, and surrounding inflammatory changes are common. Internal foci of gas may be present.

ACUTE APPENDICITIS

Acute inflammation of the appendix is characterized by a dilated (>6 mm) appendix with periappendiceal inflammation (fat stranding on CT or MRI and echogenic fat at US).[6] The appendiceal wall in appendicitis is often hyperemic and thickened. Periappendiceal free fluid and/or the presence of an obstructing appendicolith may be seen (Figure 11.13). At US, focal tenderness over the appendix and noncompressibility of the appendiceal lumen may be present.[7] The integrity of the appendiceal wall should be evaluated for gangrenous change or perforation. Associated abscess formation and/or extraluminal gas may be present in cases of appendiceal perforation, although the appendix may be perforated without these findings.

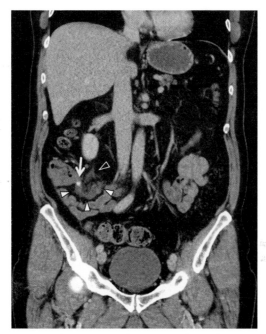

FIGURE 11.13 Acute appendicitis. Coronal contrast-enhanced CT image shows the dilated appendix arising from the cecal pole (white arrowheads). There is a hyperdense appendicolith at the appendiceal base (white arrow) with periappendiceal free fluid (black arrowhead) and fat stranding.

ACUTE DIVERTICULITIS

The presence of underlying diverticular disease is a prerequisite for acute diverticulitis. Inflammatory changes, characterized by fat stranding on CT or MRI, centered on an inflamed diverticulum with or without colonic wall thickening are typical of diverticulitis (Figure 11.14). However, one may not well see the culprit diverticulum, and a patient needs only one diverticulum to have diverticulitis. Complications may include abscesses or fistulae, including colovesicular fistula.

ACUTE CHOLECYSTITIS

Gallbladder distention is required for an imaging diagnosis of acute cholecystitis. A distended gallbladder with gallstones and either gallbladder wall thickening (>3 mm) or positive sonographic Murphy sign (arrest of inspiration with

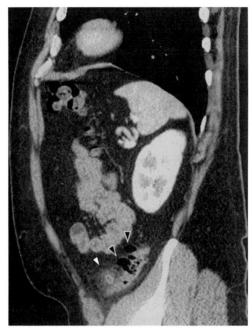

FIGURE 11.14 Acute diverticulitis. Sagittal contrast-enhanced CT image shows multiple outpouchings arising from the sigmoid colon, in keeping with colonic diverticula (black arrowheads). There is inflammatory fat stranding centered on an inflamed diverticulum (white arrowhead) in keeping with diverticulitis. Note the paucity of gas within the inflamed diverticulum, which is typical.

focal transducer pressure over the gallbladder) has high specificity (>90%) for acute cholecystitis (Figure 11.15).[8] Similar findings may be seen at CT or MRI; however, CT lacks sensitivity for biliary pathology. Nuclear medicine hepatobiliary (HIDA) scan may aid in the diagnosis of acute cholecystitis in cases with equivocal imaging findings, evidenced by lack of radiotracer uptake by the gallbladder, with reported increase in sensitivity to 97.7% versus 73.3% for US alone.[9]

ISCHEMIC BOWEL

Ischemic bowel is suggested by the presence of bowel wall thickening and loss of normal bowel wall enhancement at contrast-enhanced CT or MRI, particularly if following an expected vascular territory or corresponding to a known watershed territory. Pneumatosis and portal venous gas are highly specific signs for bowel ischemia/infarction (Figure 11.16).[10,11] Pneumatosis may be seen as air tracking along/within the bowel wall, both in the dependent and nondependent

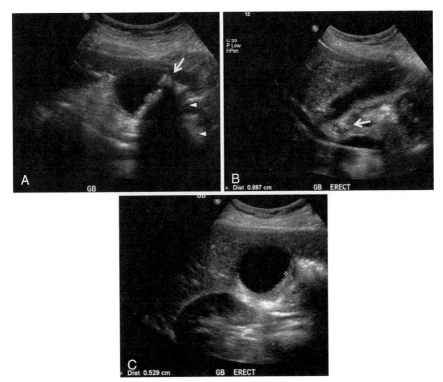

FIGURE 11.15 Acute cholecystitis. A, Grayscale ultrasound image demonstrates multiple gallstones (arrow) within the distended gallbladder. Note the posterior acoustic shadowing (arrowheads), typical of calculi. B, Grayscale ultrasound images shows a gallstone impacted in the gallbladder neck (white arrow). C, Grayscale ultrasound image demonstrates gallbladder wall thickening >3 mm (calipers). A distended gallbladder with gallstones and gallbladder wall thickening in the context of right upper quadrant pain is highly specific for acute cholecystitis.

portions, and may be circumferential. Portal venous gas in the liver may be distinguished from pneumobilia by its presence in the peripheral third of the liver.[12]

RADIOLOGIC-CLINICAL CONTEXT

An awareness of the strengths and weaknesses of imaging modalities is critical in selecting an imaging modality that will add diagnostic information and value to the patient's care. Providing the appropriate clinical context is invaluable in ensuring that the study is protocoled for best diagnostic yield and that an appropriate differential diagnosis is provided. Radiologic evaluation may reveal

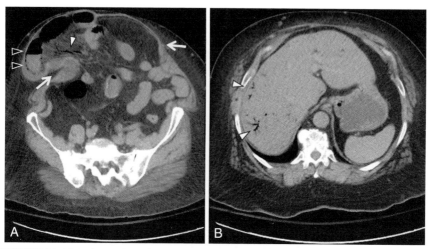

FIGURE 11.16 Ischemic bowel. A, Axial contrast-enhanced CT image demonstrates a large incarcerated ventral wall hernia (arrows). The incarcerated segment of small bowel demonstrates diminished enhancement and circumferential intramural gas (black arrowheads) consistent with pneumatosis. Gas is noted within the small portal venous branches (white arrowhead). This constellation of findings is consistent with bowel ischemia/infarction. B, Axial contrast-enhanced CT image demonstrates portal venous gas within the liver (white arrowheads). Its presence in the peripheral third of the liver parenchyma is a distinguishing factor from pneumobilia.

findings that were unexpected from the patient's initial presentation. However, it is important to remember to ensure that radiologic findings are concordant with the clinical picture. When discordant, an interdisciplinary discussion may be useful to reconcile the radiologic findings with the clinical scenario. Doing so may avoid potentially unnecessary intervention or conversely allow for treatment in a timely manner.

 P E A R L S

1. Knowing the available diagnostic studies in your armamentarium and their appropriate indications is an essential adjunct in all fields of medicine.
2. It is important to ask yourself before ordering any imaging study if this will ultimately impact your management.
3. Be sure to view all images requested, and keep practicing on how to read these images. Discussions with your seniors and radiologist can help supplement your skill level. The authors recommend this sequence: (1) review images yourself; (2) read radiology report; (3) review images again.

References

1. Laing CJ, Tobias T, Rosenblum DI, et al. Acute gastrointestinal bleeding: emerging role of multidetector CT angiography and review of current imaging techniques. *Radiographics.* 2007;27:1055-1070.
2. Smith R, Copely DJ, Bolen FH. 99mTc RBC scintigraphy: correlation of gastrointestinal bleeding rates with scintigraphic findings. *AJR Am J Roentgenol.* 1987;148:869-874.
3. Mahlon MA, Yoon H-C. CT angiography of the superior vena cava: normative values and implications for central venous catheter position. *J Vasc Interv Radiol.* 2007;18:1106-1110.
4. Goodman LR, Conrardy PA, Laing F, et al. Radiographic evaluation of endotracheal tube position. *AJR Am J Roentgenol.* 1976;127:433-434.
5. Ho RT, Blackmore CC, Bloch RD, et al. Can we rely on mediastinal widening on chest radiography to identify subjects with aortic injury? *Emerg Radiol.* 2002;9:183-187.
6. Lane MJ, Liu DM, Huynh MD, et al. Suspected acute appendicitis: nonenhanced helical CT in 300 consecutive patients. *Radiology.* 1999;213:341-346.
7. Jeffrey RB, Laing FC, Townsend RR. Acute appendicitis: sonographic criteria based on 250 cases. *Radiology.* 1988;167:327-329.
8. Ralls PW, Colletti PM, Lapin SA, et al. Real-time sonography in suspected acute cholecystitis. Prospective evaluation of primary and secondary signs. *Radiology.* 1985;155:767-771.
9. Kaoutzanis C, Davies E, Leichtle SW, et al. Abdominal ultrasound versus hepato-imino diacetic acid scan in diagnosing acute cholecystitis–what is the real benefit?. *J Surg Res.* 2014;188:44-52.
10. Wiesner W, Khurana B, Ji H, et al. CT of acute bowel ischemia. *Radiology.* 2003;226:635-650.
11. Taourel PG, Deneuville M, Pradel JA, et al. Acute mesenteric ischemia: diagnosis with contrast-enhanced CT. *Radiology.* 1996;199:632-636.
12. Abboud B, El Hachem J, Yazbeck T, et al. Hepatic portal venous gas: physiopathology, etiology, prognosis and treatment. *World J Gastroenterol.* 2009;15:3585-3590.

FOCUSED EKG PREPARATION FOR THE SURGICAL INTERN

DAVID J. SHIM, MD, PhD | ALFRED E. BUXTON, MD

The information provided by an electrocardiogram (EKG) can reveal an incredible amount of information about the cardiovascular status of a patient (eg, rhythm, hemodynamics, electrolytes) but can also be overwhelming. Earlier in your training you were taught to focus on each component individually and learn what is normal and abnormal for each aspect. The purpose of this chapter is to start transitioning you from approaching them in an isolated and systematic manner (the "trees" approach) to begin evaluating them in a purposeful manner (the "forest" approach). Above all, clinical context is paramount—T wave inversions in a patient without chest pain who is coming in for a minor elective surgery is very different from T wave inversions in someone who is postop from a major surgery, hypotensive, and having chest pain.

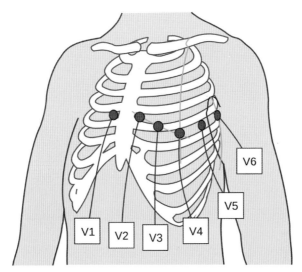

FIGURE 12.1 Standard placement of the precordial chest leads. Note V1 and V2 in the 4th intercostal space, V4 in the 5th space at the midclavicular line, and V6 at the midaxillary line, with V3 and V5 placed midway between V2 to V4 and V4 to V6, respectively. (source: Jmarchn/Wikimedia Commons/CC-BY-SA-3.0.)

The standard 12-lead EKG is obtained by recording signals from electrodes connected to each of the arms and legs (limb leads) and 6 electrodes connected to the chest (precordial leads, Figure 12.1). The printout is typically set up to show you a 10-second tracing, first from the perspective of the limb leads (I, II, III, aVR, aVL, aVF) and then from the perspective of the precordial leads (V1-V6), as well as 1 or 2 "rhythm strips" below that (Figure 12.2). Each vertically aligned QRS complex represents the *same* heartbeat, just from different perspectives. Sometimes it is helpful to scan down the leads as small components such as P waves or pacing spikes may be easier to see in one lead over another. Alternatively, a big deflection that is seen only in one lead and not any of the others may simply be an artifact.

RHYTHM

Normal sinus rhythm (Figure 12.2) is typically indicated by P waves that are upright in lead II and biphasic in lead V1 and are associated with each and every QRS complex. Often a normal QRS that appears early and is preceded by an abnormal P wave represents a conducted premature atrial complex (PAC), or an early wide QRS (duration >120 ms) represents a premature ventricular complex (PVC), and if rare and isolated are not usually clinically significant.

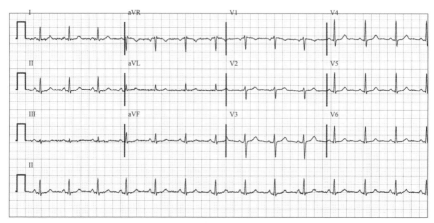

FIGURE 12.2 Normal sinus rhythm. A standard 12-lead EKG with one "rhythm strip" (in this case lead II) included in the bottom row. Note the presence of P waves that are upright in lead II, biphasic in V1, and associated with each and every QRS complex.

If a patient suddenly becomes tachycardic, obtain a 12-lead EKG (over just guessing from telemetry) to help decide in management. **Sinus tachycardia** is always a response to an underlying driver, and treatment should always be directed at that driver (eg, pain, hypotension, anemia, hypovolemia, hypoxia). Often it is the earliest sign of something more sinister (such as bleeding, heart failure, or pulmonary embolism). Alternatively, if during the tachycardia P waves are different or absent, and the QRS complexes are narrow and regular in timing, the rhythm can be a **supraventricular tachycardia** (eg, atrial tachycardia or AV nodal reentrant tachycardia). These can sometimes break on their own but are often persistent and may require interventions to break.

One of the most common arrhythmias seen in the postoperative setting is **atrial fibrillation** (Figure 12.3), characterized by the absence of clear P waves and irregular timing of QRS complexes. The initial considerations should be rate control as well as consideration of anticoagulation to reduce the risk of cardioembolic events. Antiarrhythmics or cardioversion should not be used without first considering their anticoagulation status. The same applies for **atrial flutter** (Figure 12.4), which is characterized by continuous sawtooth-appearing P waves with ventricular rates jumping between certain regular intervals, usually about 75 and 150 bpm. Rate control and anticoagulation are still the initial considerations, but this rhythm is often more difficult to control or break with medications and may require a cardioversion or an ablation procedure.

A tachycardia with wide QRS complexes should prompt consideration of **ventricular tachycardia** (Figure 12.5), especially if the complexes are regular in timing, uniform in morphology, and sudden in onset and the patient

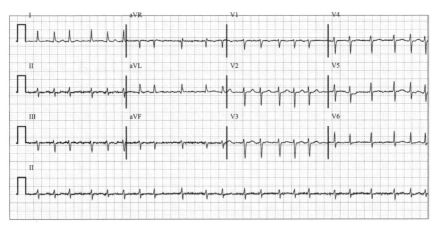

FIGURE 12.3 Atrial fibrillation. Note the absence of clear P waves in any of the leads and the irregular timing of QRS complexes.

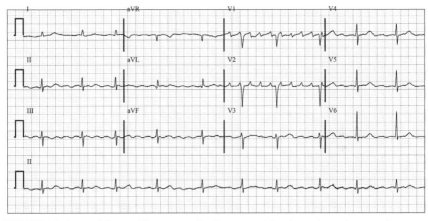

FIGURE 12.4 Atrial flutter. There is regular P wave activity throughout the recording, seen better in III/aVF, and most sawtooth appearing in V1. The QRS complexes in this case are fairly regular in timing.

is clinically symptomatic. The patient should be immediately evaluated and defibrillator pads placed. If unstable, the patient should undergo cardioversion per advanced cardiac life support (ACLS) guidelines, ensuring adequate sedation if conscious. If the patient is stable, it is extremely useful to take the time to obtain a 12-lead EKG and then consider alternative etiologies. Does the patient have a wide QRS that is identical to the baseline EKG before the tachycardia began, which can be suggestive of a **supraventricular**

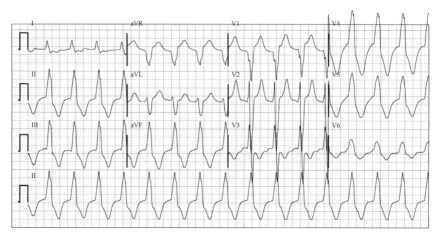

FIGURE 12.5 Ventricular tachycardia. There are wide QRS complexes that are regular in timing and uniform (or monomorphic) in appearance, seen best in the lead II rhythm strip. The deep "V" shape in lead V1 indicates a left bundle branch block pattern.

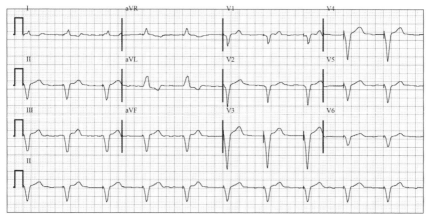

FIGURE 12.6 Paced rhythm. Similar to Figure 12.5, there are regular, uniform, wide QRS complexes, also with a left bundle branch block pattern. However, in this EKG there are also sharp vertical spikes (seen best in lead V3-V4) that precede each QRS complex indicative of ventricular pacing.

tachycardia with aberrancy? If the patient has a **pacemaker or defibrillator**, look for evidence of small sharp pacing spikes at the beginning of each QRS complex, which in most cases produce a wide QRS with a left bundle branch block pattern (deep "V" shape in V1) due to pacing from the right ventricle (Figure 12.6).

BRADYCARDIA AND CONDUCTION

The sinus node is heavily affected by autonomic input and medications, and so **sinus bradycardia** in the surgical setting is often related to these factors. Vagal activation from pain, gastrointestinal upset, bowel manipulation, and oral/tracheal suctioning can lead to sinus slowing even to the point of prolonged sinus pauses. This would be characterized by slowing in the rate of P waves with normal conduction to the QRS complex. Delays in the conduction system at the AV node can lead to **first-degree AV delay** (a lengthening of the time from the start of the P wave to the start of the QRS to >200 ms) or second degree heart block with progressive prolongation of the PR interval culminating in a P wave without an associated QRS (**Mobitz I** or Wenckebach), both of which can be due to high vagal tone or medications. More concerning is a pattern of dropped beats without any preceding change in PR interval (**Mobitz II**) or even complete dissociation of P waves and QRS complexes, with each marching along at their own rate (**complete heart block,** Figure 12.7), as these often require placement of a pacemaker.

TOXIC/METABOLIC

The QT interval (measured from the start of the QRS to the end of the T wave) represents repolarization of the heart and is prolonged by many of the common medications used on a surgical service, including antiemetics such as ondansetron,

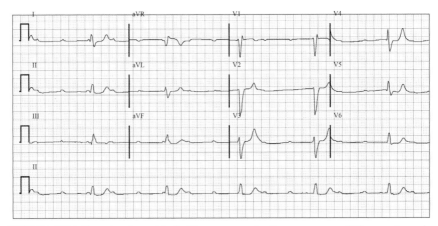

FIGURE 12.7 Complete heart block. There are regular P waves every ~600 ms and regular QRS complexes every ~1800 ms, with no clear relationship between them (seen best in the lead II rhythm strip). In some cases the P waves occur during a QRS complex and are buried or merged with them (see the beginning of the second QRS or the end of the last QRS).

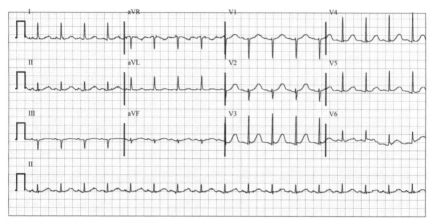

FIGURE 12.8 Prolonged QT. There is normal sinus rhythm; however, the QT interval occupies more than half the interval between 2 QRS complexes. This is less apparent in some leads but should be measured where it is longest (such as lead aVF or V1).

antibiotics such as levofloxacin, antipsychotics such as quetiapine, and pain medications such as methadone. An EKG should be obtained soon after these medications are started or uptitrated. We tend to correct the QT interval (or QTc) for a given heart rate, with normal being less than 450 ms and caution taken at or above 500 ms. A good rule of thumb is that the QT interval should occupy less than half of the time between 2 QRS complexes, or RR interval. A **prolonged QTc** interval (Figure 12.8), especially in the presence of PVCs, puts the patient at high risk of developing torsade de pointes, a type of ventricular tachycardia.

The presence of prominent and pointy T waves on many leads of the EKG should lead one to suspect **hyperkalemia**, and if found, it should be treated immediately as it could progress to more unstable arrhythmias.

ISCHEMIA

In any patient with active chest pain, a 12-lead EKG should be obtained, ideally while the patient is experiencing symptoms. One of the earliest signs of myocardial ischemia is flattening or inversion of the T wave; however, this can often be nonspecific. More concerning are very deep T-wave inversions or depressions of the ST segment, as these are more specific signs for ischemia. Any ST segment elevations (Figure 12.9), especially 1 mm or greater, should prompt immediate evaluation of the patient, as this can be a sign of myocardial infarction (complete occlusion of a coronary vessel) and the patient may need an emergent catheterization. Finally, the presence of Q waves (QRS complexes that start with a negative deflection, greater than one box wide, greater than one-third

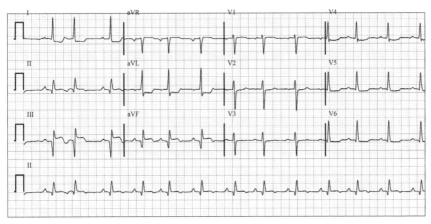

FIGURE 12.9 ST-elevation myocardial infarction. There are elevations of the ST segment in the inferior leads (II, III, aVF) with associated depressions in I and aVL. There are also Q waves in the inferior leads suggesting that the myocardial infarction is already evolving into scar. The rhythm is sinus with the second QRS occurring early and preceded by an abnormal P wave buried in the T wave (likely a PAC).

TABLE 12.1 The 12 Leads of the EKG Grouped Into the Regions of the Heart They Best Represent

Lateral	Inferior	Anteroseptal	Anterior	Anterolateral
I, aVL	II, III, aVF	V1, V2	V3, V4	V5, V6

the depth of the overall complex) indicates the presence of scar from a prior myocardial infarction.

We typically group the leads into the cardiac regions that they best represent (Table 12.1). Isolated changes (such as an elevated ST segment in lead I and lead aVF) are not typically significant, whereas concordant changes (appearing in at least 2 leads from the same territory) are more likely to represent true pathology.

In a real-world clinical setting, these EKG signs can sometimes be difficult to identify in the presence of tachycardia, patient movement, or common conditions that mimic some of these changes (pericarditis causing diffuse ST elevations or ST elevations in the setting of a left bundle branch block). As always, clinical scenario is paramount in determining what your suspicion is for ischemia or infarction. It is helpful to compare EKGs to patients' most recent baseline EKG, when they were free of symptoms. Repeating an EKG even a few minutes later, when the patient has either improvement or worsening of symptoms, can likewise be useful to evaluate evolution of these changes.

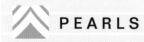 **PEARLS**

1. EKG is a relatively cheap and easy diagnostic study. Liberal use is encouraged, especially when there is a high degree of suspicion.
2. Continuous practice on reading EKGs is encouraged, and practice at recognizing arrhythmias and other conduction abnormalities is essential.
3. It is important to use EKG as an adjunct to physical examination and not in place of it.

13

MANAGING SURGICAL TUBES

CHRISTOPHER DIGESU, MD | MICHAEL S. KENT, MD

INTRODUCTION

The language of surgery is fundamentally built around the management of tubes, lines, and drains. The ability to speak the language is key to succeeding in any field and especially in surgery. This holds true no matter the field of surgery whether it is orthopedic surgery, neurosurgery, urology, or general surgery. For example, this may mean operating on "tubes," such as the bile duct or ureter, or placing a drain such as an external ventricular drain to carefully release cerebrospinal fluid in a controlled manner. Regardless, a surgeon should have a facile knowledge of the types, management, and placement of tubes, lines, and drains.

If you are working with a patient who has a tube, it is important not only to understand exactly what kind of tube that patient has but also be able to relay the information to another clinician so they can immediately understand the patient's exact status. There may be subtle differences in how a tube is described that can have profoundly different implications on a patient's clinical picture. For instance, stating a patient has a "PEG tube" (percutaneous endoscopic gastrostomy tube) when in reality the patient has a "G-tube" (gastrostomy tube that is placed open or laparoscopically) conveys a lack of understanding of what the different tubes are and the patient's anatomy and/or clinical status (ie, the patient has an esophageal stricture and an endoscope cannot be passed to place a PEG tube). In this chapter, we will re-enforce this concept and introduce the terminology and concepts necessary to communicate with your fellow surgeons and to take excellent care of your patients. We will focus on enteric tubes such as PEG tubes, G-tube, and J-tubes as well as chest tubes and tracheostomy tubes. These cover a wide breadth but are sure to be encountered by any doctor starting out on the surgery wards.

HOW TO DESCRIBE TUBES

WHAT DOES THE "FRENCH" OF A TUBE MEAN?

French (Fr) is a descriptor for the circumference of a tube, so stating "24 French" tube refers to the circumference of that tube. This is not to be confused with tubes described in millimeter (mm), as this typically refers to the diameter. In some cases, even more detail can be provided (ie, catheters used in vascular surgery), such as the inner and outer diameter in millimeters. To convert the Fr of a tube to the diameter in millimeters, simply divide the Fr by a factor of 3. Therefore, a 24-Fr tube will roughly have an 8 mm diameter. The use of French or diameter is based on the company and/or traditional measurements; however, the key is knowing what they describe and how to convert between the two.

WHAT IS THE PURPOSE OF THE TUBE?

Keep in mind that one type of tube may have different purposes in different patients. For example, we usually think of a G-tube as for nutrition in the stomach, but it could also be for drainage in a patient with a gastric outlet obstruction (a patient could have a G-tube to drain the stomach and a J-tube for nutrition). Do not assume that because you know the name of the tube, you therefore know its purpose. Be specific in your description of the tube, where it is going, how it was placed, why the patient needs the tube and for how long, how it is secured, and what would happen if the tube becomes dislodged.

TROUBLESHOOTING TUBES

You may be called on your first day on the wards to troubleshoot a tube that is malfunctioning in some way or that needs to be removed. It is important to keep in mind 3 questions when this situation arises.

WHY DOES THE PATIENT HAVE THE TUBE?

For example, in patients who had an esophagostomy and have a clogged feeding tube, it is best to recall why they have it to begin with. How are they eating? Maybe surgery was a month ago and the tube is no longer needed. So, recalling why they needed it to begin with and the status of their current clinical situation is a good fundamental principal.

DOES IT NEED TO BE REPLACED, AND CAN I DO IT SAFELY MYSELF?

A drain in an abscess that is no longer draining may not need to be replaced, but a percutaneous transhepatic biliary drain in a patient with an obstructive cholangiocarcinoma may need to be replaced. Importantly, you may have learned to place a tube such as a nasogastric tube but you may not be able to do it safely at the bedside in a fresh esophagectomy patient. Once a tube is replaced, take steps to ensure it is properly secured.

ONCE IT IS REPLACED, HOW CAN I VERIFY THAT IT IS IN THE CORRECT PLACE?

After placement of nasogastric tube, obvious gastric contents may be draining, but after placement of a feeding tube, a chest x-ray is typically required to confirm placement before feeds as the tube may be in the lungs. This is especially true in intubated patients or patients with altered mental status who may not be able to communicate effectively that the tube is in their lungs.

ENTERIC TUBES

The term G-tube is reserved for tubes placed surgically (either laparoscopically or during a laparotomy) by a surgeon under direct visualization into the stomach in an operating room. The G-tube can then be used for feeding or for draining the stomach. The key to placement is the surgeon sewing the stomach to the parietal peritoneum. Why is this important? If the tube is dislodged, enteric contents will not freely leak into the abdomen, leading to peritonitis because the stomach is sewn to the peritoneum. The stomach is not sterile, so a return to the operating room for a sterile environment is not required, and bedside placement is typically fine (ie, in the emergency room or nursing home). Once a new tube is placed, confirmation should be performed. The simple method is to aspirate. Bile return would indicate you are likely in the stomach. The definitive way is to inject contrast medium and to obtain an x-ray.

Jejunostomy tubes (J-tubes) are a similar concept to G-tubes. They are placed by a surgeon in the operating room. The jejunum is *always* tacked to the peritoneum for the same reason as with G-tubes. If the tube falls out, the jejunum is usually not leaking into the peritoneal cavity. An important difference to know is J-tubes are smaller than G-tubes because the jejunum is significantly smaller than the stomach. For reference, a G-tube is typically 20 to 24 Fr and a J-tube is typically 12 to 16 Fr. Practically, the J-tubes clog easily, and therefore, crushed medications should never be given down these tubes. If a J-tube falls out, the tract between skin and fascia may close in a very short time, so if a patient waits before replacing it after it falls out, the tube will be much harder to replace as the tract may be gone. For this reason, it is more important to confirm placement with a J-tube by using contrast. Jejunostomy tubes are used commonly when long-term enteral access is required for delivering nutrition, such as in the case of a gastrectomy, esophagectomy, short bowel syndrome, or other intra-abdominal complexity.

Percutaneous endoscopic gastrostomy (PEG) tubes involve the use of a flexible endoscope to insufflate the stomach against the abdominal wall, thereby assuming that the peritoneum is in contact with the serosa of the stomach. The stomach is then accessed percutaneously with a needle following transillumination of the abdominal wall by the endoscope. The tube is then pulled through the abdominal wall following snare of a wire or other loop placed through the large-bore needle. When the PEG tube is pulled through the abdominal wall, it is opposed to the gastric mucosa by a bumper. The key point is that there is no suturing between the stomach and the peritoneum. Ideally, by keeping the serosa of the stomach in contact with the peritoneum for some amount of time, adhesions will form and function as if sutures were placed. That time period can be from a couple of weeks to over a month. Therefore, technically, nothing is holding the PEG tube in place other than the pressure of the bumper against the inner layer of the stomach until adhesions have formed. If a PEG tube falls out, for example, the next day, it can be devastating because the stomach can communicate directly with the peritoneal cavity. It is much more emergent than a G-tube falling out (a nuisance and a bother but not an emergency). That is where the distinction between a G-tube and a PEG tube defines you as a surgeon because you must realize this difference to initiate the appropriate and safe steps to replacing the tube. A recently placed tube that is dislodged requires a phone call to the chief resident or attending, as the patient may need to go to the operating room. If a PEG tube has been put in over a long time, greater than 1 to 2 months, a Foley catheter or other convenient tube of similar or smaller size can be placed for use or for keeping the tract open until the correct tube can be replaced.

Despite the advantages of G-tubes, a PEG tube is often preferred because it is simpler than a G-tube, but there can be reasons why a PEG tube cannot be placed. Relative contraindications include previous attempts whereby the tube could not be safely placed (ie, could not transilluminate the abdominal wall), a patient with a prior upper gastrointestinal operation (such as a partial gastrectomy), or a patient with ascites.

CHEST TUBES

Chest tubes differ from enteric tubes for a few reasons. They are typically placed under sterile conditions because the pleural cavity *should* be sterile, unlike the stomach or jejunum. When placing a chest tube, you *will* prepare the patient (mask, gown, glove, skin prep, drape). The tube can then be placed in the standard fashion, being sure to dissect above the rib so as not to injure the intercostal neurovascular bundle residing on the inferior aspect of the ribs. When looking at a chest tube, there is a line that is radiopaque on it. The key thing to highlight is that the most distal hole in the tube has a line that goes right through it. Identification of the broken line, and thus the last hole in the chest tube, on a chest x-ray is used to confirm that the tube is completely in the chest cavity. The x-ray is also used to confirm the tube position (ie, apical or basilar), the adequacy of drainage of air or fluid, and the expected level of lung reinflation.

When considering replacing a chest tube, one must inquire about the initial reason the chest tube was placed. Here is a concrete example of why this makes a difference: if you are putting a tube in for evacuating fluid, it does not really matter if that final hole is in the pleural cavity or in the subcutaneous tissue—it will drain the fluid regardless of where that final hole is located. Unless a patient is super thin, the tube will be occluded by subcutaneous fat if the contents within the pleural space are being successfully drained and decreasing in volume.

However, the position of the last hole *would* matter in the case of draining air, because you cannot differentiate if the leakage of air is coming from the patient's lung or from the surrounding environment. For example, if a patient had a lung operation and he or she has an air leak from a staple line or an adhesion or an area of damaged lung, air can be sucked in from the atmosphere through the side hole and then out the chest tube. Thus, you would not know if the leakage of air is coming from the patient's lung or the atmosphere. In this situation, you do not want to push the chest tube further in, as you risk introducing bacteria to the pleural space. You will have to take it out and place a new one in. You can withdraw a chest tube, no problem, but never push one in. This scenario again demonstrates why you must know why the tube is there and its exact purpose before you take action in managing the tube.

TRACHEOSTOMY

Almost everyone will manage a patient with a tracheostomy if one spends time in the intensive care unit, so it is worth understanding how a tracheostomy is constructed, the parts of a tracheostomy tube, and why they exist, and troubleshooting when they come out. Tracheostomies typically have the following components: a clear, inflatable balloon; an inner and outer cannula; and a stylet (or obturator), which is used only when inserting the tracheostomy. Most tracheostomies have a cuff located on the outer cannula. Why would you bother putting a cuff on a tracheostomy? If a patient is on positive pressure ventilation, you have to occlude the airway to ensure that all of the air being ventilated is going into the airway. If there is no occlusion, some air is going in and some is going back out the proximal airway, thus the patient may not be adequately ventilated or oxygenated. Why do tracheostomies exist without a cuff? Noncuffed tracheostomies not only allow air to pass into the upper trachea and larynx but also allow patients to speak and cough. This is reserved for nonventilated patients or for patients undergoing operations such as a laryngectomy. Once a patient is off a ventilator or does not require the tracheostomy for a long time, a noncuffed tracheostomy may be used. The inner cannula is important because a tracheostomy can easily become inspissated and clogged with mucus. The inner cannula can be taken out, cleaned under water, and then put back in. Some tracheostomies do not have the inner cannula, but this ability to clean the tracheostomy in the future is lost. It is important to understand the exact tracheostomy tube you have chosen to use as it may have consequences down the line.

A dislodged tracheostomy can be a serious problem because it is typically the patient's only avenue for oxygen. What do you do in this situation? The number 1 priority is reestablishing an airway. Simply putting the tracheostomy back in may be easy if a patient has had it in for a long time or in patients with a relatively thin neck. If the tracheostomy is relatively new or if the patient has a thick, deep neck, it can be very difficult to put back in. Almost always, intubating orally from above is the right answer because it is a common skill and usually can be done quickly and in a safe manner. Once the airway is reestablished, there is no rush in replacing the tracheostomy. Even if you have to get an airway back into the tracheostomy site because it is not possible orally (ie, a patient with maxillofacial trauma), you should intubate the ostomy with a standard endotracheal tube instead of a tracheostomy because a tracheostomy is very short and can very easily be placed into the subcutaneous tissues above the trachea. Once the tube is replaced, you should see end-tidal CO_2 to confirm the tube is in proper position.

CONCLUSION

In conclusion, (1) practice prevention when it comes to tubes. If a tube is placed and then falls out the next day, it was likely preventable if better cared for. Take the time to ensure the tube is secured in a safe and appropriate way. (2) Always ask for help early until you are more familiar with tubes and drains. (3) If you are replacing a tube or putting one in, confirm it is in the right place. For instance, see the end tidal CO_2 once a tracheostomy is replaced or see the placement of the nasogastric tube on an x-ray. Importantly, follow up on any confirmation study you may order.

Last, be detail oriented when it comes to tubes. Know the tube (the type, the size, the components, the alternatives) and know your patient (why they have a tube and what is their current clinical status). Take notes and ask questions to fully understand each situation and you will not only perform well on your rotations but you will be a superb doctor who provides excellent care to your patients.

 PEARLS

1. Become acquainted will all the tubes, lines, and drains at your disposal. Know your armamentarium of tubes and drains well and be able to describe their various characteristics.
2. Know the most common variant of tube you use for various instances and be able to troubleshoot them appropriately. Some tubes have unique indications. Additionally, never force a "fix." Before using any force be sure to ask your senior for help.
3. Be sure to take notes daily of the drain's color, quality, and amount. In many cases, it is pertinent to know how the output changes over time. Initial intra-abdominal drains may have a high output in the first few hours and then dramatically drop. This can indicate a displaced drain or intentional complete clearance of fluid.

14

TROUBLESHOOTING FOLEY CATHETERS

DANIEL KAUFMAN, MD | RUSLAN KORETS, MD | PETER L. STEINBERG, MD

This chapter builds upon our Foley catheter insertion chapter for more advanced techniques and troubleshooting existing catheters.

DIFFICULT CATHETER INSERTION

MALES

The most common reason for inability to insert a Foley catheter is improper technique (inadequate lubrication, lack of anesthesia or incorrect catheter choice), resistance from benign prostatic hyperplasia (BPH), urethral stricture disease, bladder neck contracture or false passages in the urethra.[1] Another scenario in which catheter placement can be difficult is from inability to visualize the glans or meatus due to phimotic or edematous foreskin. It is important to take a focused urologic history ("have you seen a urologist before?" or "do you have a urologist?") and perform an examination prior to catheter placement, as this may guide your troubleshooting algorithm. Ask about prior urologic procedures, prior catheter placement attempts, medications for BPH, or prior pelvic radiation. *Review the patient's chart for any prior urology consults or operative procedures, as this can be very informative.* Examine the genitals for blood at the meatus from previous attempts at catheterization, phimosis, edema, and masses.

Lubrication will make catheter placement easier for both you and the patient. The average volume of the male urethra is 20 cc, and therefore a minimum of 10 cc of lubricant should be used. Many urologists will inject 10 to 20 cc of viscous lidocaine into the urethra before catheter placement. It is critical to tell the patient that this may burn initially but will make the procedure both more comfortable and more likely to succeed. After instillation, allow 30 to 60 seconds for the gel to contact the urethra and take effect.

In patients with BPH, the catheter tip may bounce off of the prostatic urethra and thus will not enter the bladder. The solution for this problem is to use a stiffer, larger diameter catheter or a coudé tip catheter. Larger catheters are stiffer and less prone to buckle or bend when meeting resistance at the prostate. Additionally, the use of a coudé catheter in this scenario is appropriate as the curved tip engages the prostate and follows the natural cephalad curve of the urethra. Asking the patient to void while you are advancing the catheter can also help relax the pelvic floor muscles and make catheter passage easier. *Ultimately, if you are unable to successfully place a catheter after trying a larger, stiffer catheter and/or an 18 or 20 fr coudé catheter, you should contact urology.* Although a urologist may be able to blindly place a catheter, in these scenarios, he or she often needs to place a catheter endoscopically.

In patients with urethral stricture disease, you will likely encounter resistance to catheter placement in the penile or bulbar urethra before getting to the prostate. If you notice that you cannot place much of the catheter into the penis prior to resistance, the obstruction is likely due to a urethral stricture. In this scenario, it is appropriate to try a small, stiffer catheter such as a 14fr or 12fr silicone catheter. Again, if this is unsuccessful, you should be consulting urology as the patient may require endoscopy or urethral dilation.

Sometimes exposure of the male meatus is an issue due to inability to retract the foreskin, which is called phimosis. This can occur due to scarring and recurrent infections of the foreskin or can be the result of significant edema. Sometimes, you can retract the foreskin enough to partially visualize the meatus and attempt catheter placement. To maximize success, inject viscous lidocaine beneath the foreskin in the direction of the meatus and use the tip of the catheter to try to engage the meatus beneath the foreskin. Gently advance the catheter if you think the tip is in the urethra, if it is not, you will feel resistance of the catheter curling under the foreskin. If the foreskin is so badly scarred that you are unable to retract it at all or only see a pinpoint opening, it is best to call the urology team for catheter placement as the patient may need the foreskin dilated or even cut open to allow catheter placement. Such patients may also have concurrent urethral stricture disease due to lichen sclerosis of the penis and urethra.

Many hospitalized patients suffer from penoscrotal edema due to fluid overload and lack of ambulation. The dependent tissues of the penis and scrotum can swell significantly with edema. This is more straightforward to manage than it appears, as this third spaced fluid can be redistributed by applying steady manual pressure over 5 to 10 minutes to the penis. This usually allows for foreskin retraction and catheter placement.

FEMALES

There are commonly two reasons why Foley catheter insertion in females can be difficult: obesity with poor exposure of the meatus or atrophic vaginitis with retraction and poor exposure of the meatus. *You alone cannot put a catheter in successfully in an obese female.* This requires the help of at least two other people to help retract and position the patient appropriately. You can ask your two assistants to stand on either side of the bed and hold the legs up in the air essentially in dorsal lithotomy. You can also use a pillow or towel as a bump under the patient's buttocks to elevate the pelvis off the bed. These maneuvers should allow you to visualize the urethral meatus and place the catheter easily. In a postmenopausal patient with a narrow introitus and retracted meatus, it may be impossible to visualize the urethra regardless of patient positioning. In this scenario, one solution is to insert your gloved finger into the patient's vagina and then slide the catheter anteriorly, over your finger. The urethra should be just above it. Using a coudé catheter with the tip pointed anteriorly can also aid in finding the urethral meatus.

MALFUNCTIONING CATHETERS

There will be times when you are called to assess a urinary catheter that is not working correctly. The catheter will either be correctly placed and not working, usually due to occlusion from clots or an air lock; alternatively, the catheter will not be working because it was not correctly placed. You need to determine which issue is occurring, with the former being much easier to resolve than misplacement.

Initial evaluation includes assessing the color of the urine in the drainage bag and seeing if the appropriate length of catheter is coming out of the meatus, especially in men. The majority of the catheter length in men should be inside the urethra and not visible. If there appears to be more than 15 to 20 cm of catheter outside the patient, misplacement is probable. If the catheter appears to be correctly placed then either manipulation of the drainage tubing to release an air lock and/or gentle irrigation with 120 to 250 mL of sterile water or saline should confirm appropriate patency of the catheter.

If the catheter is clearly misplaced and/or does not irrigate, then replacement is likely needed. Clues that will tip you off to a catheter that is not in the right place include lack of urinary drainage, leakage of urine or blood from the penis around the catheter, a sensation of bladder or suprapubic fullness, and overt bladder distension on examination. It is appropriate in these scenarios to first check a bedside bladder ultrasound or bladder scan. If the bladder scan shows less than 100 cc and the patient is still leaking around the catheter, this could be due to bladder spasms and it would be appropriate to initiate anticholinergics, such as oral anticholinergics or a belladonna and opium suppository, both of which help to relax the detrusor muscle of the bladder. Care must be exercised in geriatric patients, as these can induce delirium!

If a patient has a bladder scan >150 cc with a nondraining Foley catheter and blood leaking around the catheter, there is a pretty good chance that the catheter balloon has been inflated in the prostate and not in the bladder. This happens because the person placing the catheter did not advance the catheter all the way to the hub prior to inflating the balloon. The first thing you want to try to do here is to deflate the balloon completely and advance the catheter to the hub. If you do not get any significant resistance and you get spontaneous drainage of urine with advancement, you have solved the problem. Keep the catheter hubbed and reinflate the balloon. If this fails, you may attempt to gently place a stiffer and/or coudé Foley once, using the aforementioned techniques. If this fails, consult a urologist.

Another situation similar to traumatic Foley placement is a patient who pulls out his catheter with the balloon port inflated. In this scenario, you will see continuous leakage of blood from the meatus because there is bleeding from the urethra. The treatment for this is placement of a Foley catheter as this will tamponade the urethral bleeding. It is reasonable to attempt placement of an 18fr coudé catheter in this scenario prior to calling urology. Most of the time, the catheter will slide into place easily. If there is resistance to placement, urology should be called. Do not get worried if you see some ongoing bleeding around the catheter in this scenario as long as the catheter is draining clear urine as it takes some time for the urethral injury to heal. In the setting of any traumatic Foley placement or dislodgement, we typically recommend keeping the catheter in place for 7 days to allow for urethral healing.

HEMATURIA

If a patient complains of urinating blood prior and can no longer urinate, they are likely obstructed from blood clots. If you suspect the patient has bad hematuria with clots, you should try to find large diameter two-way catheter or three-way catheter for continuous bladder irrigation. At minimum, these should be 20fr in size, preferably 22fr if a three-way catheter. Once one of these catheters is in, the best thing to do is to try to get as much of the clot out as possible with hand irrigation. Get two 60 cc catheter tip syringes with saline. Get an assistant and put 120 cc of saline in the bladder and aspirated out clots until you just cannot pull them out any more. You should hand irrigate with a minimum of 500 cc total on initial presentation. Once you have cleared all of the clots, the patient may still have ongoing hematuria. If this is the case, you can initiate continuous bladder irrigation via the three-way catheter.

 PEARLS

1. Difficult insertion can be managed in a number of ways. Never apply force and "listen" to what the catheter is telling you as it is advanced. If needed, always ask for help and when appropriate consult urology.
2. Low urine output can point to a blocked catheter or low urine production. A bladder scan can be easily performed bedside and provides essential information. When in doubt, replacing a catheter is a viable option.
3. Pay close attention to the urine output and its characteristics. Frank blood should be a reason for concern.

Reference

1. Villanueva C, Hemstreet GP. *Difficult catheterizaton: tricks of the trade. AUA Update Series.* Vol 30. Linthicum, MD: American Urologic Association, Inc; 2011:chap 5.

15

SURGICAL NUTRITION

KELSEY ROMATOSKI, BA | NICHOLAS E. TAWA, JR, MD, PHD

Maintaining proper nutrition in the surgical setting is essential and should always be included on the patient's "active problem" list. Over half of hospitalized patients are nutritionally deficient as defined as consumption of less than 50% of their true caloric need. Much of this is iatrogenic (NPO for an examination that does not occur, lack of attention by the caregiver) and can be avoided. Greater than 20% weight loss correlates with increased rates of surgical complications and death. In the modern teaching hospital, the clinical nutritionist (registered dietician [RD]) has training in critical care and intravenous feeding. This person can be an excellent resource to you. The RD is responsible for "global nutritional assessment," which incorporates many objective and subjective clinical parameters. This assessment is described in readily available guidelines (ASPEN, American Association for Parenteral and Enteral Nutrition).

Nutrition support in ill patients is challenging physiologically because of their near universal inflammatory response and elevated levels of cytokines, with accompanying insulin resistance. Maintenance of blood glucose by gluconeogenesis from muscle-derived amino acids ("lean body mass") is an initial response to inadequate caloric intake. Under normal conditions of starvation, muscle protein breakdown is eventually suppressed by adaptive mechanisms and fat is increasingly utilized as an energy source. In patients with inflammation, these responses do not occur and muscle atrophy and cachexia continue. Enteral (gut) feeding can allow for net anabolism even in such sick patients and is always preferred over the intravenous route. Intravenous feeding (total parenteral nutrition [TPN]), due to issues of hyperglycemia, is best thought of as a way to retard loss of lean body mass as opposed to reversing it.

WHEN TO INITIATE ARTIFICIAL NUTRITION

Enteral feeding: Immediately if oral intake is inadequate, regardless of nutritional history, weight, or clinical status.

TPN: This is a debated topic. One approach is to prescribe TPN for patients incapable or intolerant of enteral feeding (1) immediately, if greater than 20% weight loss, or (2) after 7 to 14 days of inadequate caloric intake for most others. Another approach, especially in surgical patients, is to avoid TPN if the intestinal tract is anticipated to be a viable route for enteral nutrition within the next 5 to 7 days.

Typical scenarios where TPN is needed:

- Short bowel syndrome: Midgut volvulus, vascular accident, multiple resections
- Enterocutaneous fistula
- Gastrointestinal motility disorders, prolonged ileus
- Intractable chylous ascites
- Malabsorption
- Cancer: Treatment-related gastrointestinal (GI) dysfunction, radiation enteritis
- Chronic or acute chronic pancreatitis: However, post-pyloric tube feeding in acute pancreatitis has been shown to be safe and should be used

DEFINING TERMS

ABW = actual body weight = current admission weight
UBW = usual body weight = prehospital weight
IBW = ideal body weight

Male = 106 lb/47.7 kg + 6 lb/2.7 kg for every inch over 5 ft
Female = 100 lb/45 kg + 5 lb/2.2 kg for every inch over 5 ft

"Severe" malnutrition is defined as the ABW being 15% to 20% less than UBW over a 3-month period. Any patient living at or below their IBW should also be considered at high nutritional risk.

Caloric content: Fat 9 kcal/g, amino acids 4 kcal/g, glucose 3.4 kcal/g.

RQ = moles CO_2 produced/moles O_2 consumed.

For conversion of glucose to fat, $RQ = 8$. Therefore, a measured $RQ > 1$ implies excessive carbohydrate (CHO) provision and fat production. However, such measurements are rarely performed, even in the intensive care unit setting.

HOW TO DETERMINE IF A PATIENT IS MALNOURISHED

Clinical history and weight-based approach: The most practical and commonly used:

    Oral intake <50% of needs
    Catabolic disease (burn, sepsis, pancreatitis)
    Significant weight loss (10%-20%) or living at IBW
    More than 7 days inanition
    Nonfunctioning GI tract

Commonly accepted biochemical parameters are of little utility but include:

Nitrogen balance (inaccurate and poorly reproducible)
= Intake−loss (urine 90%, stool 5%, integument 5%)
= ([protein intake (g)]/6.25)−urinary urea (g)−2 (stool, skin)−2 (nonurea N)

Albumin<3 (t 1/2 = 14-18 days): Albumin and other serum proteins decrease in inflammatory states owing to an increased volume of distribution and decreased hepatic synthesis, and in the hospital setting, these measurements rarely reflect nutritional status alone. Prealbumin has a shorter t ½ (2 days), and a rise may reflect nutritional improvement. A transferrin <150, or decreased total iron binding capacity, is also considered a marker of risk. Of these, the prealbumin is the most useful to help assess efficacy of ongoing nutritional support in a chronically malnourished patient.

DETERMINING CALORIC GOALS

A weight-based approach (see earlier) is no less useful than other methods:
    For weight-based calculations of caloric goals:

1. Use UBW or ABW if within ±10% of IBW
2. For obesity, defined as ABW >130% IBW or BMI >27, use "adjusted IBW" = IBW + (0.25 [ABW − IBW])
3. All others, use IBW

Alternatively, various equations are available but are not superior, for example, the Harris Benedict equation:

For males: Energy expenditure in kcal = 66.5 + (13.8 × weight in kg) + (5 × height in cm) – (6.8 × age in years)
For females: Energy expenditure in kcal = 66.5 + (9.6 × weight in kg) + (1.9 × height in cm) – (4.7 × age in years)

A weight-based approach assumes a basal energy requirement of 25 kcal/kg/d, which may be increased by an "activity" factor, for example, up to +50% for a major burn. However, exceeding 40 kcal/kg/d usually will lead to hyperglycemia, particularly if administering TPN.

For example, for a 70-kg male, 70 × 25 kcal/kg × 1.25 (a common activity factor) = 2200 kcal required.

ENTERAL NUTRITION

The advantage of enteral feeding is its universal efficacy regardless of premorbid nutritional status, lower cost, avoidance of line sepsis, presumed more efficient nutrient utilization due to entry into the portal venous system, and possible preservation of gut mucosal integrity. For short-term feeding, a nasogastric tube is sufficient. The residual gastric volume is often set to <200 mL. However, more permissive values (up to 400 mL) are NOT associated with increased aspiration and often will allow reaching the full caloric goal. Placement of the tube in a postpyloric (jejunal) position will NOT lessen the risk of aspiration and is only pursued for inadequate gastric empty (high residual volumes). Most inpatients will be fed by continuous infusion versus bolus feeding. A severe ileus will limit feeding. Although hypotension or a pressor requirement are often cited as increasing the risk of jejunal injury during enteral feeding, there is little evidence to support this, except at extremely high doses of pressors that decrease splanchnic circulation. However, all tube feeds are hypertonic. Numerous options are available for percutaneous feeding tube placement, including percutaneous endoscopic gastrostomy, surgical gastrostomy, or percutaneous access by interventional radiology (IR). Although the last approach is often considered "less invasive," the IR approach carries the highest complication rate. Percutaneous jejunostomy, by whatever route, is often accompanied by issues of obstruction, volvulus, and mucosal injury and should be avoided if possible.

Most tube feeds are 1 kcal/mL, but this can rise to up to 2 kcal/mL for lipid-dense formulas. These are balanced formulas that vary most greatly in how protein is provided (eg, longer hydrolyzed protein fragments in the common "Osmolyte" versus short peptides in "elemental" formulas such as "Vivonex"). Which formula to choose is often empiric, with high-fat formulas suggested where excessive carbon dioxide production from carbohydrate is suspected in the setting of respiratory failure and ventilator dependence. A variety of approaches can improve tolerance to tube feeds, such as thickening agents (banana flakes, psyllium seeds) and/or hypomotility agents (loperamide, tincture of opium).

INITIATING TOTAL PARENTERAL NUTRITION

The indications for TPN have been discussed, with little efficacy if given for less than 7 days. Central access with the line tip in the superior vena cava is the only method to administer TPN (>900 mOsm/L). A Peripherally Inserted Central Catheter (PICC) line or central line may suffice for weeks. There is no role for so-called peripheral parenteral nutrition. The caloric sources in TPN are amino acids, fat, and glucose. Most TPN solutions are "3 in 1," that is, the lipid (Intralipid, largely soybean oil) is mixed as a micellar solution with the aqueous phase. Maintaining the correct ratios of calcium and other constituents in the solution is essential for its chemical stability, and for this reason a template-based approach to ordering is used in most institutions. For example, a final concentration of 4% to 7% AA promotes lipid solubility. It is best to consider TPN a medication. Therefore, the total volume should be minimized, and if supplemental fluid is required, this is delivered by a separate line.

Micronutrient deficiencies in parenteral nutrition are rarely observed with modern additives, which include selenium, zinc, copper, chromium, molybdenum, and multivitamins. Copper deficiency in particular can be an unrecognized cause of neutropenia.

Calcium: Maintenance 0.2 to 0.3 mEq/kg/d.

Magnesium: Maintenance 0.35 to 0.45 mEq/kg/d.

Phosphate: Maintenance 30 to 40 mmol/d.

Essential fatty acids: need as 2% to 4% total calories.

Protein guidelines: (1) Normal 1.5 to 2 g/kg/24 h. (2) Renal failure 0.8 to 1 g/kg/24 h; however, if undergoing hemodialysis may use 1.5 g/kg/24 h. (3) Liver failure 0.5 to 1 g/kg/24 h. There is no evidence to support formulas enriched in branched-chain amino acids or reduced in aromatic ones to prevent encephalopathy.

Lipid guidelines: Usually limit to 30 to 50 g/d. Use <30% total calories and <1 g lipid/kg/d. A serum triglyceride >250 to 400 is a contraindication. Give at least 50 g weekly to avoid essential fatty acid deficiency.

Dextrose guidelines: Begin with <150 g for the initial 24 hours. The final glucose infusion rate should be 4 to 8 mg/kg/min to yield maximal suppression of urea production ("protein-sparing effect"). Infusion rates >9 mg/kg/min lead to net synthesis of lipid and are to be avoided.

Sample TPN worksheet:

Step 1) Choose weight for calculation (kg): _____

Step 2) Calculate energy requirement (total calories) = Body weight in kg × (25-32 kcal/kg/24 h). Default is 25 kcal/kg/24 h

Step 3) Calculate amino acid requirement and calories provided as amino acids

   Total AA (g) = Body wt (kg) × (0.8-1.5 g AA/kg/24 h). Default is 1.5 g/kg/24 h.
   Total AA (g/24 h): ___ Amino acid calories = Total AA (g) × 4 cal/g: ___

Step 4) Calculate lipid requirement and calories provided as fat (if used)

   Calories as fat = X g fat/24 h (usually 30-50 g) × 9 cal/g: _____

Step 5) Calculate contribution from glucose

   Calories as dextrose = Total calories − amino acid calories − calories as fat.
   Calories as dextrose (kcal): _____
   Total dextrose required (g) = (Dextrose calories)/(3.4 cal/g)
   Total dextrose (g): _____

Step 6) Calculate volume and percent concentration of solutes

   Baseline fluid requirement is 25 to 35 mL/kg/24 h.
   % Concentration as used in pharmacy: Total content (g)/total vol in mL) × 100.
   AA: usually 4% to 8%; Fat: usually 3% to 5%; Dextrose: usually 10% to 25%

   Suggested Initial TPN Program

Parameter	Day 1	Day 2	Day 3
Volume (mL/24 h)	1000	1000-1500	1500-2000
Calories (% of goal)	50%	75%, may add fat	100%
Dextrose (g/24 h)	100-150	150-200	200-350
Amino acids (% of goal)	50%-100%	100%	100%, check BUN
Fat	No	Maybe	30-50 g/d
Insulin	Usually not, use SS	Add 50% to TPN	Add + 50% to TPN

Electrolytes per 24 hours:

Sodium	_____ mEq (usual 70, 40-150)
Potassium	_____ mEq (usual 20, 20-100)
Calcium	_10__ mEq (usual 10, up to 30)
Magnesium	_10__ mEq (usual 10, up to 30)
Phosphate	_30__ mEq (usual 30, up to 60)

Order chloride or acetate to balance (usually prefer Cl. Increase acetate for hyperchloremia).

MANDATORY MONITORING FOR PATIENTS RECEIVING PARENTERAL NUTRITION

Clinical: Daily I/O's, every other day body weight, evidence of infection.

Laboratory tests: Baseline: Electrolytes, blood urea nitrogen (BUN), Creatinine, Glucose, Calcium, Magnesium, Phosphate, Bilirubin, SGOT, SGPT, Alkaline Phosphatase, Triglycerides, Albumin, prothrombin time (PT)/partial thromboplastin time (PTT).

Q 6 to 12h: Glucose (Finger stick), usually for initial 3 to 5 days or until stable.

Qd until stable: Electrolytes, BUN, Creatinine, Glucose, Calcium, Magnesium, Phosphate.

Q week: Bilirubin, SGOT, SGPT, Alkaline Phosphatase, Triglycerides, Albumin, PT/PTT.

INSULIN AND TPN SOLUTIONS

When tolerance to glucose is unknown, all TPN orders should be accompanied by a sliding scale order for subcutaneous regular insulin, to coincide with Q6 h finger sticks.

If known diabetes or elevated blood sugars, start with no more than 100 g of dextrose for the first 24 hours. Initially add 10 units of regular insulin or up to one-third the usual insulin dose to the TPN.

On the second day of TPN, add ½ to ¾ the total amount of subcutaneous insulin received in the preceding 24 hours to the new TPN order. Continue this process until the patient has maintained stable blood sugars < or = 200 mg/dL.

If blood sugars remain high, consider stopping the TPN insulin and using a continuous insulin infusion. If significant hypoglycemia develops (<60 mg/dL) with insulin in TPN, administer 50 g of dextrose by bolus. Consider discontinuing TPN if hypoglycemia persists, and start 10% dextrose infusion. If TPN is continued, reduce insulin by at least 50% with next day's order.

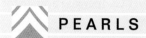 **PEARLS**

1. Assessing your patient's nutritional status is a cornerstone of management. Get familiar with equations to calculate your patient's ideal nutritional supplement. This has important implications on patient outcome.
2. When available, the enteral route is preferred. A number of formulae are available, each with their own clinical indications. Get familiar with their osmolarity, caloric values, and impact on the pulmonary, hepatic, and renal functions.
3. TPN is a last resort and should be used only when enteral access is not feasible. Calculations are an art form. Practice makes perfect. Be sure to continuously monitor electrolytes and observe for refeeding syndrome.

16

CONCERNING LABORATORY TESTS

JORDAN PYDA, MD, MPH | CHARLES S. PARSONS, MD

The appropriate laboratory study can greatly facilitate the clinical assessment of the surgical patient. Blood/serum, urine, and pleural, peritoneal, cerebral spinal fluid, among others, can be studied to assist in the identification and subsequent treatment of underlying pathological processes. The choice of the appropriate laboratory test is guided by a thorough evaluation of the patient's history and physical examination, combined with knowledge of the surgical procedure and an appreciation of its common complications. Familiarity with normal laboratory values will facilitate the recognition of abnormal values. This, in turn, will help you to identify and treat abnormal clinical states.

INDICATIONS: A GUIDE TO LABORATORY TESTS

In general, laboratory tests should be ordered if the results will influence a subsequent clinical decision. Consider if (and how) your future management of the patient, in terms of both additional clinical investigations (ie, laboratory tests, imaging) and treatment, will be affected by the results. Ordering daily laboratory tests for the sake of testing is usually an insufficient reason. However, a senior resident or an attending may disagree, and you should follow their lead.

139

BLOOD/SERUM LABORATORY TESTS

CHEMISTRY

The chemistry panel usually refers to either a basic metabolic panel (BMP) or a complete metabolic panel (CMP). A BMP typically includes 6 serum electrolytes (K^+, Na^+, Cl^-, CO_2, blood urea nitrogen, glucose) and serum creatinine (Cr). In daily practice, total (ie, bound and unbound) calcium (Ca/Ca^{2+}), magnesium (Mg^{2+}), and phosphorus (P) are often added to this laboratory order to assist with electrolyte repletion. However, striving for both good stewardship and clinical utility, these tests can often be ordered individually. A CMP usually comprises the above-mentioned blood chemistry and additionally includes alanine aminotransferase (ALT), aspartate aminotransferase (AST), total bilirubin, direct bilirubin, alkaline phosphatase ("alk phos"), and albumin and/or total proteins. The following section presents the normal concentration ranges of some commonly ordered blood chemistry tests. The most common abnormalities, their underlying causes, and possible management are presented.

CONCERNING LABORATORY TESTS

Hyperkalemia [Potassium(K^+) >5 mEq/L]

CAUSES

- Laboratory error (if hemolysis is present, repeat the blood draw)
- Potassium transiently shifts extracellularly (eg, medications, acidosis)
- Aldosterone deficiency
- Renal failure
- Medications or intravenous fluids (IVFs) (nonsteroidal anti-inflammatory drugs, beta blockers, angiotensin-converting-enzyme inhibitors, KCl)
- Crush injuries or other etiologies of rhabdomyolysis

CONCERNS (>6.5 mEq/L)

- Cardiac arrhythmias such as ventricular fibrillation (V Fib), pulseless electrical activity, or cardiac arrest
- Symptoms include musculoskeletal lethargy, nausea/emesis, diarrhea, palpitations

NEXT STEPS (>5.5 TO 6.0 mEq/L)

■ Obtain electrocardiogram (EKG) to evaluate for peaked T waves, lengthened QRS complex, or arrhythmias. Compare with earlier tests to see if changes are new. Note that EKG sensitivity is low, and the patient may have more symptomatic presentation of hyperkalemia (see earlier text under Concerns)

■ Intravenous (IV) calcium gluconate (transiently stabilizes the heart)

■ Regular insulin IV 10 units (transiently drives K^+ into the cells, dropping serum K^+ levels) and IV dextrose (50% or D50) 12.5 or 25 g (administration avoids hypoglycemia)

■ Albuterol 10 mg inhaled (inhaled beta 2 agonists are another option/administration route)

■ Order repeat laboratory tests to trend K^+ levels

TREATMENT

■ Recognizing that the aforementioned steps are temporizing measures, we must identify the underlying causes of hyperkalemia and reverse them.

■ Reducing total body K^+ can be achieved via diuretics such as Lasix (ie, furosemide) IV (onset within 1 hour) or PO/PR potassium binders.

■ Potential K^+ binders include Kayexalate (ie, sodium polystyrene sulfonate) and Veltassa (ie, patiromer), but this requires time to decrease K^+ levels and either PO/PR or PO administration, respectively.

■ Hemodialysis or continuous renal replacement therapy may be required if hyperkalemia persists, especially if cardiac symptoms are present.

Hypokalemia [Potassium(K^+) <3.5 mEq/L]

CAUSES

■ Potassium transiently shifts intracellularly (eg, medications, alkalosis)

■ Extrarenal loss ≥ Gastrointestinal (bilious emesis, nasogastric tube (NGT), diarrhea, chronic laxative use), sweating

■ Renal loss that can occur in settings of metabolic acidosis (eg, diabetic ketoacidosis (DKA), ureterosigmoidostomy) or metabolic alkalosis (emesis/NGT, diuresis) or with administration of IV NaCl 0.9% or in settings of low serum Mg^{2+}

■ Numerous other underlying comorbidities or causative medications

CONCERNS (<2.5 mEq/L)

- Cardiac arrhythmias
- Symptoms include lethargy, nausea/emesis, diarrhea, palpitations

NEXT STEPS

- Obtain an EKG to evaluate for evidence of ventricular ectopy (eg, PVCs, V Fib, V Tach), U waves, or T wave blunting (ie, opposite of the peaked T waves of hyperkalemia)
- Order repeat laboratory tests to trend K^+ levels

TREATMENT

- PO and IV potassium chloride, acknowledging that peripheral IV repletion may be caustic to veins and thus rate limited to about 10 mEq/h of potassium chloride. Higher rate of administration of 20 mEq/h, indicated in symptomatic hypokalemia, requires central IV access (eg, midline or peripherally inserted central catheter (PICC)).
- When treating hypokalemia, consider concurrent hypophosphatemia. If Phos <2.5 mg/dL, replete with potassium phosphate ("K phos"). Otherwise replete with KCl at a rate of about 20 mEq KCl IV per 0.25mEq/L below target range.
- Identify underlying pathology of potassium loss and rectify. This may include hypertensive excess of mineralocorticoids. Avoid potassium repletion in dialysis-dependent patients unless guided by nephrologist.
- Identify hypomagnesemia and replete as required.

Hypernatremia [Sodium (Na⁺) >145 mEq/L]

CAUSES

- Excess of water loss in relation to salt loss; primarily a free water problem rather than a salt problem
- Loss secondary to hypovolemic hypernatremia (eg, gastrointestinal or insensible water losses, polyuria, diuretic water loss), isovolumic hypernatremia, or hypervolemic hypernatremia (eg, iatrogenic administration of excess sodium) and in settings of excess steroid levels

CONCERNS (>160 mEq/L, PARTICULARLY IN SETTING OF HYPEROSMOLARITY >320 mOsm)

- Hypertensive, tachycardic patients (hypovolemia)
- Irritability, delirium, coma, seizure

NEXT STEPS

- Calculate the free water deficit:

Free Water Deficit = (0.6 × kg body weight) × ([(Serum Na⁺)/140]−1)

TREATMENT

- Identify and rectify the underlying disorder.
- Use D5W IV or other hypotonic fluid to replace half of the free water deficit in the first 24 hours and the remaining half in the following 48 hours.
- Avoid rapid infusion of IVF or rapid correction of hypernatremia, which may lead to cerebral edema and even uncal herniation.

Hyponatremia [Sodium (Na⁺) <135 mEq/L]

CAUSES

- Excess of free water in relation to sodium; again, primarily a free water problem rather than a salt problem
- Usually secondary to elevated levels of antidiuretic hormone, which may be in settings of hypovolemia or hypervolemia (syndrome of inappropriate antidiuretic hormone secretion, SIADH)

CONCERNS (MONITOR BELOW <130 mEq/L; SYMPTOMS APPEAR <120 mEq/L)

- Altered mental status, confusion, unconsciousness, seizures
- Headache, muscle weakness, nausea, emesis, diarrhea

NEXT STEPS

- Measure plasma osmolality and serum glucose and evaluate volume status.
- Consider hypovolemic hypotonic hyponatremia (eg, diuretics, diarrhea, pancreatitis), euvolemic hypotonic hyponatremia (SIADH, polydipsia, poor diet), and hypervolemic hypotonic hyponatremia (cirrhosis, renal failure, nephrotic syndrome).

TREATMENT

- Identify and rectify the underlying disorder.
- Fluid restriction to 1000 mL or 1500 mL of fluid per 24 hours.
- Hypovolemic hyponatremia: replete with NaCl 0.9% IVF.
- Hypervolemic hyponatremia: fluid restriction, consider diuretics with electrolyte replacement.

- Avoid rapid infusion of hypertonic saline (ie, 3% NaCl) to avoid central pontine myelinolysis. Maximum correction rate is 0.5 mEq/L/h for patients with prolonged abnormality.

Hypomagnesemia [Magnesium (Mg²⁺) <1.7 mEq/L]

CAUSES

- Gastrointestinal loss ≥ diarrhea, emesis, fistula with biliary drainage
- Urinary loss ≥ diuresis
- Postoperative ≥ Parathyroidectomy
- Medications ≥ loop diuretics, cyclosporine; gentamycin, streptomycin, tobramycin, and other aminoglycoside antibiotics

CONCERNS

- Symptoms include altered mental status, seizures, lethargy, tremors, tetanus

NEXT STEPS

- Obtain an EKG to evaluate for PR and QT interval elongation, widening of QRS, noting concern for ventricular arrhythmia

TREATMENT

- Replete with IV $MgSO_4$ (ie, magnesium sulfate) using the typical orders of 1, 2, or 4 g IV. Approximately 1 g will raise the serum Mg by 0.1 mEq/L.
- PO magnesium oxide is a common option but leads to significant diarrhea.

Hypoglycemia (Glucose <70 mg/dL)

CAUSES

- NPO status (without glucose containing IVF) with continued insulin administration in a diabetic patient
- Repeat insulin administration without appropriate interval

CONCERNS

- Symptoms include altered mental status, lethargy, or unconsciousness
- Prompts stress response hormones (eg, cortisol), which inhibit wound healing, etc.

NEXT STEPS

- Administration of 15 to 25 g of glucose orally usually as juice or soda
- Alternatively, administration of 25 g IV glucose as 50% dextrose IV
- Recheck fingers stick glucose (FSG) q15-30 minutes until normal

TREATMENT

- Adjust insulin dose to prevent recurrent hypoglycemic episodes.
- Note that FSG goals on inpatient floor are usually around 100 to 140 mg/dL but 120 to 180 mg/dL in the intensive care unit (ICU). The strategy behind permissive borderline hyperglycemia (less strict glycemic control) in the ICU setting is to minimize hypoglycemic episodes, which have been correlated with increased mortality.
- Consider insulin IV drip if unable to control hyperglycemia; may require transfer to ICU or step-down unit.

Lactic Acidosis (Normal Range 0.5 to 1 mmol/L)

CAUSES

- The switch from aerobic to anaerobic metabolism results in lactic acid production; this is often the result of inadequate tissue oxygenation from decreased circulation, sepsis, ischemia, or respiratory failure.
- Liver usually metabolizes lactic acid; buildup is the result of decreased tissue clearance (ischemia) or inadequate metabolism (liver disease).
- Surgical patients such as the bleeding trauma patient, a septic patient, or a patient with suspected ischemic bowel may have elevated lactic acid. Levels can help guide fluid resuscitation.
- Medications: linezolid, metformin (eg, metformin is often held for surgical inpatients).

CONCERNS (>1 MMOL/L)

- Organ malfunction or ischemia (ie, bowel)
- Possible malignancy

TREATMENT

- Resuscitation with IVF or blood product
- Resolution of primary underlying etiology (eg, bowel resection or treatment of sepsis)

BLOOD LABORATORY TESTS

COMPLETE BLOOD COUNT

A complete blood count is primarily drawn to evaluate the white blood cell (WBC), hemoglobin and hematocrit (HGB/HCT or "H&H"), and platelet counts. In referring to these laboratory tests, we often use the term "levels." However, these values are, more precisely, concentrations.

Noting elevations in WBCs may help in the identification of underlying infections or to monitor success of antimicrobial treatments. Broadly, normal values of WBC are 4 to 10 K/μL. Transient elevations in WBC may be secondary to the postoperative stress response or to certain medications such as steroids. For example, an elevated WBC result on postoperative day 1 after an elective procedure is usually monitored unless there are other signs of an infection.

An HGB or HCT is indicated if anemia or hemorrhage is suspected. Normal values of HGB are 11.5 to 16 g/dL for a woman and 13 to 18 g/dL for a man. Broadly, transfusions are considered for patients with a hemoglobin value of between 7 and 10 g/dL. Age, comorbidities, and baseline levels, among other factors, may influence the interpretation and significance of the laboratory result. For example, a normal HGB or HCT in an acutely hemorrhaging patient may be obtained and may remain elevated and be falsely reassuring. Because both the HGB and HCT values are intravascular concentrations, the intravascular fluid (ie, blood) requires adequate time to equilibrate (via fluid shifts) in order for the laboratory tests to be clinically interpretable.

Platelet levels are often noted during the preoperative assessment. Acceptable levels are dependent on the overall clinical situation and the proposed operation. Broadly, normal levels are 150 to 400 K/μL. Thrombocytopenia requiring platelet transfusions is usually defined below 50 K/μL. Note that, although platelet levels may appear normal, platelets may have inhibited function owing to use of common medications (eg, aspirin or clopidogrel/Plavix).

ARTERIAL BLOOD GAS

Arterial blood gas (ABG) is useful in identifying acid-base derangements and elucidating the underlying causes and can guide treatment or resuscitation.

ABGs usually require an arterial puncture to collect arterial blood. The radial or ulnar artery is commonly used, but the femoral artery can be used in trauma patients as well.

Normal Arterial Blood Gas

$$pH = 7.40 / PaCO_2 = 40 / PaO_2 = 60 - 100 /$$
$$HCO_3 = 24 / \text{Base Deficit or Base Excess} = 0$$

Nota bene: The normal partial pressure of oxygen (PaO2) declines with increasing age. The bicarbonate ("bicarb") or HCO3 from an ABG is a calculated value, whereas the HCO3 from a metabolic panel is a measured level and thus more accurate.

Primary Acid-Base Derangements

Disorder	Process	pH	HCO_3	$PaCO_2$
Metabolic acidosis	Excess H⁺, decreased HCO_3	–	–	–
Metabolic alkalosis	Excess HCO_3, decreased H⁺	+	+	+
Respiratory acidosis	Hypoventilation	–	+	+
Respiratory alkalosis	Hyperventilation	+	–	–

URINE LABORATORY TESTS

Urinalysis (UA) is most commonly ordered for the general surgical patient to assess for a urinary tract infection (UTI). In some instances, interpretation may seem to be subjective. However, keep in mind that different tests are sometimes referred to as a UA; these include screening tests such as the dipstick test or more advanced analysis such as urine microscopy. Usually you will be evaluating the results of a urine test to identify a UTI.

First, determine if the urine sample is a "clean catch" by noting if the number of epithelial cells is normal. Epithelial cells are indicative of contact with the skin and thus skin flora making the sample uninterpretable owing to contamination. Next, note if the enzyme leukocyte esterase or if nitrites are present. The presence of leukocyte esterase suggests that WBCs are present in the urinary tract and thus possibly an infection. The WBCs should be evaluated and counted with urine microscopy. Nitrites in urine are a more specific sign of a UTI, as nitrites are made only by enzymes present in *E. coli*. Findings suggestive of a UTI will often prompt a "reflex" order of a urine culture. Typically, management consists of concurrent administration of empiric antibiotic therapy until the micro-organism can be identified and then antibiotics are tailored. Erythrocytes (RBC) in the urine may be indicative of urinary tract pathology, trauma, contamination, or an infection. Note that asymptomatic pyuria in elderly females is not evidence of a pathogen and instead often represents asymptomatic colonization.

OTHER FLUIDS

Pleural, peritoneal, and cerebrospinal fluids may be drawn to evaluate for specific clinical abnormalities. Pleural fluid is usually sent at the time of pleural catheter or chest tube insertion. Relying on Light criteria, the fluid can be identified as exudative or transudative. These criteria compare the levels of protein and lactate dehydrogenase between the serum and the pleural fluid. Cultures are often sent at the same time. Peritoneal fluid can be examined for bacterial content to evaluate for spontaneous bacterial peritonitis or for RBC via a deep peritoneal lavage. In specific clinical scenarios, peritoneal fluid or abdominal fluid collections may be evaluated for bilirubin to evaluate for a biliary leak, lipase to evaluate for a pancreatic duct leak, or a creatinine level may be drawn to evaluate for a urine leak. Cerebrospinal fluid is usually obtained by lumbar puncture by colleagues either from the medical or neurosurgical service.

TROUBLESHOOTING

Recognizing abnormalities or derangements in laboratory test results requires properly drawn laboratory tests. Abnormalities that complicate or make interpretation impossible may include hemolyzed or diluted blood samples. Hemolysis can be pathological, but in terms of laboratory error, it occurs during the drawing or the handling of the blood specimen. Additionally, sometimes samples for laboratory tests are incorrectly drawn downstream from an intravenous infusion. This may result in abnormally elevated electrolyte levels if the patient is receiving a concurrent (upstream) repletion. Similarly, an infusion of heparin will affect a nearby partial thromboplastin time draw. Lastly, dilutional effects should be considered if the patient is undergoing fluid resuscitation. For example, a concurrent drop in WBC count, hematocrit (HCT), and platelet count after the administration of a few liters of IVF bolus is suggestive of a dilutional effect.

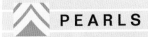

PEARLS

1. Familiarity with normal laboratory values will facilitate the recognition of abnormal values. Recognize when variation may be normal or expected. For example, a "normal" serum creatinine concentration in an elderly, frail patient may still represent acute kidney injury. These patients often have a low lean muscle mass and lower baseline serum creatine concentrations before the kidney injury.

2. Misnomers are common in medicine. Try to identify and avoid them as they can be confusing to you and others. For example, although AST and ALT are commonly included in the group of laboratory tests termed liver function tests, they do not reflect liver function. Instead, abnormally elevated levels of AST and ALT suggest liver (ie, hepatocyte) injury. Liver synthetic function is better assessed by coagulation studies, specifically prothrombin time/international normalized ratio, and by serum albumin levels.

3. Laboratory values are often only one piece of evidence in a clinical evaluation. Do not treat patients based on a single laboratory test abnormality if the sum of the other clinical evidence weighs against the abnormality. Consider other reasons the laboratory test result does not fit the overall picture.

Suggested Reading

1. Maithel SK, Critchlow J. *Critical Care Quick Glance: Physiology and Management.* New York: McGraw-Hill; 2006.
2. McLathchie G, Borley N, Chikwe J, eds. *Oxford Handbook of Clinical Surgery.* 3rd ed. New York: Oxford University Press, Inc; 2011.
3. Preston R. *Acid-Base, Fluids, and Electrolytes Made Ridiculously Simple.* 2nd ed. Miami: MedMaster, Inc; 2011.
4. Sabatine M, ed. *Pocket Medicine.* 4th ed. Philadelphia: Lippincott Williams and Wilkins; 2011.
5. Stehr W, ed. *The Mont Reid Surgical Handbook.* 6th ed. Philadelphia: Saunders Elsevier; 2008.
6. Wall DB, Klein SR, Black S, et al. A simple model to help distinguish necrotizing fasciitis from non-necrotizing soft tissue infection. *J Am Coll Surg.* 2000;191(3):227-231.
7. Yaghoubian A, de Virgilio C, Dauphine C, et al. Use of admission serum lactate and sodium levels to predict mortality in necrotizing soft-tissue infections. *Arch Surg.* 2007;142(9):840-846. doi:10.1001/archsurg.142.9.840.

17

SEPSIS AND SHOCK

PETER A. SODEN, MD | STEPHEN R. ODOM II, MD

Sepsis is a leading cause of admission to intensive care units (ICUs) and mortality of ICU patients around the globe. Sepsis is defined as a loss of regulation of the inflammatory response as a result of infection. Sepsis is part of a continuum that includes severe sepsis and septic shock. The incidence of sepsis has been on the rise over recent years, in part because of better diagnosis after consensus on definitions, as well as aging populations who are more susceptible to sepsis and multidrug resistant infections.

DEFINITIONS

The International Sepsis Definition Conference in 2001 refined prior work to more clearly define sepsis, severe sepsis, and shock.

The systemic inflammatory response syndrome (SIRS) is a dysregulation of the inflammatory response to a variety of noninfectious stimuli. SIRS is present when two or more of the following conditions are present:

1. Temperature greater than 38°C or less than 36°C
2. Heart rate greater than 90 beats/min

3. Hyperventilation, with respiratory rate greater than 20 breaths/min or $PaCO_2$ lower than 32 mm Hg
4. White blood cell (WBC) count less than 4000 cells/mm³, greater than 12,000 cells/mm³, or more than 10% bands

Sepsis is the presence of two or more SIRS criteria resulting from infection. Severe sepsis occurs when this response results in hypoperfusion or organ dysfunction. Septic shock is when persistent hypotension occurs despite adequate fluid resuscitation. Hypotension is defined as systolic blood pressure (SBP) less than 90 mm Hg or a mean arterial pressure (MAP) less than 70 mm Hg. Organ dysfunction is diagnosed in many ways depending on organ system.

DIAGNOSIS

The diagnosis of sepsis starts with a complete history and physical examination, looking for sources of infection. This should result in focused laboratory and imaging studies to support a suspected infection. There is no singular confirmatory test for sepsis, which has led to underdiagnosis in the past and the need for international standards to help better identify this entity. Common serum biomarkers used to support sepsis are WBC and lactic acid levels. Additionally, other biomarkers are available and are being studied at this time to better diagnose sepsis, such as C-reactive protein, procalcitonin, and interleukin-6. Research to date is inconclusive on the utility of these biomarkers, and more work remains on efficiently separating noninfectious SIRS from sepsis, which will help better define antibiotic selection and duration. Importantly, confirmatory testing is not required to diagnose sepsis if the suspicion for infection is high enough.

MANAGEMENT

Early and aggressive therapy gives patients the best chance of survival. Out of this came early goal-directed therapy (EGDT), as published by Rivers and colleagues, which showed improved outcomes for patients arriving to the emergency department in sepsis who underwent EGDT. This method focused on tasks to be completed within the first 6 hours of hospitalization for patients with suspected sepsis. These included a series of laboratory studies, initiation of broad-spectrum antibiotics, placement of a central venous catheter, and use of this central venous line (CVL) to monitor hemodynamic parameters (such as MAP, central venous pressure (CVP), and central venous oxygen saturation) to guide fluid resuscitation. Many emergency departments have incorporated the EGDT concepts into sepsis bundles. There have been recent trials, ProCESS, ARISE, and ProMISe, that have not shown mortality benefit with EGDT, but the overall concept of early resuscitation is still widely accepted.

The initial management should include a quick assessment of the patient's airway, breathing, and circulation. Additionally, appropriate intravenous access must be secured, and the patient should be directed to the correct level of care, often the ICU. However, resuscitation should not wait until the patient arrives in the ICU, it should start as soon as sepsis is suspected. Isotonic crystalloid fluid boluses should be administered and in patients with signs of hypovolemia, an initial bolus of 20 mL/kg should be trialed and the patient assessed for an appropriate response, with a MAP >65 mm Hg or urine output >0.5 mL/kg/h, before a second bolus amount is determined. Urine output, MAP, CVP, or mixed venous oxygen saturation can be measured to guide ongoing resuscitation. If lactate levels were initially elevated, then this should also be rechecked to assess the level of tissue hypoperfusion with resuscitation. Transfusions should be limited to those with hemoglobin less than 7 g/dL, except in those with active bleeding, myocardial ischemia, or refractory hypoxemia.

Broad-spectrum antibiotics should be administered as soon as possible in all patients suspected of sepsis. When possible, cultures should be obtained prior to administration of antibiotics. But the need to obtain cultures should not significantly delay administration of antibiotics as prior studies have shown an increase in mortality with every hour that antibiotic administration is delayed. Local resistance patterns and patient-specific culture history should help guide selection of initial broad-spectrum antibiotics. Empiric antifungal therapy should be considered in immunocompromised patients, such as those on chemotherapy, steroids, or other immunosuppressing medications, as well as those on total parenteral nutrition.

Identification of the source of an infection is critical for improved survival in sepsis and septic shock. Interventions to obtain source control should not be delayed in the patient with sepsis. This may include percutaneous or surgical drainage of infected collections or debridement of necrotizing soft-tissue infections.

Hemodynamic support is also often needed in the patient with septic shock. Norepinephrine should be the first agent trialed in septic shock. Importantly, this is not necessarily the optimal medication for hemodynamic support in other forms of shock. Vasopressin can be added if the patient needs a second agent. Other agents, such as epinephrine, dobutamine, milrinone, and dopamine, may be used in special circumstances.

Appropriate monitoring is also critical to ensure real-time feedback on resuscitation and perfusion efforts. Noninvasive measures, such as telemetry, pulse oximetry, and blood pressure cuff measurements should be routine.

In addition, CVLs can measure CVPs and central venous oxygen saturation, although many are moving away from using CVP to guide resuscitation. Multiple noninvasive devices including the Vigileo and PICCO monitors are commonly used in septic critical care patients to guide therapy. Tissue oxygen saturation is also emerging as a potential noninvasive transcutaneous method for quantifying tissue perfusion. Ultrasonography is becoming common practice to assess both venous return and cardiac function at the bedside.

ADDITIONAL MANAGEMENT

Nutrition should be started in all patients with sepsis unless there is a contraindication, such as bowel obstruction. Enteral nutrition is still heavily preferred. For patients unable to eat themselves, there is no standard for selection of enteral nutrition. To date, there is no strong evidence to support use of glutamine-rich or immunomodulatory enteral formulas in septic patients.

Chemical prophylaxis against venous thromboembolism (VTE) is important in patients with sepsis. Inflammation and immobility put these patients at higher risk for VTE. Low-molecular-weight heparin or unfractionated heparin should be used with pneumatic compression devices.

Both low and high blood glucose levels should be avoided in patients with sepsis. Target glucose control should be between 140 and 180 mg/dL. The use of glucocorticoid therapy in sepsis is controversial despite being studied extensively. Patients with hypotension refractory to fluid resuscitation and vasopressor medications may be candidates for a hydrocortisone trial, but this should be tapered as soon as possible.

Patients with sepsis who require mechanical ventilation are at risk for developing acute respiratory distress syndrome (ARDS). As a result, patients with sepsis should initially be on ARDS ventilator strategies, which limit volume and pressure settings.

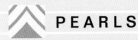

PEARLS

1. Sepsis, severe sepsis, and septic shock are a continuum of a dysregulated inflammatory response due to infection.
2. A high index of suspicion is needed to correctly diagnose sepsis.
3. Diagnosis does not require confirmation of infection, and once sepsis is suspected early and aggressive resuscitation, as well as antibiotic therapy, is critical for improving mortality from sepsis.

Suggested Readings

1. Dellinger RP, Levy MM, Rhodes A, et al. Surviving sepsis campaign: international guidelines for management of severe sepsis and septic shock: 2012. *Crit Care Med.* 2013;41(2):580-637.
2. Investigators A, Group ACT, Peake SL, et al. Goal-directed resuscitation for patients with early septic shock. *N Engl J Med.* 2014;371(16):1496-1506.
3. Mouncey PR, Osborn TM, Power GS, et al. Trial of early, goal-directed resuscitation for septic shock. *N Engl J Med.* 2015;372(14):1301-1311.
4. ProCESS Investigators; Yealy DM, Kellum JA, Huang DT, et al. A randomized trial of protocol-based care for early septic shock. *N Engl J Med.* 2014;370(18):1683-1693.
5. Rivers E, Nguyen B, Havstad S, et al. Early goal-directed therapy in the treatment of severe sepsis and septic shock. *N Engl J Med.* 2001;345(19):1368-1377.
6. Cameron JL, Cameron AM, eds. *Current Surgical Therapy.* 11th ed. Philadelphia, PA: Elseiver; 2014.

TOP 10 FLOOR PAGES

GABRIELLE E. CERVONI, MD | CHARLES S. PARSONS, MD

The greatest and most intense challenge of the general surgery internship year is to establish an equilibrium between your learning and the safe care of the patients in your charge. The purpose of this chapter is to present you with the most common scenarios with which new interns are frequently confronted, in the hope of giving you a practical leg-up in both learning the appropriate way to approach these problems, as well as providing optimal care to your patients.

As you have likely already realized, much of the "art of medicine" requires a strong background knowledge with superimposed pattern recognition and algorithm development. While these 10 scenarios will in no way substitute your own real-life algorithm development on the wards, their purpose is to provide you with the opportunity to practice the thought processes which result in successful patient care.

We encourage you to address each scenario by first establishing a broad list of differential diagnoses. You should then plan an approach that helps you define and treat the specific underlying disease process in your patient while concurrently using assessment tools to rule out other disease processes, with priority given to ruling out the most life-threatening disease processes first. There are several clinical pearls that you should remember in *every* scenario:

- You should always go see and examine your patient; there is no substitute for your own in-person assessment

- Review your patient's vital signs, ins/outs, recent labs/imaging, and recent medications
- Clarify the operative details for your patient—Are they pre- or post-op? Were there complications? Were there variations from standard operative procedure?
- Involve your patient's nurse; the nurse will often have very useful information and can be instrumental in effecting interventions quickly
- Briefly document your clinical assessment, differential diagnoses, and the management steps you are taking
- When unsure or in doubt, call for help

We fully expect that you will eventually hone your own patient management strategies in accordance with your own internship experiences, but we anticipate that this will provide a practical place to start.

PATIENT IS IN 10/10 POSTOPERATIVE PAIN

In the case of a patient with poorly controlled postoperative pain, symptoms can often be broken down into three categories: (1) poor control of expected postoperative pain, (2) abnormal pain, resulting from a postoperative complication, and (3) abnormal pain, unrelated and incidental to the operation. In distinguishing among these categories, the exact nature and duration of the patient's symptoms become very important. The patient should be examined first, and their pain medication regimen should be reviewed.

While the most frequently encountered situation in this case is an undermedicated patient, we cannot disregard the more concerning possibility of abnormal pain postoperatively, which often requires more aggressive intervention. Abnormal vital signs can be appreciated in all patients with poorly controlled postoperative pain; however, the patterns observed differ depending on the clinical status of the patient. While all patients experiencing severe pain will demonstrate mild to moderate sinus tachycardia, those who are simply undermedicated may demonstrate *hyper*tension, while patients with other, hemodynamically disruptive underlying processes will often be *hypo*tensive, and may further exhibit low urine output, mental status changes, and other clinical findings not anticipated postoperatively. These are the patients who warrant further workup and immediate notification of the team. In the case of a stable, hemodynamically appropriate (if somewhat tachycardic) patient in whom there is low suspicion for unexpected underlying cause of their pain, a reasonable initial course of action is to administer an additional dose of pain medication and to observe.

Patients with poor control of expected postoperative pain should indicate a physical location of their pain consistent with the nature of the operation and at their incision(s). Patients who have undergone laparoscopy will often complain of referred pain, usually to the upper back or shoulders, which usually resolves within a few hours. Patients who complain of pain not clearly referable to their operation should undergo the anatomically relevant workup; for example, chest pain following a laparoscopic appendectomy is not typical and should elicit a swift cardiopulmonary workup to rule out a more ominous etiology. When the nature of a patient's pain does not clearly indicate one cause over another (eg, the patient is not clearly distinguishing whether they have epigastric pain versus chest pain), a conservative approach should be employed such that the most concerning items on the differential are eliminated first.

A patient's postoperative pain may be undertreated for a variety of reasons, and recognition of these requires taking a thorough history, interviewing the patient's nurse, and sometimes soliciting help from the inpatient pharmacist. Among the most common reasons for poor pain control are inappropriate dosing of pain medication, preexistence of unidentified narcotic tolerance in the patient, failure to optimally administer nonnarcotic medications (such as acetaminophen or NSAIDs) where appropriate, patient incapability of correctly using a patient-controlled analgesia (PCA) device, and failure of regional anesthesia (such as a poorly placed epidural).

High yield:

- *DDx: Expected pain versus unexpected pain (may be related/unrelated to surgery)*
- *Initial interventions: Clinical assessment, add nonnarcotics, alter medication dosing*

PATIENT IS AGITATED, CONFUSED, PULLING AT LINES, AND ROAMING THE HALLS NAKED

In this scenario, you are presented with a patient exhibiting an altered mental status (AMS). Given the patient's abnormal behavior, your principle concern, even prior to developing a differential diagnosis, is to confirm the physical safety of both the patient and the staff (including you!). This requires an expedient examination of the patient and a conversation with nursing staff, including the floor resource nurse. Should the patient display aggression or physical violence, you should not hesitate to call hospital security; it is always preferable to involve security staff early if there is any question of a threat to safety. Even if you determine that the patient and staff are safe, you should ensure that physical restraints are easily accessible should the patient's behavior acutely become violent.

Once safety is addressed, your patient should be disconnected from any unnecessary devices or lines. If they no longer need a urinary catheter, for example, this should be discontinued. Necessary devices or drains should be secured under their garments and an abdominal binder to prevent the patient from inadvertently pulling them out. The patient should be offered a quiet space, preferably without a hospital roommate, and should be reoriented by a friend or family member (when available), or a familiar staff member.

Once these preliminary measures are undertaken, patient context and history become critically important in effectively managing the situation. A patient's AMS may be the consequence of underlying (sometimes previously undiagnosed) dementia or other mental health pathology. Alternatively, particularly in patients over the age of 65, an acutely AMS can indicate an underlying disease process or—in many cases—it may simply be the result of hospital delirium for which there is no single treatable explanation. Acute hospital delirium in elderly patients is frequently referred to as "sundowning," for the reason that it typically occurs in the evening or during the overnight shift.

Given the possible etiologies of AMS in your patient, your strategy should involve ruling out underlying organic factors; you should perform a basic infectious workup (complete blood count [CBC], urinalysis [UA], urine culture, blood culture, CXR), an electrolyte evaluation (Chem 10 panel), and a focused examination of the patient's drains and incisions for signs of infection. You should also perform a medication reconciliation to ensure that the patient has been receiving all of their home psychotropic medications; the patient should resume their home psychotropic regimen as soon as safely possible in the postoperative period. Particularly in elderly patients, certain medications have been noted to worsen confusion, and these should be avoided; these include anticholinergic agents (eg, diphenhydramine, scopolamine, TCAs) and benzodiazepines. In the instance of a violent patient who requires restraint, chemical restraints (eg, quetiapine, olanzapine, haloperidol) or physical restraints (eg, mitts, wrist bands, ankle bands) are available. Chemical restraints are generally very effective; haloperidol, however, can be sedating in the elderly and should be reserved for situations in which the patient must be rapidly subdued. Note that most chemical restraints can prolong the Qtc interval and should be used cautiously in patients with underlying cardiac arrhythmias. Physical restraints when used alone can increase agitation and aggression and, as such, should be reserved for situations in which chemical restraints are insufficient or contraindicated.

High yield:

- *DDx: Underlying psychiatric Dx, sundowning, medication effects, evolving sepsis*
- *Initial interventions: Address safety, reorient, consider chemical versus physical restraints, AMS workup: CBC/diff, blood chemistry, blood culture, UA/urine culture, fingerstick blood glucose (FSBG), arterial blood gas (ABG)*

PATIENT HAS CHEST PRESSURE, TIGHTNESS, OR PAIN

This scenario should automatically raise concern for an acute cardiac or pulmonary disease process and requires immediate attention to rule out these items. While these diagnoses are actually less common than more benign explanations—including musculoskeletal pain, gastroesophageal reflux disease (GERD), and anxiety—they have the potential to be rapidly fatal and thus must be ruled out in *every* case. You should immediately examine the patient and review their vital signs; in the meantime, you should initiate a complete, expeditious cardiopulmonary workup that includes a 12-lead ECG, CXR, CBC/chemistry, and troponins/CK/CK-MB. In a patient whom you believe is likely exhibiting acute coronary syndrome (ACS), you should alert your team and initiate preliminary intervention measures, which you can remember by the acronym "MONA" and which are shown in Table 18.1.[1]

TABLE 18-1 Initial Interventions for Suspected Acute Coronary Syndrome.

Therapy:	Morphine (M)	Oxygen (O)	Nitroglycerin (N)	Aspirin (A)
Dosing:	2-4 mg given IV push every 5-15 min	Up to 6 L/min via nasal cannula or face mask, titrating to $SPO_2 > 94\%$	0.3-0.4 mg SL every 5 min up to three doses	325 mg PO x1, chewed
Details:	Decreases pain if not alleviated by nitroglycerin; Should avoid if patient is hypotensive	Use in patients with SOB, heart failure, or hypoxia ($SPO_2 \leq 94\%$)	Arterial/venous dilation, decreases myocardial demand; should avoid if patient is hypotensive	Decreases platelet aggregation

SOB, shortness of breath.

Your degree of suspicion for a cardiac or pulmonary disease process will be based upon patient history and their overall clinical picture. The patient may disclose a history of angina, prior myocardial ischemia, heart failure (HF), previous cardiac surgery, pneumonia, chronic obstructive pulmonary disease (COPD)/emphysema, asthma, GERD, gastritis, costochondritis, or mechanical injury to the chest. The presence or absence of these factors may help inform your clinical suspicions. The patient's hemodynamic status should be considered, as acute *hypo*tension and tachycardia in the appropriate clinical context may imply an evolving ACS or pulmonary embolism (PE). Hypoxia should prompt you to draw an ABG from your patient to help identify a large PE or pneumonia, keeping in mind that a more definitive way to rule out a PE is with a computed tomography angiography (CTA) chest (PE protocol). D-dimer can be considered but is rarely useful in a postoperative patient. Importantly, hemodynamic stability does not preclude a cardiopulmonary etiology.

When examining your patient, you should clarify the character, duration, location, and reproducibility of their chest pain. Cardiac pain tends to be irreproducible, substernal, and "pressurelike" while primary pulmonary processes often result in pleuritic chest pain. These characteristics can be a helpful rule of thumb; however, they are not absolute, and a high clinical suspicion for these processes should be maintained.

High yield:

- *DDx: ACS, PE, HF decompensation, COPD/asthma/emphysema exacerbation, pneumonia, GERD, gastritis, musculoskeletal*
- *Initial interventions: ECG, CXR, troponins/CK/CK-MB, MONA; consider CTA PE protocol*

PATIENT HAS LOW URINE OUTPUT

For this scenario, you can conceptually organize changes in urine output as the result of (1) prerenal, (2) intrarenal, or (3) postrenal etiologies. Prerenal physiology refers to the importance of adequate kidney perfusion; hypovolemia, bleeding, and renal arteriolar vasoconstriction represent prerenal causes of poor urine output. Intrarenal pathology refers to intrinsic kidney malfunction which is frequently the consequence of nephrotoxic medications, acute tubular necrosis (ATN), or acute kidney injury (AKI) resulting from systemic illness. Postrenal pathology refers to mechanical urinary obstruction; postoperatively, this is frequently the consequence of a clogged urinary catheter, benign prostatic hypertrophy (BPH), or detrusor muscle dysfunction resulting from bladder overfilling.

In order to formulate a differential diagnosis in the above conceptual framework, you will need several additional pieces of information. You should evaluate the patient's fluid balance for the day including all intake (oral, intravenous) and output (urine, drains, stool, emesis). If the patient has a urinary catheter in place, you must ensure that the catheter is draining properly and may need to be flushed. If there is no urinary catheter present, you should interview the patient and their nurse to exclude undocumented voids or incontinence, and you should obtain a bladder scan to exclude urinary retention. You should calculate the predicted urine output for your patient (0.5-1 cc/kg/h in adults) with the expectation that patients age 65 and older may have diminished urine output relative to their younger counterparts due to loss of functioning glomeruli over time. If the patient is status post an operation, you should compare pre- and postoperative urine output of that patient to help ascertain whether there has been a significant change.

If indeed your patient does demonstrate a significant reduction in their urine output not referable to urinary retention or poor documentation, you should consider this a reflection of poor urine production. This in the postoperative patient results from hypovolemia or kidney malfunction. Intravascular hypovolemia can be the result of bleeding, underresuscitation, or sepsis. While kidney malfunction may exist at baseline in the patient, it may also be the result of diuretic-dependence, administration of a nephrotoxic agent, or intraoperative underperfusion injury. Examination of the patient can be very helpful in this circumstance. A patient who is hypovolemic will often demonstrate tachycardia, hypotension, and dry mucus membranes while a patient with a primary intrarenal etiology will not demonstrate these signs. The patient's drain output should be examined for overt signs of bleeding that may account for their hypovolemia. A patient who appears hypovolemic should be given 1 to 2 boluses of 500 cc crystalloid fluid and their urine output response monitored. A patient's failure to respond to these boluses implies that either hypovolemia is not the correct underlying diagnosis or that there is a source of ongoing volume loss (such as bleeding) at a rate which is hemodynamically significant.

In the event of a patient suspected of having a primarily renal problem or with suspected hypovolemia who has failed to respond appropriately to crystalloid resuscitation, a reasonable next step is to obtain a blood chemistry panel and urine electrolytes, which will allow you to calculate FENa and BUN:creatinine ratio. The urgency of this workup is dictated by the degree of hemodynamic instability in the patient. A postoperative patient who is hemodynamically labile and who demonstrates other clinical findings such as fever, AMS, or ileus may warrant a complete infectious workup to rule out impending sepsis as the underlying cause of their oliguria.

High yield:

- *DDx: Prerenal (poor perfusion), intrarenal, postrenal (obstructive)*
- *Initial interventions: Assess catheter, bladder scan, consider fluid challenge, blood chemistry, urine chemistry*

PATIENT IS NAUSEATED AND VOMITING

In a postoperative general surgery patient, this scenario underscores how important it is for you to know exactly what *type* of surgery your patient underwent and how *long* it has been since their operation. You may initiate antinausea therapy as you formulate your differential. You should make sure that the patient is NPO and administer a 4 mg one-time IV dose of ondansetron. Second-line agents include metoclopramide, scopolamine, compazine, and lorazepam. Ondansetron and metoclopramide can be QTc-prolonging, so a baseline QTc should be obtained with a 12-lead ECG if you anticipate needing to give additional doses.

It is important to remember that nausea, particularly in female patients, can frequently be an initial symptom of an ACS. You should prioritize ruling this out early with a focused history, cardiopulmonary physical examination, and an ECG. While nausea and vomiting are more often the consequence of a gastrointestinal process, failure to diagnose and treat an ACS can be deadly.

In a patient who has undergone an operation in the preceding 12 to 24 hours, it is reasonable to expect some nausea and even emesis as the result of general anesthesia. This is usually self-limited. You should interview the patient and, if possible, examine the vomitus to determine whether it is bloody, bilious, and/or high volume. Any of the preceding descriptors imply an underlying gastrointestinal cause. Common gastrointestinal causes may include mechanical obstruction, postoperative ileus, gastroenteritis, pancreatitis, and food allergy/intolerance; in postoperative patients, however, mechanical obstruction and postoperative ileus are the most likely culprits.

You should consider the patient's oral consumption pattern, abdominal examination, and bowel function; for example, a patient who has not resumed eating for several days postoperatively and who remains distended and without passage of flatus is likely experiencing an ileus and should be kept NPO until bowel function returns. A patient who remains distended and nauseated following high-volume or bilious emesis should undergo nasogastric tube placement and decompression with low continuous wall suction. If a mechanical obstruction is suspected, placement of a nasogastric tube is appropriate and may improve the likelihood of resolving the obstruction without surgery. If your patient remains nauseated, vomits multiple times, or exhibits hemodynamic changes or persistence of the above symptoms despite nasogastric decompression and antiemetics, you should immediately alert your team; it may be appropriate at this point to obtain imaging of the abdomen and pelvis (either CT or plain X-ray) to rule out a high-grade or closed-loop bowel obstruction.

High yield:

- *DDx: Anesthetic effects, obstruction, ileus, gastritis/gastroenteritis*
- *Initial interventions: Make NPO, serial clinical examinations, antiemetics, consider nasogastric tube, kidney, ureter, and bladder (KUB) XR, or CT arterial portography (AP)*

PATIENT'S K⁺ IS 6.4

Patients who have undergone surgery, particularly gastrointestinal surgery, often present electrolyte abnormalities. If alerted to a single electrolyte abnormality by nursing staff, your first course of action should be to examine a complete (current) chemistry panel for the patient. In some cases, a specimen will be noted by the lab to be "hemolyzed" in which case you should expect the potassium to be spuriously high. If a patient's chemistry panel demonstrates several deranged values, this may be due to an error in the blood draw or in the lab handling. In an otherwise asymptomatic patient, the above situations all warrant the redraw of a complete chemistry panel.

Once you have verified that your patient is actually hyperkalemic, you should examine their previous medical history and lab values. If your patient has a known history of hyperkalemia or of chronic kidney disease, their baseline potassium level is likely elevated relative to the normal patient population. For any potassium level greater than 5.5 to 6.0 mEq/L in a patient whose baseline potassium is normal, you should obtain a 12-lead ECG. Inspect the ECG for (1) peaked T waves and/or (2) a widened QRS interval. Either finding may imply impending arrhythmia and warrants further prompt intervention.

In a patient whose ECG demonstrates changes referable to their hyperkalemia, your first step should be to speedily administer 2 g IV calcium gluconate. This does not treat the hyperkalemia itself but serves to stabilize the cardiac cell membranes and decrease the likelihood that your patient will develop an arrhythmia; this effectively buys you some time to treat the hyperkalemia. You should ensure that the patient is not receiving any potassium in their IV fluids or receiving any medications that decrease potassium excretion (eg, nonsteroidal anti-inflammatory drugs [NSAIDs], angiotensin-converting-enzyme [ACE] inhibitors, potassium sparing diuretics). You may administer insulin (10-20 units humalog) with an ampule of 50% dextrose (D50), which will transiently reduce intravascular potassium by sequestering it intracellularly; importantly, this is an additional measure that will buy you time, but it will not enhance potassium removal from the body. Treatments which enhance the removal of potassium from the body include loop diuretics (if your patient is producing urine normally), oral sodium polystyrene, and finally hemodialysis. Most patients can be treated effectively with a loop diuretic (with or without a normal saline bolus) or sodium polystyrene, and their potassium level can be reassessed via serial chemistry lab draws. You should consider your patient's overall clinical status and confer with your team before deciding upon a therapy strategy. Hemodialysis (HD) is a measure of last resort.

High yield:

- DDx: Hyperkalemia
- Initial interventions: Verify lab values, ECG; consider IV calcium gluconate, insulin/dextrose, albuterol to buy time; consider loop diuretics, sodium polystyrene, and HD for removal of potassium

PATIENT'S TELEMETRY IS SHOWING ATRIAL FIBRILLATION (A-FIB) WITH A HR 160

In this situation, you are given the correct diagnosis up front—usually by the patient's nurse who has witnessed the telemetry change—and you need to make management decisions. You should expediently obtain a 12-lead ECG to confirm the diagnosis, which is defined by the absence of individual p waves.

Your first objective should be to quickly establish whether this patient is hemodynamically stable or unstable; namely, you want to know if the patient's systolic cardiac function is so compromised as a result of their rapid ventricular response (RVR) that they have become *hypo*tensive or have developed an AMS. If this is the case, you should immediately call a rapid response. Provided that the A-FIB is indeed a *new* finding, initiation of ACLS protocol and cardioversion are required. In an unstable patient, you should quickly examine the patient and ascertain whether they have any history of A-FIB (whether paroxysmal) or have been treated for this problem before. If the patient has a known history of A-FIB, you should verify that they are being prescribed their home antiarrhythmic medication regimen.

New onset A-FIB is an arrhythmia which is often inflammatory or—though much less often—ischemic in nature. It occurs commonly in the 24 to 48 hours following thoracic surgery but may occur after any operation as the result of a transiently proinflammatory physiologic state. It should be emphasized that chest pain or ST-segment changes on an ECG in this context should raise suspicion for cardiac ischemic injury and should precipitate a complete cardiology evaluation. New-onset A-FIB may also result from overstretching of the right atrium secondary to volume over-load; the net fluid balance of the patient is important as it is informative in this regard.

In a hemodynamically stable patient presenting with new-onset A-FIB and RVR, medical therapy is attempted before cardioversion. The first-line agent is IV metoprolol, which should be given as bolus doses of 5 mg, with each dose administered (typically by you) slowly, over the course of 2 minutes. You should flush 5 cc of normal saline after each dose and wait 5 to 8 minutes to observe any change your patient's blood pressure. You should always have a bedside telemetry monitor anytime you are bolus administering antiarrhythmic agents. You may give up to a total of 5 to 20 mg IV metoprolol, depending on your patient's hemodynamic response. If your patient fails to convert to sinus rhythm with the above measures but remains hemodynamically stable, you should administer IV diltiazem as bolus doses of 10 mg, up to 20 mg of IV diltiazem. As with administration of IV metoprolol, you should wait 5 to 8 minutes between doses to ensure that the patient does not become hypotensive.

If your patient converts to sinus rhythm, you can stop administering antiarrhythmic agents; in the case of postoperative new A-FIB, further therapy is seldom required. If your patient fails to convert to sinus rhythm despite optimal use of IV metoprolol and IV diltiazem, your team should be notified. In some cases, your patient may become "rate-controlled," which means that the A-FIB persists but that their heart rate has dropped into a near-normal range; in an otherwise healthy patient, A-FIB with a maximal HR of 110 to 115 is acceptable, and this can be maintained with low-dose IV metoprolol given every 4 to 6 hours.

If your patient fails to convert to sinus rhythm and cannot be rate-controlled with the abovementioned measures, you should again notify your team and make arrangements for transfer of your patient to the intensive care unit (ICU) for treatment with a continuous IV antiarrhythmic agent, such as amiodarone. Consultation with a cardiologist is often required in this instance.

High yield:

- *DDx: Atrial fibrillation*
- *Initial interventions: Very A-FIB by ECG; if unstable, call rapid response for cardioversion; if stable, IV metoprolol or IV diltiazem*

PATIENT HAS A POSTOPERATIVE FEVER

This is a scenario in which clinical context is of primary importance. You should clarify several points prior to formulation of your differential diagnosis; you should verify the exact timing and grade of the fever, the amount of time elapsed since surgery, what *type* of operation was done, and what (if any) antibiotics have already been given. While normal human body temperature is usually 98.6°F (37°C), an elevated temperature is not generally regarded as a fever until it is 100.5°F (38°C) or higher. You may use antipyretic agents (eg, acetaminophen, NSAIDs) to treat a fever to enhance patient comfort; you should not fear "masking" a fever with medication as persistent fevers will manifest regardless of medication.

The classic teaching of the "Rule of 4 Ws" while imprecise can be a useful reminder of the variety of things that can result in postoperative fever. Within 12 to 24 hours following invasive surgery, patients frequently experience elevated body temperature >100.5°F, which is most often the result of the proinflammatory physiologic state of the patient due to the surgery itself. While such occurrences are usually self-limited, any very elevated temperature (above 102°-103°F) or accompanying unexpected symptoms should prompt further investigation.

In the days to weeks which follow surgery, regardless of exact timing, any fever >100.5°F in the absence of other symptoms should trigger an infectious workup. A complete infectious workup should include a UA, urine culture, blood culture, CBC with differential, CXR, and sputum culture (if applicable). The most common infectious culprits of fever in the postoperative patient include cystitis, pyelonephritis, pneumonia, peritonitis, and infected indwelling IV access. If a patient presents with specific symptoms accompanying their fever (eg, dysuria), it is reasonable to pursue a targeted workup prior to obtaining a comprehensive infectious workup (eg, obtain UA and urine culture first for a patient with dysuria).

If your patient has undergone a gastrointestinal tract operation featuring a resection and reanastomosis of bowel, you should strongly consider the possibilities of anastomotic leak and/or an intra-abdominal abscess as the source(s) of their fever. These patients will frequently present with worsening abdominal pain, bloating, and ileus resulting from the leakage of succus or stool into the peritoneum. Untreated, they will develop sepsis and shock. A similar clinical picture can be seen in patients following biliary tree surgery, in which case a bile leak should be suspected. In terms of noninvasive imaging, the biliary tree is generally best interrogated with abdominal ultrasound (US), whereas an anastomotic leak is best identified with a CT of the abdomen and pelvis featuring intraluminal contrast (whether per oral or per rectum).

Particularly in patients who are at risk for hypercoagulability, you should strongly consider the possibility of venous thromboembolism (VTE) as the underlying etiology of their fever. D-dimer values are typically *not* useful, as we anticipate their elevation in nearly all surgical patients. If you suspect an extremity deep vein thrombosis (DVT) in your patient, you should obtain a venous duplex ultrasound. If your patient is inexplicably hypoxic or tachycardic in the setting of a fever, you should minimally obtain an ABG and alert your team such that a CTA chest (PE protocol) can be considered.

An uncommon cause of postoperative fever is a medication reaction. Certain medications such as inhalational anesthetic or succinylcholine can result in the development of malignant hyperthermia in patients who have inherited a rare susceptibility to this problem. This usually presents intraoperatively, immediately following administration of the anesthetic, and is managed by emergency administration of dantrolene and hemodynamic support with discontinuation of the offending agent. In contrast, neuroleptic malignant syndrome can present as high fevers, muscle rigidity, severe dysautonomia, and altered mentation following the administration of antipsychotic agents. This can occur anytime the agent is given and can be life-threatening; treatment involves immediate discontinuation of the agent and hemodynamic support, with dantrolene and benzodiazepines used as needed.

High yield:

- DDx: *Postoperative fever, infection, VTE, anastomotic leak, medication reaction*
- *Initial interventions:* UA/urine culture, blood culture, CBC/diff, CXR/sputum culture, consider CTA chest (PE protocol)

PATIENT IS HYPOTENSIVE

This scenario should evoke a similar algorithmic thought process to that of low urine output. Particularly in a postoperative patient, hypotension can result from the following general categories of disease processes: (1) intravascular hypovolemia ("the tank is empty"), (2) cardiac pathology ("pump failure"), and (3) neurogenic dysautonomia. The degree of hypotension and overall clinical picture dictate the urgency of the situation. A patient who displays a single depressed blood pressure in the setting of normal heart rate and mental status is much less concerning than a patient who is tachycardic, oliguric, or who has altered mentation.

The patient should always first be placed on a telemetry monitor and their vital signs examined. Their fluid balance should be calculated. Adequate IV access should be established including at least one but preferably two large bore peripheral IVs.

In a patient with an epidural in place, neurogenic dysautonomia as the cause of hypotension should be an early consideration. If turning off the epidural results in an improved blood pressure, this is likely the etiology.

Tachycardia may be present in both an intravascularly hypovolemic patient and a patient with cardiac failure; however, patients with neurogenic hypotension may have a normal or even depressed heart rate. A primary cardiac etiology may include HF (new or preexisting) or ischemic injury to the cardiac muscle; such pathologies severely compromise the ability of the heart to pump effectively and hinder the generation of an appropriate blood pressure. A primary cardiac etiology is suggested by a patient with a significant history of cardiac disease, telemetry changes, or symptoms of new chest pain or shortness of breath. Any of the above items should prompt a full cardiac workup including a 12-lead ECG, troponins/CK/CK-MB, and cardiology evaluation.

A postoperative patient may have intravascular hypovolemia resulting from evolving sepsis (so called "leaky capillaries"), bleeding, or underresuscitation. All of these entities can feature hypotension in the setting of tachycardia and oliguria. In addition, all of the above entities should demonstrate a response to IV crystalloid resuscitation unless the underlying pathophysiology is very advanced; it becomes important, therefore, to evaluate the entire clinical picture of such a patient. Fever, inexplicable pain, or suspected infectious source all imply early or evolving sepsis. If sepsis is suspected, an infectious source should be sought. Underresuscitation should be discernible by calculating the total fluid balance of the patient and ruling out postoperative bleeding. As mentioned in the oliguria scenario, postoperative bleeding is suggested by increased bloody drain output, a declining hematocrit value, and escalating pain at the surgical site where such bleeding might be expected.

Regardless of the etiology of the hypotension in your patient, it is to your (and your patient's) benefit to alert your team to the situation early. Particularly if your patient fails to respond to early resuscitative efforts or demonstrates symptoms of end-organ underperfusion (eg, AMS or oliguria), they may end up requiring transfer to the ICU for hemodynamic monitoring and treatment with vasopressor medications. It is never wrong to call for help early when caring for an unstable patient about whom you are concerned.

High yield:

- *DDx: Intravascular hypovolemia (bleeding, underresuscitation), cardiac failure, neurogenic dysautonomia*
- *Initial interventions: ECG, CBC, assess drains and fluid balance, consider fluid challenge*

PATIENT'S WIFE IS CALLING FROM HOME WITH QUESTIONS

When a patient or their family member calls from home with a concern, you should return the call as soon as possible. In these types of interactions, you should bear in mind that regardless of how straightforward the question may seem, you are *always* disadvantaged by not being able to interview and examine the patient in person. Sometimes patients will call by mistake or with logistical questions (eg, "Where is my appointment tomorrow?"); you can easily assist them in these situations. When a patient calls with a *clinical* question—whether regarding a change in their symptoms or a prescription request—you should confer with your team and clearly document your phone interactions.

A wise strategy is to take as complete a history as you can over the phone with the patient; whenever possible, it is best to speak with the patient directly rather than a friend or family member. If the patient has undergone an abdominal operation, you should ask the same questions you might ask at a follow-up clinic appointment: How do they feel? What is their pain level? What are their eating patterns like? Do they experience regular passage of flatus and stool? Are they still taking pain medications? You should obtain a review of systems. As you cannot physically examine the patient over the phone, you should ask the patient to self-examine their abdomen and surgical wounds and report their findings to you.

Once you have obtained the above information, you may alert your team to the situation. Your chief resident may want to speak with the patient directly or they may work with you to formulate a patient plan about which you can then call the patient back. A good rule of thumb is: when in doubt, direct the patient to come to the emergency department so they can be evaluated by a physician. This will minimize the number of missed diagnoses and poor patient outcomes.

If for any reason you suspect a patient to be in extremis, you should instruct the patient or their family member to immediately dial emergency medical services (EMS) at 911. Patients with acute respiratory decompensation or chest pain, for example, should be brought to the hospital via EMS as soon as possible. You may also offer to call EMS on behalf of the patient but should make sure the patient understands your plan and has provided you with the correct street address and contact information. Again, you should always document these interactions in the official medical record.

High yield:

- *DDx: Depends on information from the patient*
- *Initial interventions: Obtain focused history, communicate with your chief resident, document encounter*

While the above scenarios in no way represent all of the situations you will face as a general surgery intern, they may provide a reasonable scaffold on which you can begin to develop your own problem-based patient management strategies. These examples should illustrate that optimal patient care generally comes as the result of developing a broad list of differential diagnoses and effecting interventions which allow you to rule out dangerous pathologies without delaying the treatment of more common ones. As you progress through your internship year, we encourage you to keep a written record of the challenging patient problems that you encounter and your resultant decision-making; this will gradually help you construct your own patient care algorithms which you will continue to hone over the course of your surgical career.

 PEARLS

1. Always answer your pager promptly. Be ready to assess your patient bedside and do not make any assumptions.
2. Contact your senior as needed without hesitation. Be sure to communicate your concerns clearly and ask for support when needed.
3. Become familiar with the presentation of some of the most common emergencies and develop a systematic approach to your management.

Reference

1. O'Connor R, Brady W, Brooks SC, et al. Part 10: acute coronary syndromes. 2010 American Heart Association guidelines for cardiopulmonary resuscitation and emergency cardiovascular care. *Circulation.* 2010;122:787-817.

19

NASOGASTRIC AND NASOJEJUNAL TUBE PLACEMENT

SAYURI P. JINADASA, MD, MPH | EMILIE B. D. FITZPATRICK, MD | WEI WEI ZHANG, MD

Nasogastric tubes (NGTs) and nasojejunal tubes (NJTs) are tubes that are inserted through a nare, passed through the esophagus into the stomach or jejunum, respectively. NGTs are available in several diameters, measured in French, with varying designs and functions. These tubes can be used for both enteral access for feeding and gastrointestinal (GI) decompression. The most common nasogastric tube used for decompression is the Salem Sump tube. You may encounter a variety of commercially available NJTs used for enteral nutrition. Dobhoff and Corpak are two of the most widely available.

TYPES OF NASOGASTRIC TUBES

Salem Sump tubes are colloquially known as NG tubes and are rarely referred to by their trade name. These tubes are popular because they can be used for either decompression or feeding and can be either placed in a nostril as an NGT

171

or passed through the oral cavity as an orogastric tube (OGT). Salem Sump tubes have two lumens; the larger, main lumen acts as a conduit for delivery or removal to/from the stomach, whereas the smaller side port acts as a sump. The sump allows air to be drawn from the outside into the tube. This is important when the NGT is put to suction as it allows for equalization of pressure between the stomach and the atmosphere, which prevents tube adherence to the wall and possible injury to the gastric wall.

In contrast to Salem Sump tubes, Dobhoff tubes (DHTs) are fine-bore tubes that can be used only to administer medications or tube feeds. The smaller and more pliable DHT does not allow for suction decompression of the stomach or intestinal tract but is more comfortable to have in place than the large, stiff Salem Sump tube. Given the pliability of DHTs, a guidewire is used for initial placement of the DHT, which is removed after successful placement is verified with a chest or abdominal x-ray. The presence of the guidewire increases ease of DHT placement; however, it also increases the risk of causing a pneumothorax if mistakenly passed into the airway. The tip of the DHT is weighted; this in combination with its finer diameter allows it to be passed beyond the pylorus for small bowel access.

INDICATIONS

FEEDING/MEDICATION ADMINISTRATION

Salem Sump and Dobhoff tubes can be used for direct access to the GI tract to administer medication or tube feedings to a functional GI tract. Enteral access is often needed in patients who are intubated and sedated, in patients with impaired swallowing mechanisms, or in patients with a dysfunctional intestinal tract.

An intubated and sedated patient may receive feeds through an orogastric Salem Sump tube (OGT). This method of feeding confers several advantages. First, because of the larger diameter of the Salem Sump tube, it allows for easy delivery of enteric feeds and medication without becoming obstructed or "clogged." Salem Sump tubes can often accommodate crushed oral medications and viscous liquids without an issue. Another advantage of using the Salem Sump tube for feeding is that you can place the tube to intermittent suction to check for gastric residuals. High residuals are a sign of impaired gastric emptying and poor tube feed tolerance. Residuals are usually checked every 4 to 8 h, and enteric feeding is often held if the residual amount is deemed high by the clinician, usually between 200 and 500 mL. Although this practice is easy to perform and thought to minimize the risk of aspiration, there is debate in the nutrition and critical care literature as to whether checking for residuals actually prevents pulmonary complications (eg, aspiration).

Awake patients (who are not intubated) do not tolerate orogastric tubes and should have a feeding tube placed nasally. DHTs are often used in this case for increased patient comfort. DHTs can be used to feed the stomach or advanced past the pyloric or ligament of Treitz in patients with mechanical or functional gastric outlet obstructions. Post pyloric tube placement can be achieved at the bedside or under fluoroscopic or endoscopic guidance. Because of their thin caliber, DHTs are more prone to clogging and need frequent flushing to remain patent. This becomes especially problematic when a DHT is placed post pyloric, as it is often difficult to replace. Various methods are available to declog a nonfunctioning DHT, including infusion of coca cola, meat tenderizer, pancreatic enzyme with bicarbonate, and wire manipulation.

DECOMPRESSION

The NGT (Salem Sump) can be used for gastric decompression in patients who have an intestinal obstruction or ileus. Once the NGT is in position, it is placed to low intermittent or continuous suction to facilitate removal of enteric contents. This minimizes recurrent vomiting and aspiration risk, improves patient comfort, and allows for monitoring for resolution of the obstruction or ileus. When an NGT is used for decompression, it is important to periodically flush the main lumen with normal saline or water and sump lumen with air to keep the system patent and functioning. This ensures adequate drainage of gastric contents and avoids suction injury to the gastric mucosa. It is your responsibility to ensure that an NGT on suction is actually functioning properly. Make it a habit to check it every time you enter the room of a patient with an NGT.

LAVAGE

NGTs are at times utilized in the diagnosis of upper GI bleeds through gastric lavage. This is performed by instilling 50 to 200 mL of irrigation through the main lumen of the Salem Sump tube, then aspirating or placing the tube to suction. If there is blood in the initial aspirate or the aspirate after water instillation, this confirms that there is a gastric bleed. However, a nonbloody aspirate does not rule out an intermittent gastric bleed. If bilious, nonbloody aspirate is obtained, then at least the proximal duodenum has been sampled, but it still does not definitely rule out an upper GI bleed. The routine use of gastric lavage during GI bleed is controversial because its clinical benefit has not been proven. The process does facilitate clearing of the stomach of gastric contents, food, and old clot, making subsequent endoscopy easier to perform.

STEPS FOR NASOGASTRIC TUBE PLACEMENT

1. Gather supplies:
    a. Extension tubing (if using NGT for gastric decompression)
    b. Wall canister (if using NGT for gastric decompression)
    c. Plastic connector
    d. NGT or DHT
    e. Lubricant (with lidocaine if possible)
    f. Ice water with straw
    g. 60-mL Toomey syringe
    h. Stethoscope
    i. Silk tape
    j. Emesis bin

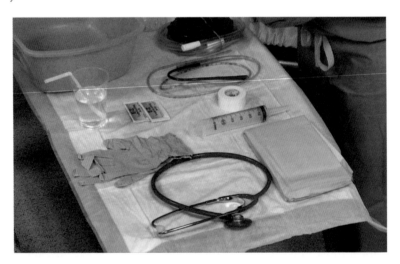

2. Describe the procedure to the patient; relay to the patient that the procedure will be uncomfortable and that their cooperation with sipping fluid is paramount.
3. If using NGT for gastric decompression, place the wall canister in the wall bracket and connect the vacuum suction tubing from the wall to the canister; connect the extension tubing to the wall canister and assure that the vacuum is working properly.

4. Rip two pieces of silk tape and place them in an easily accessible location for after placement of the tube.

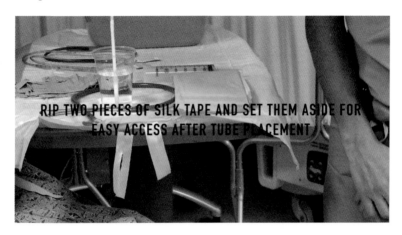

5. Put gloves on.
6. Measure the approximate length that the NGT must be inserted to reach the stomach; hold the tip of the NGT midway between the xiphoid process and umbilicus, measure the distance to the earlobe and then from the earlobe to the tip of the nostril. This distance is usually 50 to 60 cm.

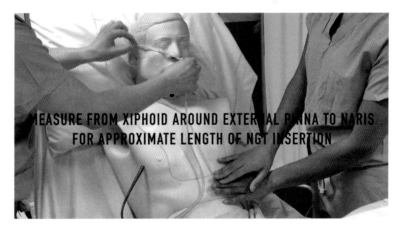

7. Assess the patient's nostrils and select the side that is more patent; inject lubricant into that nostril and ask the patient to sniff.

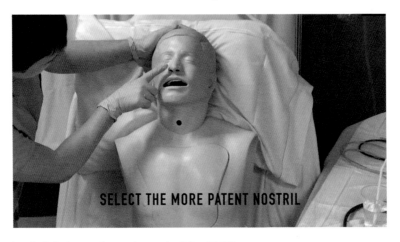

SELECT THE MORE PATENT NOSTRIL

8. Apply lubricant along the end of the NGT.
9. Ask the patient or the nurse/assistant to hold the cup of water and emesis bin close to the patient; ask the patient to tilt the chin toward the chest.
10. Insert the NGT into the nostril; after a few centimeters, resistance will be felt when the NGT tip hits the posterior aspect of the nasopharynx; apply gentle pressure so that the tube turns inferiorly and continues to advance with less resistance.
11. Ask the patient to sip water while advancing the NGT to the predetermined measurement.
    a. If the patient coughs continuously, the tube is likely inserted into the trachea; promptly withdraw the tube.
    b. If the NGT is placed for obstruction or ileus, gastric or bilious reflux out of the NGT is often seen as the tube is passed into the stomach, before it is placed to suction.

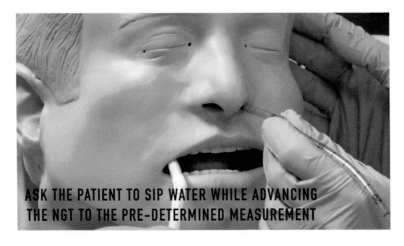

ASK THE PATIENT TO SIP WATER WHILE ADVANCING
THE NGT TO THE PRE-DETERMINED MEASUREMENT

12. Holding the NGT in place, ask the nurse/assistant to connect the 60-mL Toomey syringe filled with air to the proximal end of the tube.
13. Place the stethoscope along the patient's left upper quadrant and ask the nurse/assistant to inject the air into the NGT; if the passage of air is heard through the stomach, proper placement is likely.

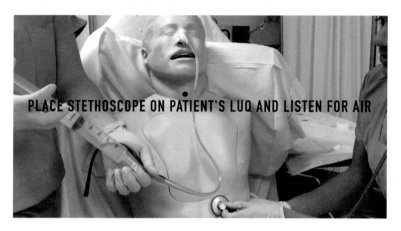

PLACE STETHOSCOPE ON PATIENT'S LUQ AND LISTEN FOR AIR

14. Attach the plastic connecter at the end of the NGT; either clamp the tube or, if using the NGT for gastric decompression, connect the extension tubing attached to the wall connector.
15. Use the silk tape pieces to secure the NGT to the patient's nose.
16. Order a chest x-ray (CXR) to assess proper placement of the NGT.
17. Look at the CXR yourself to assure proper placement of the NGT.

NEXT STEPS

1. Always obtain a CXR to verify that the NGT is in the appropriate position if the tube is used for enteric feeding. **NEVER start tube feedings before appropriately verifying appropriate positioning.** If feedings or medications are given into the lung, this can be fatal.

NGTs for decompression can be used if proper placement is confirmed with gastric auscultation and reflux of enteric contents. If the NGT was difficult to place or if there is a question regarding tube location, an x-ray is always a good idea. Some institutions advocate for CXR for all NGT placements to confirm that the tube is not coiled and that complications such as pneumothorax did not occur.

1. If the tube is not in the correct place, retract the tube to attempt adjustment or remove completely and start placement again from the first step.
2. If a DHT was placed and appropriate positioning is verified, remove the wire from the tube.

COMPLICATIONS

Salem Sump or Dobhoff tube placement can be very uncomfortable for patients, especially for those who are awake and not sedated. Proper placement technique, topical anesthetics, and adequate patient preparation may alleviate some patient anxiety and discomfort. In addition, NGT placement is not without its risks, with complications ranging from epistaxis to respiratory tree intubation and esophageal perforation. Because it is not benign, NGT should be placed only when necessary and removed as soon as possible. The routine use of NGTs has fallen out of favor postoperatively in recent years, especially with the rise in popularity of enhanced recovery after surgery protocols that favor early feeding. Despite this trend, NGTs remain essential in the treatment of many surgical patients and a surgeon should be adept at the bedside placement and management of an NGT.

NGT complications include:

Upper airway irritation/trauma:
Epistaxis
Rhinitis/sinusitis
Laryngospasms

Misplacement/traumatic placement:
Intracranial insertion
Submucosal passage
Pneumothorax
Esophageal perforation
Intrapulmonary feeding

Chronic NG intubation:
Aspiration
Mechanical occlusion
Dislodgement
Cracking/breakage

Gastric erosion, ulceration, bleeding
Aortoesophageal fistula
Esophageal stricture

 PEARLS

1. To soften or harden the NGT tip for patient comfort and/or ease of placement, place the tip in either hot water or cold water, respectively. Lidocaine gel can be placed intranasally and used as an NGT lubricant to decrease patient discomfort.
2. Always interrogate an NGT to ensure it is functioning. This is the responsibility of the junior resident on the team.
3. Familiarize yourself with the different nasogastric tubes and their relative indications and uses.

References

1. Kuppinger DD, Rittler P, Hartl WH, Rüttinger D. Use of gastric residual volume to guide enteral nutrition in critically ill patients: a brief systematic review of clinical studies. *Nutrition.* 2013;29(9):1075-1079.
2. Fakhry S, Rutherford E, Sheldon G. Routine postoperative management of the hospitalized patient. In: Souba W, Fink M, Jurkovich G, et al, eds. *ACS Surgery Principles & Practice.* New York, NY: WebMD; 2005:87.
3. Pallin DJ, Saltzman JR. Is nasogastric tube lavage in patients with acute upper GI bleeding indicated or antiquated? *Gastrointest Endosc.* 2011;74:981-984.
4. Prabhakaran S, Doraiswamy VA, Nagaraja V, et al. Nasoenteric tube complications. *Scand J Surg.* 2012;101:147-155.

20

PHLEBOTOMY

SAYURI P. JINADASA, MD, MPH | STEPHEN R. ODOM II, MD

Blood draws are performed in both routine care and under urgent and emergent scenarios. They are performed by a variety of health care workers, including physicians, nurses, phlebotomists, and nursing technicians. The specific person who draws samples for laboratory tests depends on the setup of a given hospital system. However, this skill is essential for trainees to master, as having these skills will allow for expedited care, especially in situations in which there is no time to wait.

Common sites for drawing l samples for laboratory tests include the antecubital fossa (cephalic vein, brachial vein, median cubital vein), the forearm (cephalic vein), or the hand. There are increasing numbers of nerve endings the more distal you go on the upper extremity, and therefore, the hand will usually be more sensitive to pain than the antecubital fossa.

The current consensus is to avoid performing blood draws from an extremity that has or will soon be used for an arteriovenous (AV) graft or fistula.

INDICATIONS

Indications for blood draw include obtaining a blood sample for testing, including blood culture, electrolyte panel, complete blood count, and toxicology screen (Table 20.1).

TABLE 20-1 Common Blood Tests

Name	Tests	Tube Type
Coagulation study	International normalized ratio (INR), partial thromboplastin time (PTT), prothrombin time (PT)	Citrate
Complete blood count	White blood cell (WBC), hemoglobin (Hgb), hematocrit (Hct), platelets (Plt)	EDTA
Liver function test	Alanine aminotransferase (ALT), aspartate aminotransferase (AST), total bilirubin, direct bilirubin, alkaline phosphatase	Serum separator
Chemistry panel	Sodium, potassium, chloride, bicarbonate, blood urea nitrogen (BUN), creatinine, glucose, phosphorus, calcium, magnesium	Serum separator

STEPS

1. Gather supplies:
   a. Gloves
   b. Alcohol/chlorhexidine pads
   c. Tourniquet
   d. Collection tubes
   e. Butterfly needle
   f. Connector
   g. Gauze pads
   h. Band-Aid or medical tape
   i. Chux pad (optional)
   j. Patient label

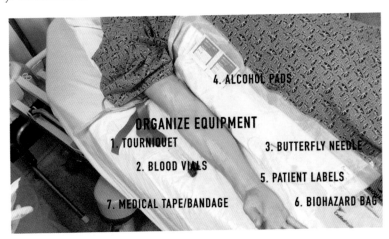

2. Wash hands or clean hands with alcohol.

3. Position patient and bed to position that is comfortable to the patient and the person drawing samples.
4. Arrange all equipment in order of use:
   a. Alcohol pads, tourniquet, butterfly needle and connector, collection tubes, gauze pads, Band-Aid/tape
5. Attach connector to butterfly.
6. Ask the patient if there is a preferred site; if not, identify a suitable site.
   a. Do not draw from an arm with an AV fistula, a site close to a running intravenous (IV) tube.
   b. The veins in the antecubital fossa are the usual choice; the next choice would be veins along the ventral aspect of the arms or dorsum of the hand.
7. Place the chux pad under the patient's arm/hand.
8. Tie the tourniquet 3 to 4 inches above the site of venipuncture.
   a. Tie loop that allows for easy one-handed release.

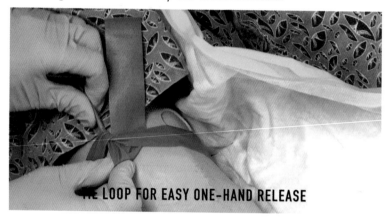

TIE LOOP FOR EASY ONE-HAND RELEASE

9. Look for and palpate the vein; observe the trajectory of the vein.
   a. Sometimes gentle tapping and/or application of a warm compress can help make the vein more prominent.

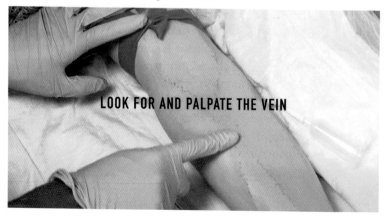

LOOK FOR AND PALPATE THE VEIN

10. Put on gloves.
11. Clean the area to be punctured with the alcohol/chlorhexidine pad; let air dry.
12. Hold the butterfly at a 15° to 30° angle with the bevel up.

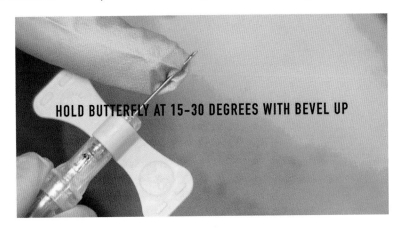

13. Grasp the patient's arm firmly using thumb of nondominant hand to draw the skin taut and anchor the vein.

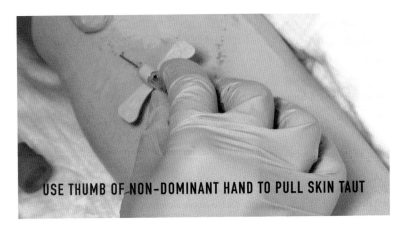

14. Deliberately insert the needle until you see a flash of blood.
15. Connect the collection tube to the butterfly connector.

16. Collect an adequate amount of sample.

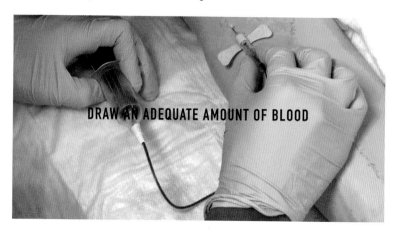

17. Disconnect the collection tube.
18. Release the tourniquet with one hand while holding the needle steady in the other.
19. Place gauze over the puncture site and hold gentle pressure as the needle is removed.
20. Click the button to retract the needle.

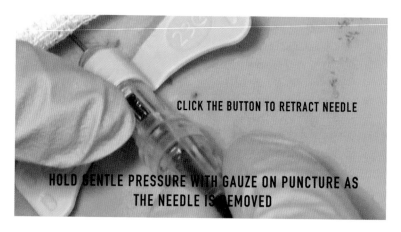

21. Place a Band-Aid or tape to hold the gauze in place.
22. Place the patient label on the tube(s).
23. Appropriately dispose of needle and all other supplies.

COMPLICATIONS

Complications include bleeding and hematoma, which should be treated with compression. Thrombophlebitis is another potential complication, which is inflammation of the vein secondary to a clot. This should be treated with warm compresses, elevation, and nonsteroidal anti-inflammatory drugs.

In the case of a needle stick, assure that the needle and all sharps are secure, wash hands immediately, and refer to your institution's procedures to be evaluated for postexposure treatment.

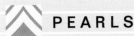 **PEARLS**

1. Always ask patients where they prefer to be "stuck" as they often know both the most successful and most comfortable place. Always make sure you are positioned comfortably while performing this and any other procedure.
2. In inpatients, look for clues of prior successful sites (areas of needle sticks) and prior sites that were not successful (hematomas, bruises). Try not to draw close to an IV infusion site.
3. Always label patient tubes soon after drawing blood and double check that the label represents the correct patient.

Suggested Readings

1. Norsayani MY, Hassim IN. Study on incidence of needle stick injury and factors associated with this problem among medical students. *J Occup Health*. 2003;45:172-178.
2. Centers for Disease Control and Prevention TNIfOSaH. Available from https://www.cdc.gov/niosh/topics/bbp/sharps.html.

21

INTRAVENOUS LINE PLACEMENT

SAYURI P. JINADASA, MD, MPH | STEPHANIE B. JONES, MD

Intravenous (IV) lines can be placed by a variety of health care providers, including physicians, nurses, and technicians. Who routinely places IV lines is usually institution specific, but having this skill as a trainee is essential, especially if urgent intervention is required.

IV catheters come in sizes that range from 14 to 24 gauge (as gauge size increases, diameter of catheter decreases). Smaller IV lines (24 gauge) are most commonly used in the pediatric population. Larger IV lines (14-18 gauge) are considered in adult patients who require emergent or urgent resuscitation. In adult patients receiving nonurgent resuscitation or medications, mid-sized IV catheters are typical (18-22 gauge).

Common sites for placement of IV lines include the antecubital fossa (cephalic vein, brachial vein, median cubital vein), the forearm (cephalic vein), or the hand. If these sites are difficult to cannulate, the external jugular vein can be considered as a site for peripheral IV placement. Another alternative is placement of a central line.

Currently, the consensus is to avoid placing an IV in an arm that has or will soon be utilized for an arteriovenous (AV) graft or fistula or in an arm ipsilateral to a full axillary node dissection.

INDICATIONS

IV lines are placed to provide peripheral vascular access for infusion of fluids, blood products, or parenteral medications. The size that is selected is dependent on the patient and the urgency with which treatment interventions need to be provided.

STEPS

1. Gather supplies:
   a. Gloves
   b. Alcohol/chlorhexidine pads
   c. Tourniquet
   d. Over-the-needle safety IV catheter (14-24 gauge, size dependent on indication and patient)
   e. IV tubing connector
   f. Sterile saline flush in 10-mL syringe
   g. Gauze pads
   h. Clear adhesive dressing (eg, Tegaderm), medical tape
   i. Chux pad (optional)

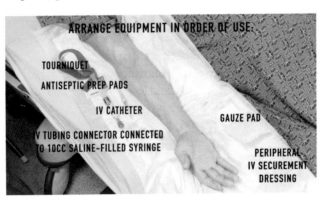

2. Wash hands or clean hands with alcohol cleanser.
3. Place patient and bed in a position that is comfortable for the patient and the person placing the IV.
4. Invert saline syringe and eliminate all air within the syringe.
5. Attach sterile saline syringe to IV tubing connector.
6. Inject saline through IV tubing connector to eliminate air along the tubing.
7. Arrange all equipment in order of use:
   a. Tourniquet, alcohol pads, IV catheter, IV tubing connector connected to saline syringe, Tegaderm (opened), gauze pads, Band-Aid/tape

8. Ask the patient if there is a preferred site and/or a site previously used with success; if not, identify a suitable site.
   a. The veins in the antecubital fossa are the usual choice; the next choice would be veins along the ventral aspect of the arms or dorsum of the hand.
   b. Avoid sites that are in the same location as another recent IV or show signs of infection, ipsilateral arm in patients with AV grafts, areas with valves, sclerosed veins, and areas with bruises or hematomas.
9. Place the chux pad under the patient's arm/hand.
10. Tie the tourniquet 3 to 4 inches above the site of IV placement site.
    a. Tie with a loop for easy one-handed release.

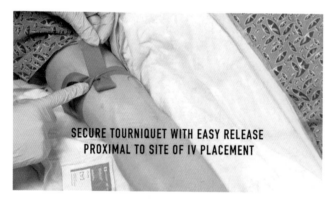

SECURE TOURNIQUET WITH EASY RELEASE
PROXIMAL TO SITE OF IV PLACEMENT

11. Look for and/or palpate a prominent vein; observe the trajectory of the vein.
    a. Sometimes gentle tapping and/or application of a warm compress can help make the vein more prominent.

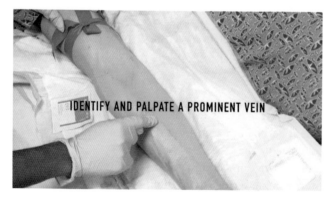

IDENTIFY AND PALPATE A PROMINENT VEIN

12. Put on gloves.
13. Clean the area to be punctured with the alcohol/chlorhexidine pad; let air dry.

14. Remove the cap on the IV catheter needle, push the catheter hub slightly off and back on the needle to ensure that the catheter is loosely on the needle.

15. Grasp the patient's arm firmly using thumb of nondominant hand to draw the skin taut and anchor the vein.

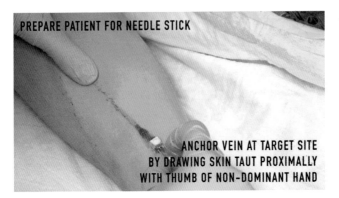

16. Hold the needle-catheter at a 15° to 30° angle with the bevel up.

17. Deliberately insert the needle through the skin into the vein, reducing the angle of the needle as it is advanced into the vein until you see a flash of blood.

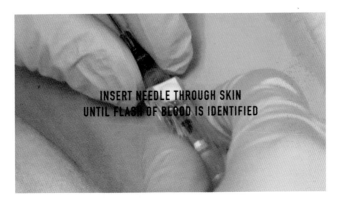

18. Once a flash is detected, advance the needle a few more millimeters into the vein.

    a. If the vein is missed, draw the needle-catheter tip back to the level of the skin and redirect the needle.

b. If the vein is missed multiple times, abort IV placement attempt: remove tourniquet, place gauze at the insertion site, apply gentle pressure while activating the needle safety mechanism (if applicable) and removing the needle-catheter. Tape the gauze pad with a Band-Aid or medical tape.

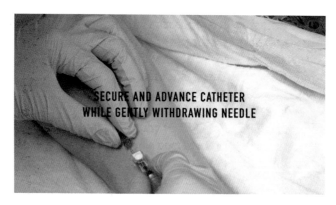

19. With the dominant hand that is on the needle-catheter, use the index finger to advance the catheter into the vein until the hub is at the skin.
20. Using the nondominant hand, unfasten tourniquet and occlude the vein several centimeters above the insertion site.
21. Apply the needle safety mechanism (as applicable) and pull *only* the needle back, leaving the catheter in place.

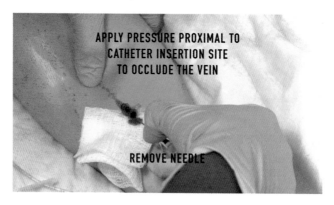

22. Screw on the IV tubing connecter that is connected to the saline syringe.
23. Continue stabilizing the IV catheter with one hand while holding the syringe with the other hand.

24. Holding the syringe such that any residual air bubbles do not enter patient, push several milliliters of saline into the vein to assure a well-placed IV in a patent vein. Look for swelling or resistance to flow to indicate a malpositioned IV.

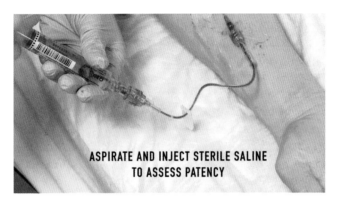

ASPIRATE AND INJECT STERILE SALINE
TO ASSESS PATENCY

25. Secure the catheter using a Tegaderm; make a loop with the IV tube connector and secure it with medical tape.
26. Appropriately dispose of needle and all other supplies.

COMPLICATIONS

Complications of IV placement are similar to those encountered when drawing blood and include bleeding, hematoma, and thrombophlebitis. In addition, the IV line may cause discomfort for the patient. This may be due to positioning or irritation from infused medications. The patient can be asked to keep the extremity straight if the IV line is in the antecubital fossa. Other possible options include removing the tape, adjusting the position of the IV line, and replacing the tape. Placing a hot pack on the area may decrease the discomfort. Finally, if the discomfort or pain appears to be because of a complication such as infiltration or thrombophlebitis, the IV line should be removed and replaced in an alternate location.

In the case of a provider needle stick, ensure that the needle and all sharps are secure, wash the area of injury immediately, and refer to institutional procedures to be evaluated for postexposure treatment.

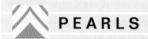

PEARLS

1. If there is difficulty in identifying a vein for IV placement, consider using an ultrasound to assist in identification and placement in a vein.
2. Prepare all the equipment you need, and make sure both yourself and the patient are comfortable before starting.
3. Know the various calibers of lines and choose the correct line based on its indication.

Suggested Readings

1. Panebianco NL, Fredette JM, Szyld D, Sagalyn EB, Pines JM, Dean AJ. What you see (sonographically) is what you get: vein and patient characteristics associated with successful ultrasound-guided peripheral intravenous placement in patients with difficult access. *Acad Emerg Med.* 2009;16:1298-1303.
2. Joing S, Strote S, Caroon L, et al. Ultrasound-Guided peripheral IV placement. *N Engl J Med.* 2012;366:e38.

22

FOLEY CATHETER PLACEMENT

DANIEL KAUFMAN, MD | PETER L. STEINBERG, MD |
SAYURI P. JINADASA, MD, MPH | RUSLAN KORETS, MD

As a surgical intern, you will be the point of first contact for a nurse who is having difficulty placing a urinary drainage catheter. With a basic understanding of genitourinary anatomy, pathology that causes difficult catheter placement, and the different types of catheters at your disposal, you will be able to avoid urology consultation in the great majority of circumstances. This chapter will review basic urethral anatomy, the most common types of urinary drainage catheters, and proper technique for insertion of urinary catheters.

URETHRAL ANATOMY

The female urethra is approximately 4 cm in length. The urethral meatus lies anterior to the vaginal opening and posterior to the clitoral hood. The urethra can be recessed in elderly females with atrophic vaginitis. In obese women, the medial thigh pannus can obscure the urethral meatus as well, making it difficult to visualize the urethral meatus for catheter placement. The female urethra is relatively straight in its course from meatus to bladder, but can curve anteriorly as it approaches the bladder neck.

The male urethra measures approximately 20 cm in length, with variability depending on stretched penile length. The male urethra is divided into five segments. From distal to proximal: fossa navicularis, pendulous, bulbar, membranous, and prostatic urethra. The anterior urethra includes the fossa navicularis, pendulous or penile urethra, and the bulbar urethra; the posterior urethra includes the membranous and prostatic urethra. With the penis on stretch, the male urethra is straight and of similar caliber until the proximal bulbar urethra where it widens and turns cephalad toward the bladder at the bulbomembranous junction. The membranous urethra spans the external urinary sphincter, just distal to the prostate. The prostatic urethra is surrounded by the transitional zone of the prostate, which can be enlarged and cause urethral obstruction in males with benign prostatic hyperplasia (BPH). The bulbar urethra and posterior urethra are often the site of difficulties with Foley catheter placement in males.

CATHETERS

The first urinary drainage catheter was introduced in 1930 by Frederic Foley,[1] hence the name Foley catheter. Urinary catheters come in a variety of styles, shapes, sizes, and materials; however, adult catheters are usually 40 to 45 cm long. There are specialized pediatric length catheters and shorter nonindwelling catheters for use in women, but these are beyond the scope of this chapter and the sphere of knowledge you need as a surgery intern. The following will be a brief discussion of the most common types of catheters that will be at your disposal.

All indwelling urinary catheters have, at minimum, the following components: tip, balloon, balloon port, and urinary outflow port. The catheter tip sits in the bladder and allows urine to flow through the "eye" of the catheter down the lumen of the catheter. The catheter balloon is situated just proximal to the tip and inflates, preventing catheter dislodgement by sitting at the bladder neck. The balloon port has a valved plastic tip that connects to the balloon to allow inflation with fluid. The outflow port drains urine by gravity to a urimeter or drainage bag and can be used for manual irrigation, if needed. The majority of indwelling catheters are typically made of either latex or silicone, range in caliber from 12 to 26 French, and have either a straight or curved tip (coudé catheter).

The standard Foley catheter insertion kit consists of either a 14fr or 16fr, latex two-way Foley catheter (Figure 22.1A). Standard catheter kits have what is called a closed drainage system, meaning that the catheter is attached to the

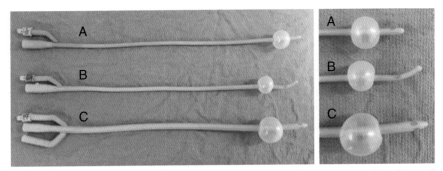

FIGURE 22.1 A, Standard 16fr two-way Foley catheter. B, 18fr two-way coudé catheter. C, 24fr three-way catheter (hematuria catheter).

drainage bag during sterile packaging. Unless a nonstandard catheter is needed for use, this connection should not be broken, as it has been shown to decrease catheter-associated urinary tract infections (CAUTIs).[2,3]

Coudé catheters have curved tips (Figure 22.1B). These catheters are helpful in select patient populations, most commonly in men with BPH and women with a recessed urethral meatus. The upward curve of the coudé catheter mimics the anatomic cephalad curve of the bulbar and posterior urethra in men. As with standard catheters, coudé catheters can be two-way or three-way, made from latex or silicone, and come in a variety of sizes. Coudé catheters *are meant to be placed with the curved tip pointing upward toward the ceiling! This allows the catheter to traverse the curved aspects of the male urethra.*

Silicone catheters are slightly stiffer than standard latex catheters and are also available in a range of sizes and styles. They should be used in patients with latex allergies, and given their stiffness, they can be helpful in patients with urethral stricture disease or BPH, as they can often traverse the urethra more readily than a latex catheter.

Three-way catheters have a third port, in addition to the balloon port and outflow port. This is a smaller lumen port that can be used for introduction of fluid into the bladder for continuous irrigation and subsequent drainage via the large caliber outflow port (Figure 22.1C). This third port can be clamped or capped, resulting in a three-way catheter functioning like a standard two-way catheter. These catheters are typically used in certain patients after transurethral urologic surgery or in patients with significant hematuria. Of key importance is the fact that a three-way Foley's lumen is *smaller* than a two-way Foley of the same French size, because the infusion port occupies some space that would solely be reserved for drainage in a two-way catheter.

PROPER INSERTION TECHNIQUE

Preparation: Universal precautions should be followed for placement of all urinary catheters, as there is potential for contact with blood or bodily fluids. Sterile technique is used as well. As with any procedure, you can optimize your chances of success and increase your efficiency with proper preparation and use of appropriate equipment.

The following is a list of equipment that should be used for standard Foley placement and is included in a standard Foley insertion kit:

- Sterile gloves
- Sterile drapes
- Betadine solution
- Cotton swabs
- Disposable plastic forceps
- 10 cc sterile water in syringe for Foley balloon inflation
- Lubrication (either in packet or additional plastic syringe)
- Foley catheter
- Urinary drainage bag and tubing (preconnected to the catheter for closed drainage system)
- Lidocaine jelly

Prior to starting the procedure, you should ensure you have all equipment in the room. It is critical to have a nurse or other nonsterile assistant with you in case you start the procedure and have forgotten some necessary equipment. As with all procedures, first explain who you are to the patient, what the procedure is, and why it is necessary. Written consent is not usually required, but this discussion functions as informed consent in most centers. Allow the patient to ask questions prior to beginning. Place the patient supine. In men have their legs slightly spread, and in women place their feet/heels together in "frog leg" position. Examine the patient and identify the urethral meatus: retracting the foreskin in males and spreading labia majora in females is needed. You may also need additional help with exposure in obese men (on the abdominal pannus) and obese women (medial thigh pannus).

Technique: Open the catheter kit and catheter in sterile fashion (Figure 22.2). Put on sterile gloves and drape the patient placing the sterile fenestrated drape over the patient's genitals (Figure 22.3). Prepare your equipment by pouring the betadine/cleaning solution on the cotton balls, emptying the

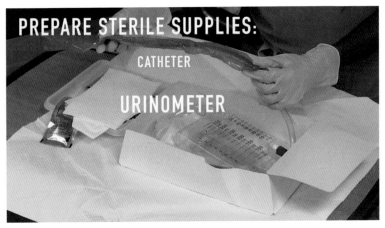

FIGURE 22.2 Put on your sterile gloves and prepare your tray.

lubrication into the plastic tray and taking the plastic sheath off the catheter (Figure 22.4). You can place the catheter tip into the lubrication on the tray (Figure 22.5). This will keep it from flopping around and will prelubricate the catheter prior to insertion. ***Do not test the Foley balloon, and do not break the connection between catheter and drainage bag***.

Begin the procedure by using your nondominant hand to expose the urethral meatus by retracting and holding the labia or retracting the foreskin and holding the penis on stretch (perpendicular to the patient's body with upward

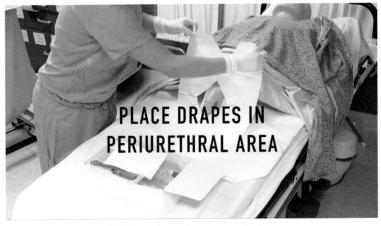

FIGURE 22.3 Apply your sterile drapes.

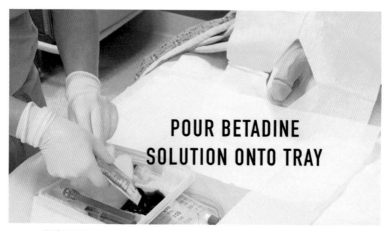

FIGURE 22.4 Empty your betadine and lubricant onto the tray.

traction) (Figure 22.6). Use your still sterile dominant hand to prep the meatus with the forceps and betadine-soaked cotton balls (Figure 22.7). If you have lidocaine jelly (and you should for men), inject the viscous lidocaine jelly into the urethra, gently pinching the glans to prevent backflow. Now insert the pre-lubricated tip of the catheter into the urethral meatus and advance (Figure 22.8). *For females, advance the catheter 2 to 3 inches beyond the point at which urine is noted prior to inflating the balloon. For males, advance the catheter until the hub of the catheter reaches the meatus.*

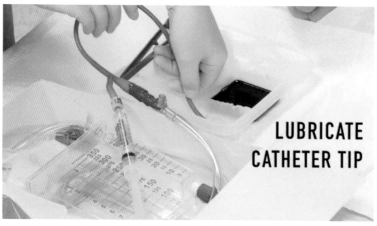

FIGURE 22.5 Generously lubricate the catheter tip.

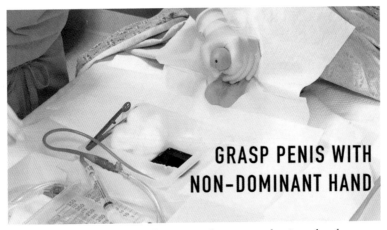

FIGURE 22.6 Grasp the penis with your non-dominant hand.

While keeping the catheter hubbed and *only after seeing urine in the drainage tubing*, inflate balloon with 10 cc of sterile water (Figure 22.9-10). After balloon inflation, gently pull the catheter back until you feel slight resistance, ensuring that the balloon has settled against the bladder neck. In some cases, liberal use of lubricants will occlude the catheter temporarily and urine may not flow: this can be gently irrigated away via the drainage port if needed. If the catheter is not already attached to a drainage bag, now

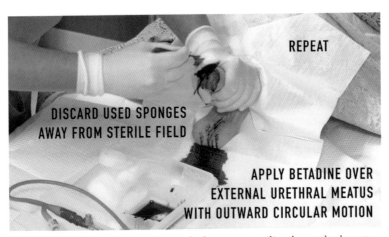

FIGURE 22.7 Using the betadine soaked sponges sterilize the urethral meatus.

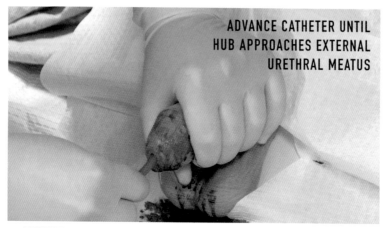

FIGURE 22.8 Gently advance the catheter taking note of any resistance.

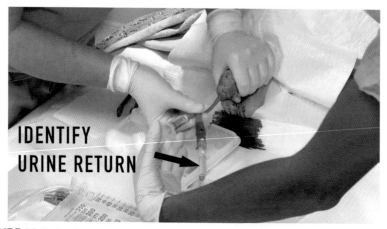

FIGURE 22.9 Gentle pressure in the suprapubic area may be necessary to see a return of urine.

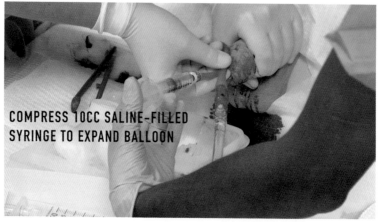

FIGURE 22.10 Fill the balloon with the 10 cc pre filled syringe.

is the time to do so. Always secure the catheter to the upper thigh with some slack. This prevents discomfort from tension during patient movement/ambulation. Properly dispose of all equipment and gloves, and clean excess betadine from the patient. *Always remember to replace the foreskin in uncircumcised men to prevent paraphimosis.*

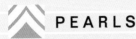 **PEARLS**

1. Have all equipment ready and available, make sure both you and the patient are comfortable prior to starting.
2. Ask for help or assistance especially when dealing with difficult anatomy or patient body habitus.
3. Be vigilant of the initial urine return and if there is any associated bleeding.

References

1. Tennyson L, Kafka I, Averch TD. *Stents and catheters – what's new? AUA Update Series.* Vol 34. Linthicum, MD: American Urologic Association, Inc.; 2015:26.
2. Kunin CM, McCormack RC. Prevention of catheter induced urinary-tract infections by sterile closed drainage. *N Eng J Med.* 1966;274:1115-1161.
3. Gillespie WA, Lennon GG, Linton KB, Phippen GA. Prevention of urinary tract infection by means of closed drainage into a sterile plastic bag. *Br Med J.* 1967;3(5557):90-92.

23

WOUNDS AND DRESSINGS

BRIAN MINH NGUYEN, MD | ANN MARIE FEINSTEIN, RN, BSN, CWOCN | THERESE PARE, RN, BSN, CWOCN

INTRODUCTION

A wound is any disruption of the normal skin structure and function. It can be the result of trauma to the skin, such as a bite or a stab wound, or from surgery. Acute wounds heal through a predictable progression.

TYPICAL STAGES OF WOUND HEALING

Hemostasis: This occurs within minutes. Platelets begin to adhere to the injured site, promoting clotting and activating fibrin.

Inflammation: Phagocytosis occurs to remove damaged/dead cells, bacteria, and other pathogens.

Proliferation: This refers to the growth of new tissue. There is angiogenesis, collagen deposition, and granulation tissue formation. Reepithelialization begins.

Maturation: Collagen is realigned. Type III collagen is replaced with type I collagen, increasing the wound's tensile strength. The maximum strength of a healed wound is approximately 80% of strength of unwounded skin.

TYPES OF SURGICAL CLOSURES

PRIMARY CLOSURE

- Wound edges are sutured together to close the defect.
- Wound heals quickly with less pain and scarring than other types of closure.
- Contraindications to primary closure: Acute wound >6 hours old, wounds with foreign debris, too much tension, or if there is concern about infection.

SECONDARY CLOSURE

- The wound is left open and allowed to heal by forming a granulation tissue matrix that begins to fill in and contract the wound.
- This technique is used for wounds that cannot be brought together, typically as a result of excess tension or infection.
- The wound typically with take longer to heal.
- Results in a larger scar.

DELAYED PRIMARY CLOSURE

- This technique is a combination of primary and secondary wound closure.
- It is used in wounds that are heavily contaminated.
- The wound is cleansed and watched for days until wound appears void of infection or debris.
- Once the wound is thought to be clean, it is then closed primarily.

INDICATIONS

It is essential that all wounds are cared for appropriately. For wounds that have been primarily closed, an occlusive dressing provides protection from trauma and should be impermeable to bacteria.

For open wounds that will heal by either delayed-primary or secondary closure and other large open wounds, wet-to-dry dressings have been traditionally used; however, the recent literature has recommended a shift in ideology to promote optimal wound healing and closure. Dressings that are able to maintain a moist environment have been shown to increase the rate of epithelialization and promote the inflammatory phase by establishing low oxygen tension. Gauze that has dried can actually damage tissues when it is removed because it may disrupt the healing process of the wound when the dry gauze is removed.

There are many types of dressings that are suitable for managing open wounds. Semipermeable dressings, such as Tegaderm, consist of a sterile polyurethane-coated plastic that is impermeable to water and bacteria but is permeable to water vapor and air. These films are flexible and are good for dressing wounds over joints or other difficult locations.

Hydrocolloids (eg, Comfeel, DuoDERM, Aquacell) are a combination of carboxymethylcellulose, gelatin, pectin, elastomers, and adhesives bonded to a carrier, such as foam or semipermeable film, that provide a moist healing environment by forming a gel over the wound surface. This gel is impermeable to water vapor and air and is used to rehydrate necrotic tissue and promote autolytic debridement.

Hydrogels (eg, Intrasite, Aquaform) are a combination of polymers and water that can provide a moist environment by delivering water molecules to the surface of the wound. They provide debridement by promoting autolysis of necrotic tissue and are used for sloughy or necrotic wounds without evidence of infection.

Alginates are derived from naturally occurring salts in brown seaweed. They can absorb up to 20 times their weight in fluid and are typically used for wounds with a significant amount of exudate. They should be avoided in low-exudative wounds as they can adhere to the wound surface and cause damage or pain.

Antimicrobial dressings are typically impregnated with silver or iodine and used for infected or colonized wounds. Metronidazole gel is particularly useful in the treatment of fungating malignant wounds.

TECHNICAL STEPS

MOIST DRESSING

1. Locate supplies: Depending on the size of the wound, you will need gauze bandages (2 × 2, 4 × 4, or 4-inch rolls [Kerlix], normal saline, and tape).
2. Remove previous dressing.
3. Measure and document the dimensions of the wound, including depth.
4. Examine the bed of the wound to determine if there is a need for debridement.
5. You can use a saline-moistened gauze to clear the surface of the wound from debris or exudate.

6. If using gel such as Intrasite or Aquaform, apply a generous amount evenly onto the surface of the wound.
7. You may cover the gel with a layer of gauze and tape or with a semipermeable film such as Tegaderm.
8. Depending on the type of dressing, make sure to change dressing at an appropriate frequency to prevent drying out of the wound or infection.

NEXT STEPS

1. Continue dressing changes until wound has healed.
2. Keep in mind that the type of dressing may need to be altered over time to optimize healing, depending on the appearance and size of the wound.

COMPLICATIONS

INFECTION

For wounds that have been closed primarily, if there are signs of infection, such as fever, chills, worsening pain, erythema, swelling, warmth, or purulent drainage, the wound should be opened to allow drainage of any underlying fluid collections. The wound should then be allowed to heal by secondary closure.

MACERATION

For wounds that have significant drainage, this can damage the surrounding skin if it is exposed to this fluid for a prolonged period of time. Highly absorptive dressing or skin protecting emollients can be used to avoid this complication.

DRYING OUT OF THE WOUND

If a wound becomes completely dry, this may delay or halt the healing process. For a dry wound, the use of a highly absorptive dressing may further dry out the wound and may lead to disruption of healing tissue. It is imperative to keep the wound in a moist healing environment.

ALLERGIC REACTIONS

If a patient develops an allergic reaction to the wound dressing product or tape, remove the dressing immediately and avoid the offending agent on subsequent dressing changes. Depending on the extent of the reaction, topical steroids may be needed to treat the allergy.

 PEARLS

1. Wounds that are grossly contaminated (eg, bite wounds, infections) should not be closed primarily. If there are any signs or symptoms of infection (foul odor, increased drainage, erythema, fevers, or chills) the dressing should be taken down and wound evaluated.
2. When placing a dressing on an open wound, make sure to cover the entire wound while avoiding the adjacent epithelialized skin to prevent maceration.
3. Make sure to choose the appropriate type of dressing for the type of wound. If you have any questions or concerns, it is best to ask your senior or consult a wound care specialist for assistance or recommendations to allow for optimal wound healing.

Suggested Readings

1. Duttaroy DD, Jitendra J, Duttaroy B, et al. Management strategy for dirty abdominal incisions: primary or delayed primary closure? A randomized trial. *Surg Infect.* 2009;10:129-136.
2. Jones V, Grey JE, Harding KG. Wound dressings. *BMJ.* 2006;332:777-780.
3. Ovington LG. Hanging wet-to-dry dressings out to dry. *Home Health Nurse.* 2001;19(8):1-11.
4. Mulder GD. Cost-effective managed care: gel versus wet-to-dry for debridement. *Ostomy Wound Manage.* 1995;41(2):68-76.

24

SPLINTING

STELLA J. LEE, MD | EDWARD K. RODRIGUEZ, MD, PhD

INTRODUCTION

A splint is a device that provides *relative* immobilization of an injured bone or joint. In contrast to a cast, a splint is noncircumferential. This allows for continued swelling of the injured region without compromising blood flow to the limb.

A splint offers stability, which in turns minimizes pain, stabilizes and enhances clot formation, reduces local inflammation, limits further soft tissue injury, reduces the risk of further fracture displacement and potential vascular injury, and reduces the risk of compartment syndrome. Splinting of large bones also contributes to minimize escalation of the systemic inflammatory response that contributes to acute respiratory distress syndrome or other systemic organ failure.

INDICATIONS

1. Fracture
   a. Definitive nonoperative treatment in the splint
   b. Temporary immobilization while awaiting surgery
   c. Temporary immobilization while awaiting evaluation by an orthopedic surgeon (such as at a community hospital transferring to a tertiary center)

2. Soft tissue injury
   a. Immobilization following an orthopedic or plastic surgery procedure
   b. Nonoperative treatment of soft tissue infections (eg, cellulitis) with antibiotics
   c. Nonoperative treatment of sprains, strains, and other soft tissue injuries

SPLINT TYPES

1. Plaster splints

   Plaster-of-Paris (the same material that is used for papier-mâché projects) is the most traditional material used for custom splinting, whereby the splint is molded around the injured limb. The main advantage of the plaster splint is that it sets relatively slowly, allowing sufficient time for molding. The subsequent technique sections will be devoted to preparing plaster splints.

2. Prepadded splints

   Prepadded splints are used in some emergency departments and urgent clinics. It is preferred by some emergency physicians because it can be made very quickly. However, a major disadvantage of the plaster splint is that it sets quickly, allowing little time to adequately mold the splint. In addition, there is minimal padding, which can lead to pressure ulcers. Use of this type of splint should be limited to temporary immobilization before evaluation by an orthopedic surgeon.

3. Prefabricated splints

   Prefabricated splints are available for certain injuries of the thumb, wrist, knee, foot, and ankle. These include thumb spica splints, volar wrist splints, knee immobilizers, and walking boots. In general, a fracture that is at risk for displacement or a joint injury that is at risk for dislocation should be immobilized in a well-molded plaster splint, rather than in a prefabricated splint.

PLASTER SPLINTING TECHNIQUE

EQUIPMENT NEEDED (FIGURE 24.1)

- Cotton padding
- Plaster gauze bandages (4-inch bandage works for most splints)

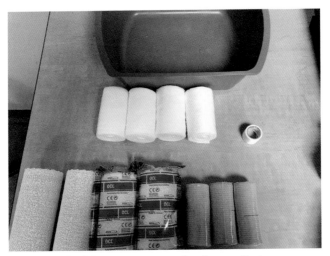

FIGURE 24.1 Equipment for plaster splinting.

- Elastic bandages (3 inch for hand and forearm, 4 inch for arm and leg, 6 inch for thigh)
- Tape
- Large bucket

STEPS

1. If splinting will involve significant manipulation of the injured area, ensure patient has adequate pain control.
2. Gather all necessary materials.
3. Fill a large bucket with lukewarm water.
4. Recruit an assistant to help position the affected limb.
5. Measure the appropriate length of the plaster slabs on the affected limb.
6. Fold the plaster slab into an accordion style, with a thickness of 8 to 10 layers for upper extremity splints and 10 to 12 layers for lower extremity splints (Figure 24.2).
7. Wrap the limb with cotton padding with a minimum of three to four layers, with more layers at pressure points, such as the heel, elbow, or knee.
8. Dip the plaster slabs into the water, while securing both ends of the slab, then squeeze out as much water as possible.
9. Laminate the plaster bandage by smoothing the plaster until all the holes in the gauze are filled with plaster material (Figure 24.3).
10. Lay the plaster flat against the affected extremity.

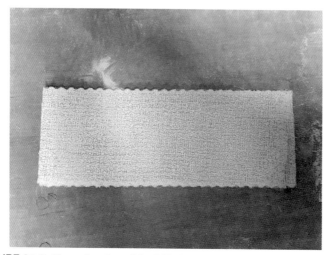

FIGURE 24.2 Plaster bandage slabs folded to appropriate length and thickness.

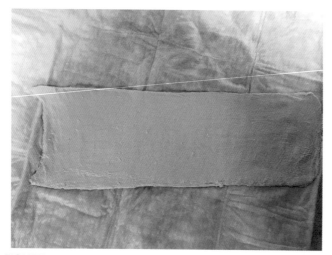

FIGURE 24.3 Plaster bandage after dipping in water and laminating.

11. Secure the plaster with elastic bandages, overlapping 50% of the previous layer each time.
12. Secure the edge of the elastic bandage with tape.
13. Keep the limb immobilized until the plaster hardens completely. This may take up to 20 minutes. Patients should report warming of the plaster, followed by cooling, which indicates the plaster is adequately set.

SPLINTING DESIGN

In general, splinting of a diaphyseal or metaphyseal fracture should immobilize the joint above and below the fracture. For example, splinting of a tibia fracture should immobilize both the ankle and knee. Splinting of a periarticular fracture should immobilize the bone above and below the involved joint. For example, splinting of an elbow fracture should cover the entire arm and forearm. Subsequently, splints are not commonly used for shoulder, hip, or femur injuries, with exceptions for pediatric injuries.

COMMON SPLINTS

1. Forearm sugar-tong splint

    Sugar-tong splints are used for wrist injuries and forearm fractures. The arm is positioned with the forearm in neutral rotation and the elbow in 90° of flexion. The position of the wrist depends on the injury. A single slab of plaster is positioned starting from the dorsal aspect of the metacarpophalangeal (MCP) joints of the hand, wrapping around the elbow, then extending to the volar aspect of the MCP joints (Figure 24.4). Make sure that the plaster fits snugly around the elbow and that the plater does not extend too distally, restricting MCP movement.

2. Posterior elbow splint
    Posterior elbow splints are used for elbow fractures and dislocations. The arm is positioned with the forearm in neutral rotation and the elbow in slight extension beyond 90°; flexion past 90° can compromise blood flow in the setting of soft tissue swelling. A slab of plaster is positioned starting just distal to the axilla, extending along the posterior arm and elbow, then ulnar border of the forearm to the wrist (Figure 24.5). An alternative method of splinting involves preparation of a padded plaster slab, which is applied directly to the skin.

3. Ankle stirrup splint
    Ankle stirrup splints are used for ankle fractures, distal tibia fractures, and certain fractures of the foot. The splint can be extended proximally for tibia shaft fractures and proximal tibia fractures. The leg is positioned with the ankle in neutral dorsiflexion; prolonged immobilization in plantarflexion can lead to Achilles contractures. A posterior slab is positioned along the posterior leg, heel, and plantar foot (Figure 24.6). A second stirrup slab is positioned perpendicular to the first, starting laterally, fitting snugly around the arch of the foot and both malleoli, then extending to the medial aspect of the leg.

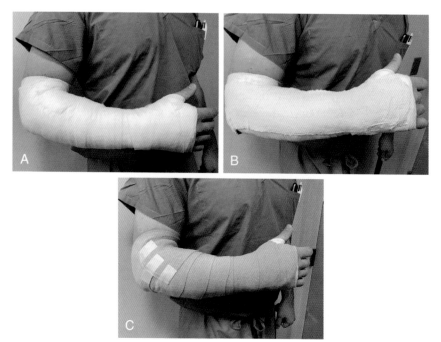

FIGURE 24.4 Forearm sugar-tong splint. (A) Cotton padding wrap. (B) Plaster slab placement. (C) Elastic bandage wrap.

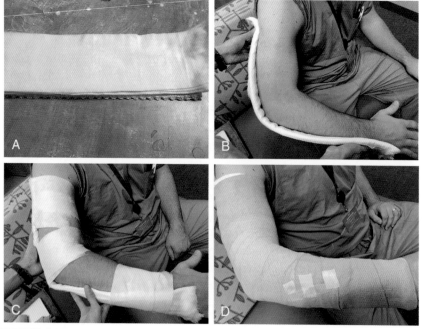

FIGURE 24.5 Posterior elbow splint. (A) Padded plaster splint. (B) Padded plaster slab placement. (C) Provisional wrap with cotton padding wrap. (D) Elastic bandage wrap.

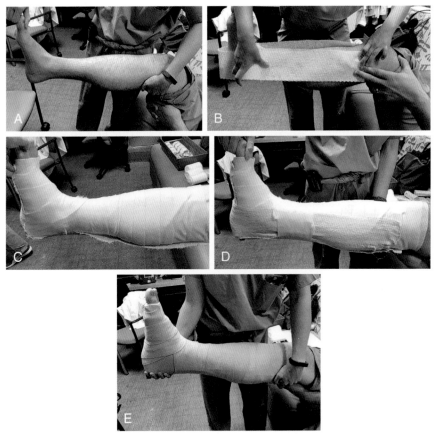

FIGURE 24.6 Ankle stirrup splint. (A) Limb positioning. (B) Measurement of plaster slab length. (C) Cotton padding wrap. (D) Plaster slab placement. (E) Elastic bandage wrap.

OTHER SPLINTS

Other splints include the thumb spica splint, which is used for scaphoid fractures and injuries of the thumb; the ulnar gutter splint, which is used for fifth metacarpal fractures and other injuries involving the ulnar aspect of the hand; and the volar resting splint, which is used as part of the nonoperative treatment of hand infections. These are beyond the scope of this manual and can be found in other resources.

COMPLICATIONS AND PITFALLS

1. Inadequate padding

   Prolonged immobilization with inadequate padding can result in pressure ulcers. Make sure that edges of the plaster are fully covered with padding.

Pressure points such as heels, elbows, and knees should be covered with additional layers of padding. Particular attention should be paid in patients with neurologic injuries, such as those with diabetic peripheral neuropathy, who may not sense an evolving pressure ulcer.

2. Thermal injury

Plaster "setting" is an exothermic process, transferring heat to the soft tissues, and this can potentially lead to burns. Using more than 25 layers of plaster can result in burns. Therefore, a splint design that requires two slabs of plaster should have no more than 12 layers per slab. Use of hot water, rather than lukewarm water, can also result in burns. Particular attention should be paid to anesthetized or nonverbal patients, who cannot verbalize pain from an ongoing thermal injury.

 PEARLS

1. Know the various types of splints that can be used, as each has its own unique indications and advantages.
2. Prepare all materials you need in advance. Make sure both the patient and you are comfortable to proceed with the procedure.
3. Have a strong understanding of the potential complications and pitfalls so that you can take precautions prior or spot them early in their course.

25

DRAWING AN ARTERIAL BLOOD GAS

SAYURI P. JINADASA, MD, MPH | MYLES D. BOONE, MD, MPH

Arterial blood gas (ABG) is a blood test that is drawn specifically from an artery. An ABG is essential in assessing a patient's acid-base balance and oxygenation and ventilation as it measures pH, bicarbonate (HCO_3^-), and partial pressure of oxygen (PaO_2) and partial pressure of CO_2 ($PaCO_2$) dissolved in the blood.

This chapter focuses on drawing blood for an ABG. Interpretation of ABGs is important; however, it is beyond the scope of this chapter. Please refer to the references for more resources on ABG interpretation.

INDICATIONS

ABGs are often drawn in urgent and critical care scenarios where an acid-base abnormality or an impairment in oxygenation and/or ventilation is suspected. Serial ABGs are often drawn in the critically ill to titrate specific interventions such as mechanical ventilation.

STEPS

1. Gather supplies:
   - Gloves
   - Alcohol/chlorhexidine pads*
   - A 23-gauge needle attached to a 2-mL syringe with heparin*
   - Syringe cap*
   - Gauze pads*
   - Band-Aid or medical tape*
   - Chux pad (optional)
   - Patient label
   - Ice (depends on institution)

   * Often provided in one ABG draw kit.

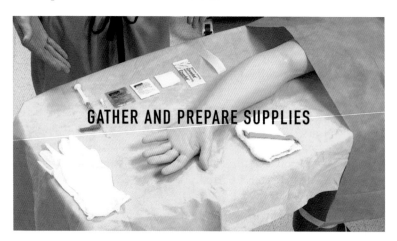

GATHER AND PREPARE SUPPLIES

2. Wash hands or clean hands with alcohol.
3. Place patient's wrist in an extended position and adjust bed to position that is comfortable to the patient and the person drawing the ABG.
4. Place the chux pad under the patient's arm/hand.
5. Arrange all equipment in order of use:
   - Alcohol pads, heparin syringe with needle attached, gauze pads, Band-Aid/tape
6. Locate the target artery by palpation.

7. Put gloves on.
8. Circumferentially clean the area to be punctured with the alcohol or chlorhexidine pad.
9. Remove the cap to the needle.
10. Using your nondominant hand, palpate the pulsations of the radial artery.

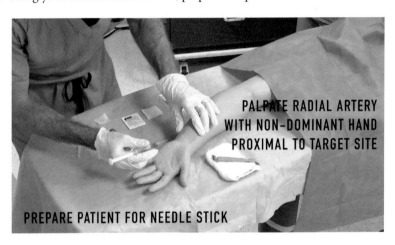

11. Insert the needle at a 30° to 60° angle to the skin at the point of maximal pulsation; advance the needle until a flash of blood is noted in the syringe.
    - If blood return is not achieved, withdraw the needle to skin level, reangle the needle toward the artery, and reinsert the needle.

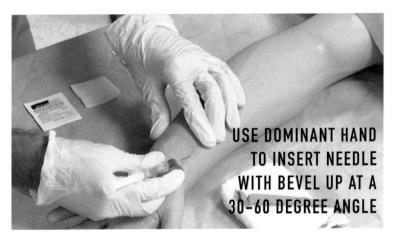

12. Wait until the syringe is filled.

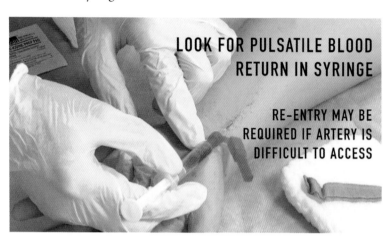

13. Place gauze over the puncture site and hold firm pressure as the needle is removed.

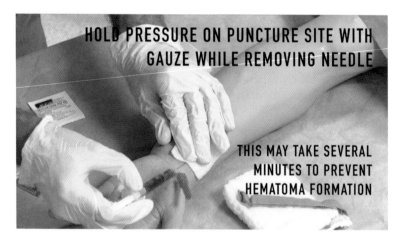

14. Continue holding pressure at the puncture site while applying the needle safety to cover the needle.
15. After 1 to 5 minutes of holding pressure to the puncture site, place a Band-Aid or tape to hold the gauze in place as a pressure dressing.
16. Remove the needle from the syringe and place the syringe cap onto the syringe.

17. Push out excess air within the syringe.
18. Place the patient label on the syringe and immediately place on ice; make sure the laboratory requisition form is noted with the time of the draw, the patient's oxygen support, and the patient's SpO_2.
19. Appropriately dispose of needle and all other supplies.

COMPLICATIONS

- Bleeding
- Hematoma
- Arterial occlusion from clot
- Arterial vasospasm
- Vessel laceration
- In the case of a needle stick, assure that the needle and all sharps are secure, wash the area of injury immediately, and refer to your institution's procedures to be evaluated for postexposure treatment.

 PEARLS

1. If a radial pulse is difficult to palpate or a patient's body habitus makes it difficult to identify the location of the artery, consider using ultrasound to guide the insertion of the needle.
2. If a radial arterial line is not possible, consider drawing from the femoral artery.
3. Practice reading multiple ABG results to know the unique metabolic acid-base disorders, their causes, and their management.

Suggested Readings

1. Kaufman D. *Interpretation of ABGs.* Available at http://www.thoracic.org/professionals/clinical-resources/critical-care/clinical-education/abgs.php.
2. Williams AJ. ABC of oxygen: assessing and interpreting arterial blood gases and acid-base balance. *BMJ Br Med J (Clin Res Ed).* 1998;317:1213.

26

CENTRAL LINE PLACEMENT

SAYURI P. JINADASA, MD, MPH | STEPHEN R. ODOM II, MD

Central venous lines (CVLs) are single- or multilumen catheters that are placed into the central venous system, as opposed to intravenous lines, which are placed peripherally. Locations for CVL placement are the following in the order of least to greatest risk of infection: subclavian vein, internal jugular vein (IJV), and femoral vein (FV).

Although the subclavian vein site is the most sterile, the vein is not compressible if bleeding complications were to occur, whereas the IJV and FV are compressible. A careful assessment of a specific patient and his/her risk factors is required before selecting the site for CVL placement. For example, if a patient is coagulopathic, one might consider placing the CVL in the IJV or FV in case of bleeding complications. If a particular site is infected, the contralateral side or a different site should be selected. If a patient has injury or reduced mobility in the neck, consider a site other than the IJV. If a patient would not be able to tolerate Trendelenburg position (eg, patient has elevated intracranial pressure), consider placing the line in the FV. If a patient already has a pneumothorax with a chest tube in place, place the line in the ipsilateral subclavian or IJV to prevent potential pneumothorax to the "good lung."

INDICATIONS

There are a multitude of indications for CVL placement. CVLs provide large-bore, multilumen, central access. Caustic medications such as chemotherapy, hypertonic saline, high-concentration potassium chloride, and vasopressors require central access for delivery. CVLs allow for administration of total parenteral nutrition. CVL placement allows for central venous pressure monitoring. Dialysis access and plasmaphoresis also require central access.

STEPS

1. Gather supplies:
   - CVL placement kit (antiseptic preparation, local anesthetic, small-gauge finder needle, 14- to 18-gauge introducer needle, J-tip guidewire, dilator, multilumen CVL, 11-blade scalpel, gauze, sterile dressing)
   - Sterile drapes
   - Ultrasound machine, high-frequency linear probe (if available)
   - Personal protective equipment (cap, eye wear, mask, sterile gown, sterile gloves)

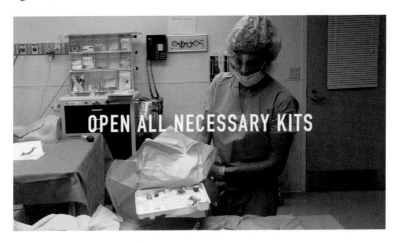

2. Obtain consent if needed.

3. Turn on bedside audio on bedside electrocardiogram monitor (to listen for ectopy during placement).
4. In patients at risk for thrombosed central veins, if available, use ultrasound to scan target vessel for patency.
5. Position patient (Trendelenburg for IJV or subclavian vein, nasal cannula for nonintubated patients who will be under sterile drapes, position head).
6. Wash hands.
7. Open sterile equipment and put on sterile gown and gloves.
8. Clean skin surface with antiseptic; use chlorhexidine if available.

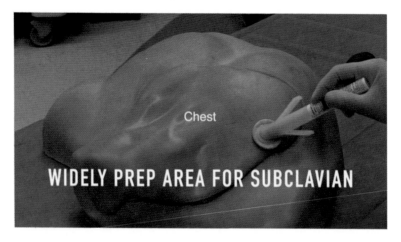

9. Drape patient.

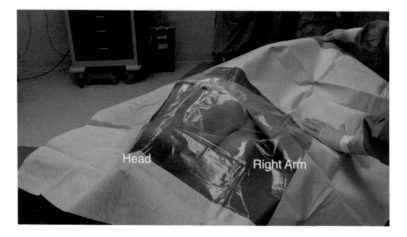

10. Flush and close all ports except the one that the wire will come out of with sterile saline.

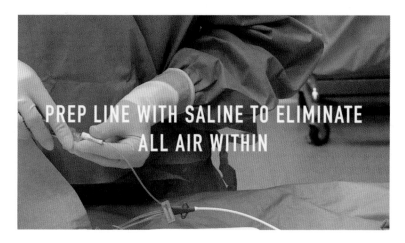

11. Lay out equipment in order of use.
12. Perform a "time out" before any needle stick.
13. Inject local anesthetic (skin, subcutaneous tissue; periosteum of clavicle for subclavian lines).
14. Use introducer needle while constantly applying negative pressure by pulling back on the plunger of the syringe to puncture the target central vein.

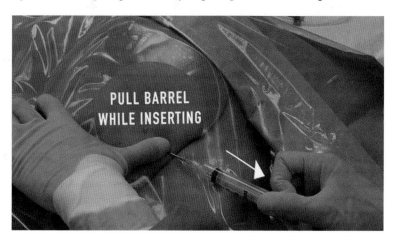

15. Once blood flash is obtained, stabilize needle and remove syringe.
16. Thread wire; always hold onto the wire.

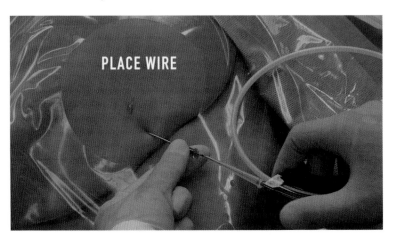

17. Listen for ectopy while threading the wire.
18. Remove the introducer needle over the wire.
19. Nick the skin with 11-blade scalpel at wire entry site.

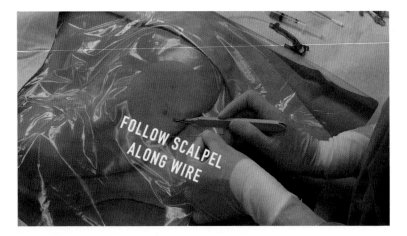

20. Pass dilator over wire once and remove dilator.

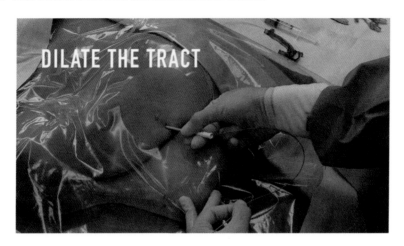

21. Pass central line over wire.

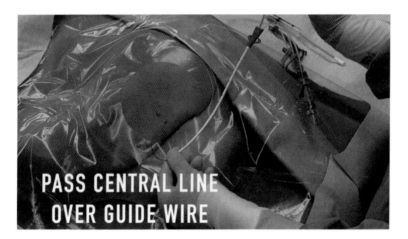

22. Remove wire.

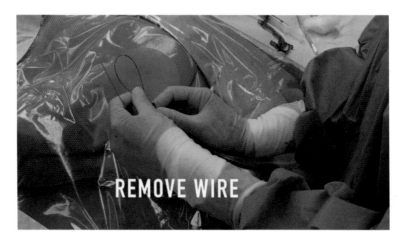

REMOVE WIRE

23. Draw back all air, flush lines with sterile saline.
24. Suture central line in place.
25. Place sterile dressing.
26. Obtain postplacement chest x-ray to confirm proper placement (tip should be at the cavoatrial junction) and check for complications (such as pneumothorax).
27. Try to remove catheters as soon as possible.

SITE-SPECIFIC APPROACHES

SUBCLAVIAN VEIN, INFRACLAVICULAR APPROACH USING LANDMARKS

- Insert introducer needle 1 to 2 cm lateral to the bend of the clavicle.
- "Walk" needle down under the clavicle.
- Redirect the needle in the direction of the sternal notch.
- Advance needle parallel to clavicle until subclavian vein (SCV) is punctured.

INTERNAL JUGULAR VEIN, APPROACH USING LANDMARKS

- Insert introducer needle at apex of the angle formed by the two heads of the sternocleidomastoid, lateral to the carotid artery pulsation at an angle approximately 30° from the skin.

- Direct the needle toward the ipsilateral nipple.
- Advance needle until IJV is punctured; prevent pneumothorax and/or carotid artery cannulation by avoiding passage of the needle beyond a depth of 1 to 2 cm.
- Assure that the carotid artery is not punctured by assessing pulsatility and color of blood; send an ABG to assess pO_2 if further clarification is needed.

INTERNAL JUGULAR VEIN, APPROACH USING ULTRASOUND GUIDANCE

- Place the ultrasound transducer between the two heads of the sternocleidomastoid muscle.
- Identify the IJV (larger, compressible, no pulsations) and the carotid artery (difficult to compress, pulsating).
- Puncture the skin holding the introducer needle at a 45° angle, and advance the needle until IJV is punctured.

FEMORAL VEIN, APPROACH USING LANDMARKS

- Palpate the femoral artery.
- Puncture the skin holding the introducer needle at a 30° to 45° angle 1 to 2 cm below the inguinal ligament and just medial to the femoral artery.
- Assure that the femoral artery is not punctured by assessing pulsatility and color of blood; send an ABG to assess pO_2 if further clarification is needed.

FEMORAL VEIN, APPROACH USING ULTRASOUND GUIDANCE

- Place the ultrasound transducer 1 to 2 cm below the inguinal ligament.
- Identify the FV (larger, compressible, no pulsations) and the femoral artery (difficult to compress, pulsating).
- Puncture the skin holding the introducer needle at a 30° to 45° angle and advance the needle until the FV is punctured.

How to Distinguish Venous from Arterial Puncture

There are a number of ways to ensure you have accessed a vein *before* dilation:

- Dark, nonpulsatile flash
- Ultrasound view of wire in vein

- Transduce a pressure to determine if your pressure is a central venous pressure (CVP) or mean arterial pressure (MAP)
- Blood gas (pO_2 should be low, not arterial)
- Wire on right side of chest in superior vena cava (eg, during fluoroscopy for a port-a-cath insertion)

COMPLICATIONS

Immediate: Air embolism, arrhythmia, arterial puncture, hemorrhage, pneumothorax, hemothorax, malposition

Late: Central line–associated bloodstream infection, myocardial perforation, venous thrombosis

PEARLS

1. If there is any concern for arterial puncture, DO NOT dilate the vessel. Some ways to assess for venous versus arterial puncture include assessing pulsatility and color of blood, using ultrasound to assess which vessel the wire is in, transducing the needle, sending a blood gas to assess pO_2.
2. Always obtain a chest x-ray to assure that the CVL is in the correct place, that it is not kinked or coiled, and that no iatrogenic complications, such as pneumothorax, occurred.
3. Ask for help if you need it!

Suggested Readings

1. Bannon MP, Heller SF, Rivera M. Anatomic considerations for central venous cannulation. *Risk Manag Healthc Pol.* 2011;4:27-39.
2. Pronovost P, Needham D, Berenholtz S, et al. An intervention to decrease catheter-related bloodstream infections in the ICU. *N Engl J Med.* 2006;355:2725-2732.
3. Segal JB, Dzik WH. Paucity of studies to support that abnormal coagulation test results predict bleeding in the setting of invasive procedures: an evidence-based review. *Transfusion.* 2005;45:1413-1425.
4. Weigand K, Encke J, Meyer FJ, et al. Low levels of prothrombin time (INR) and platelets do not increase the risk of significant bleeding when placing central venous catheters. *Med Klin (Munich).* 2009;104:331-335.

27

CHEST TUBE PLACEMENT

SAYURI P. JINADASA, MD, MPH | SIDHU P. GANGADHARAN, MD, MHCM

Chest tubes are placed through the chest wall between rib spaces into the pleural cavity to drain air or fluid such as blood, pus, or bile or instill therapeutic agents. Standard chest tubes range in size from 12F to 40F, with the size selected depending mostly on the viscosity of what is expected to be drained. For example, a tube placed for drainage of a pneumothorax does not need to be as large as one that is placed for drainage of blood, which can clot.

INDICATIONS

Chest tubes are placed to drain air or fluid, such as a pneumothorax, hemothorax, or large pleural effusions, that affects a patient's ability to breathe. These scenarios are often encountered in trauma and post cardiac and thoracic surgery; however, they are certainly not restricted to these situations.

Not all pneumothoraces require placement of a chest tube; they are generally placed when a pneumothorax takes up at least 20% of the pleural space or if serial films show increasing size or persistence of the pneumothorax.

An exception to this rule of thumb is when a patient is to be placed on invasive ventilation, in which case the positive pressure provided through a ventilator could exacerbate a pneumothorax.

Less often, chest tubes are placed to instill agents to treat empyema, retained hemothorax, or for chemical pleurodesis.

STEPS

1. Gather supplies:
   - Personal protective equipment (cap, eye wear, mask, sterile gown, sterile gloves)
   - Chest tube drainage system
   - Suction tubing
   - Chlorhexidine or betadine solution
   - Sterile drapes or towels
   - Lidocaine
   - A 25-gauge needle
   - Scalpel with 10 blade
   - Kelly clamp
   - 0 or 1-0 silk suture
   - Needle driver
   - Scissors
   - 4 × 4 drain sponge
   - Tegaderm or tape

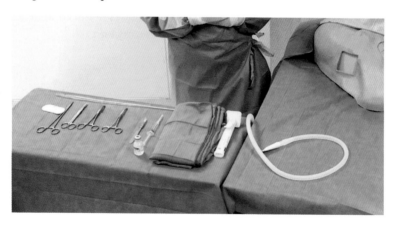

2. Obtain consent if chest tube placement is nonemergent.

3. Place the patient in supine position with the arm ipsilateral to the side of placement out of the field.
4. Identify the site for placement; this should be in the midaxillary line at the level of the fourth intercostal space, which can be approximated by the level of the nipple.

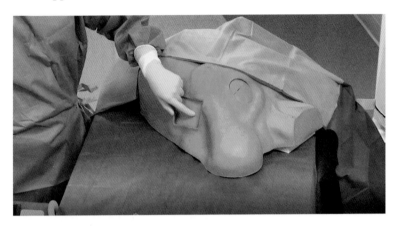

5. Prep the area with chlorhexidine or betadine.
6. After waiting the appropriate time for drying, drape the area with sterile drapes or towels; make sure to keep the nipple exposed.
7. Inject lidocaine under the skin, along the subcutaneous tissue, and along the periosteum of the rib along which the chest tube will go.
8. Make a transverse incision about 2 to 3 cm in length through the skin and subcutaneous tissue to the periosteum; a hemostat can be used to dissect through the subcutaneous tissue and chest wall musculature to reach the rib.

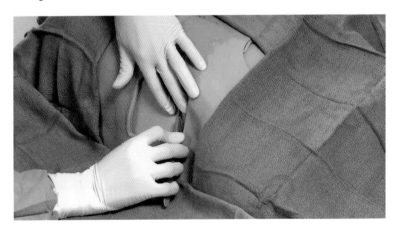

9. Using the index finger, guide the tips of the Kelly clamp through the incision to the superior border of the fourth rib; use the tips of the Kelly clamp to carefully poke through the pleura, making sure that you have a way to brake the instrument's trajectory into the chest once it traverses the parietal pleura.

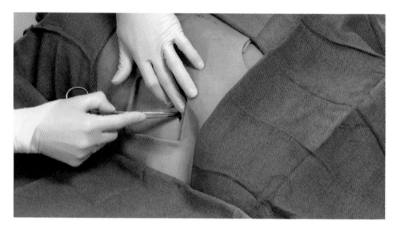

10. Use the index finger to sweep along the inside of the pleura to assure that there is no lung that is adherent to the pleural cavity.
11. Place a Kelly clamp on the tip of the chest tube (the side with the side holes) and use the instrument to guide the tube into the pleural space, aiming it posteriorly toward the apex; make sure all the side holes are in the pleural space when you are done advancing the tube.

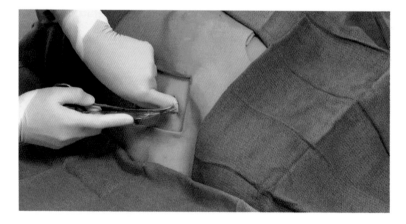

12. Have your assistant connect the chest tube to the chest tube drainage system while you are suturing the chest tube to the skin.

13. Dress the wound. Although an occlusive seal around the site may be useful in a very thin patient or one in whom a larger incision was required, most smaller incisions are fine with a drain sponge and tape.
14. Take note of the amount of blood or other fluid that drains upon initial placement.
15. Obtain a chest x-ray (CXR) to verify appropriate placement.

NEXT STEPS

- Always obtain a CXR after placement of a chest tube to verify placement.
- Monitor output from the chest tube. This is the most likely reason you placed the tube.
- Monitor for air leaks on a frequent basis to assess whether the chest tube may be removed. Effluent quality (eg, blood, bile, pus) will also inform this decision.
- There is controversy as to whether a chest tube should be removed at peak inspiration or peak expiration. Some sources report that the important thing about chest tube removal is for the patient to perform a Valsalva maneuver regardless of the part of the respiratory cycle.

COMPLICATIONS

Complications from chest tube placement include infection; bleeding; malposition (kinking, getting dislodged); injury to the lungs, great vessels, or heart; creation of a false tract; and patient discomfort.

 PEARLS

1. Chest tubes are indicated for drainage of air or fluid and for instillation of treatments needed in the pleural cavity.
2. Consider placement of a pigtail catheter in patients for whom a large-bore chest tube is not needed. There is growing evidence that even a traumatic hemothorax can be effectively evacuated with a pigtail catheter.
3. If a patient with a chest tube in place has acute decompensation, consider problems with the chest tube, including kinking or malposition. Obtain an urgent CXR STAT to diagnose the problem if an issue with the chest tube is suspected.

Suggested Readings

1. ATLS Subcommittee; American College of Surgeons' Committee on Trauma; International ATLS Working Group. Advanced trauma life support (ATLS(R)): the ninth edition. *J Trauma Acute Care Surg.* 2013;74:1363-1366.
2. Cameron JL, Cameron AM. *Current Surgical Therapy: Expert Consult.* Elsevier Health Sciences; 2010:917.
3. Bell RL, Ovadia P, Abdullah F, Spector S, Rabinovici R. Chest tube removal: end-inspiration or end-expiration? *J Trauma.* 2001;50:674-677.

28

CRICOTHYROIDOTOMY

SAYURI P. JINADASA, MD, MPH | ALOK GUPTA, MD

Cricothyroidotomy is an emergency procedure that involves placing a tube through the cricothyroid membrane to obtain an airway for oxygenation and ventilation. It is performed in the setting of failed attempt at establishing a definitive orotracheal or nasotracheal airway. Although this procedure is performed emergently, it is important for the operator to consider whether placement of a cricothyroidotomy would effectively achieve an airway: an obstruction in the distal trachea would not be alleviated by a cricothyroidotomy.

Although there is controversy surrounding the true risk for tracheal stenosis, it is recommended that an emergency cricothyroidotomy be converted to a formal tracheostomy within 1 to 2 days of initial placement to reduce this risk.

INDICATIONS

This method is performed in the setting of a failed airway when orotracheal or nasotracheal intubation cannot be achieved owing to scenarios such as obstructing mass, upper airway stenosis, massive hemorrhage, trismus, or severe maxillofacial trauma.

There are two main techniques for performing a cricothyroidotomy, including the Seldinger wire-guided technique and the open technique, both of which are explained in the subsequent text.

STEPS

OPEN SURGICAL TECHNIQUE

1. Gather supplies:
   - Personal protective equipment (cap, eye wear, mask, sterile gown, sterile gloves)
   - Povidone/iodine (or chlorhexidine, whichever is faster)
   - Scalpel
   - Hemostat
   - Tracheostomy tube or 6.0 endotracheal tube
   - Cloth tie or sutures

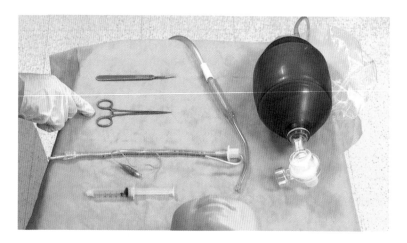

2. Place the patient in supine position and extend the neck (unless patient is on cervical spine precautions).
3. While the operator and patient are being prepped, make sure that the patient is being preoxygenated with bag-valve mask.
4. Prep the patient's neck with povidone/iodine or the fastest available prep. Time is of the essence.

5. Put on all the personal protective equipment.
6. Identify the relevant anatomy by palpating the thyroid and cricoid carti- lages and the cricothyroid membrane that lies in between.

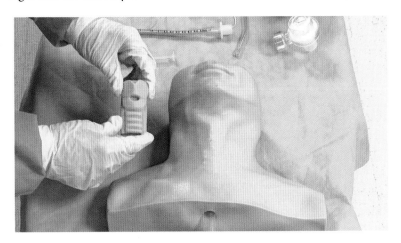

7. Stabilize the larynx with the nondominant hand.
8. Make a 2- to 3-cm vertical incision through the skin and subcutaneous tis- sue above the area of the cricothyroid membrane.

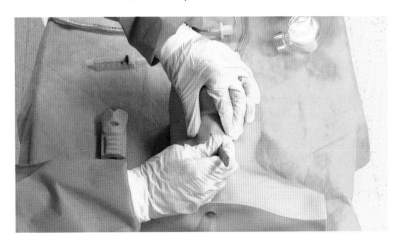

9. Stop bag-valve masking once incision is made, as this can cause blood splat- ter or subcutaneous emphysema in subsequent steps.

10. Palpate the cricothyroid membrane; make a 1-cm horizontal incision in the membrane.

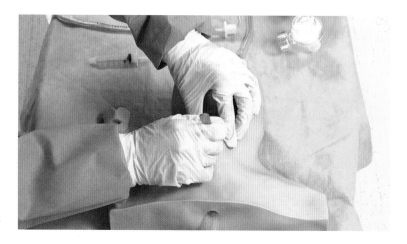

11. Place the index finger of the nondominant hand into the incision as the incision is made.

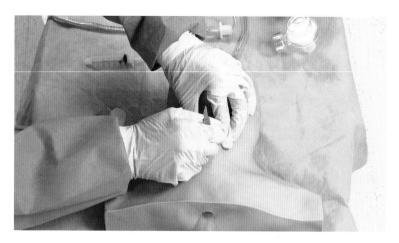

12. Insert the hemostat to replace the finger; dilate the incision in the vertical direction.

13. Place the tracheostomy or endotracheal tube through the incisions into the trachea and direct it inferiorly.

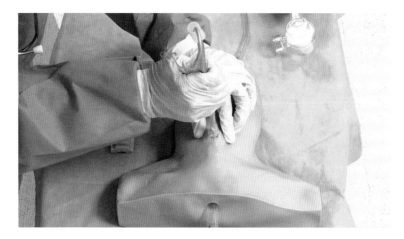

14. Remove the tube obturator.
15. Inflate the cuff of the tube and connect to the ventilator while holding the tube in place.
16. Auscultate the lungs and assess chest rise for appropriate bilateral ventilation. Use colorimetric or quantitative end-tidal CO_2 monitor to confirm position.

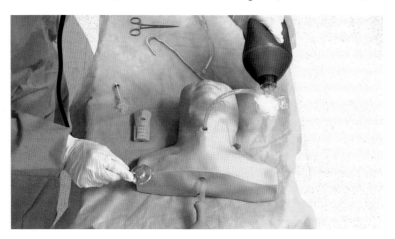

17. Secure the tube in place using the cloth tape or sutures.
18. Obtain a chest x-ray (CXR) to assess placement and for any iatrogenic complications.

SELDINGER WIRE-GUIDED TECHNIQUE

1. Gather supplies:
   - Personal protective equipment (cap, eye wear, mask, sterile gown, sterile gloves)
   - Povidone/iodine (or chlorhexidine, whichever is faster)
   - 12- or 14-gauge, 8.5-cm over-the-needle catheter attached to a 10-mL syringe containing 5 mL of sterile water (can also use existing lidocaine if faster)
   - Wire
   - Scalpel
   - Tissue dilator-airway catheter
   - Tracheostomy tube
2. Place the patient in supine position and extend the neck (unless patient is on cervical spine precautions).
3. While the operator and patient are being prepped, make sure that the patient is being preoxygenated with bag-valve mask.
4. Prep the patient's neck with povidone/iodine or the fastest available prep. Time is of the essence.
5. Put on all the personal protective equipment.
6. Identify the relevant anatomy by palpating the thyroid and cricoid cartilages and the cricothyroid membrane that lies in between.
7. Stabilize the larynx with the nondominant hand.
8. Puncture the skin in the midline directly over the cricothyroid membrane with the over-the-needle catheter connected to syringe.
9. Direct and advance the needle at a 45° angle inferiorly while drawing back on the syringe.
10. Once air is aspirated, which signifies entrance into the trachea, stop advancing the needle.
11. Remove the syringe and needle, leaving the catheter behind.
12. Insert the wire into the catheter in an inferior direction.
13. Remove the catheter while holding the wire in place.
14. Incise the skin at the entrance of the wire to allow for tissue dilator-airway catheter insertion.
15. Thread the tissue dilator-airway catheter over the wire and advance into the trachea in an inferior direction; a firm motion is necessary.
16. Remove the dilator and wire while holding the airway catheter in place.
17. Inflate the cuff of the tube and connect to the ventilator while holding the tube in place.

18. Auscultate the lungs and assess chest rise for appropriate bilateral ventilation. Use colorimetric or quantitative end-tidal CO_2 monitor to confirm position.
19. Secure the tube in place using the cloth tape or sutures.
20. Obtain a CXR to assess placement and for any iatrogenic complications.

NEXT STEPS

A CXR should be obtained after the procedure is performed to assure that the tube is in the right place, that it is not too far in or not far in enough, and that no complications such as pneumothorax were caused.

A cricothyroidotomy should be converted to a formal tracheostomy within 1 to 2 days from placement to minimize the risk for development of tracheal stenosis.

COMPLICATIONS

Complications of emergency cricothyroidotomy include inadequate ventilation, aspiration of blood, esophageal laceration, hematoma, posterior trachea perforation, subcutaneous or mediastinal emphysema, thyroid injury, pneumothorax, creation of false tract, and subglottic stenosis.

 PEARLS

1. If there is any difficulty or doubt while performing the procedure, ask for help.
2. It is imperative that this procedure be done swiftly as a delay in appropriate oxygenation and ventilation can lead to cerebral ischemia and/or death.
3. Spend time in the simulation laboratory practicing so you are ready when the real case presents itself.

Suggested Readings

1. Talving P, DuBose J, Inaba K, Demetriades D. Conversion of emergent cricothyrotomy to tracheotomy in trauma patients. *Arch Surg.* 2010;145:87-91.
2. ATLS Subcommittee; American College of Surgeons' Committee on Trauma; International ATLS Working Group. Advanced trauma life support (ATLS(R)): the ninth edition. *J Trauma Acute Care Surg.* 2013;74:1363-1366.
3. Elliott D, Baker P, Scott M, Birch C, Thompson J. Accuracy of surface landmark identification for cannula cricothyroidotomy. *Anaesthesia.* 2010;65:889-894.

ADMISSION ORDERS

ALISON M. PEASE, MD | SYLVESTER A. PAULASIR, MD

INTRODUCTION

All patients in the hospital need a set of "orders." These are the instructions that reflect the practical aspects of the surgical team's plan for the patient. Examples of orders could include the chosen drug, dose, and frequency of antibiotics; the recording of urine output every 4 hours; ensuring the patient has nothing to eat by mouth before surgery; and so on. Accordingly, "admission orders" are the initial orders that are written upon a patient being admitted to an inpatient service. Thoughtful and thorough admission orders will ensure that the patient receives all aspects of the care that you intend and allow nursing staff to begin implementing the care plan once the patient arrives to the inpatient floor.

There is more than one way to plan out admission orders, but it helps to have a framework in mind. Mnemonics have long been used to ensure that the admission orders address all relevant aspects of patient care. Perhaps the most popular of these is "ADC VAANDIMLS" (with VAAN-DIMLS read phonetically). Another option is a problem-based framework, in which each medical or surgical issue is considered and all relevant orders entered before moving on to the next problem. Fortunately, with the modern-day use of computerized admission order sets, it is easier than ever to ensure that essential basic orders, such as the frequency of vital signs or use of deep venous thrombosis prophylaxis, are not forgotten. Nevertheless, not all admission order sets will include all aspects of care, and it remains important to review the set of admission orders with at least one of the above-mentioned frameworks in mind before considering the admission orders complete. Electronic medical record systems may also be temporarily offline for maintenance, underscoring the importance of having a framework in mind.

INDICATIONS

Admission orders are necessary for all patients being admitted to an inpatient service. Patients may come in as direct admissions (from the outpatient clinic or from home), through the emergency department, intensive care unit, or post-operatively from the recovery room.

STEPS

1. Gather information about the patient:
   - See the patient if he or she is already in the hospital.
   - Determine if important historical information such as an updated home medication list is already entered in your electronic medical record, is available in the paper chart (often the case if the patient is transferred from another facility), or will need to be gathered de novo from the patient. Reviewing a preprinted list is often easier and more accurate than asking about the name and dose of each home medication. Confirm accuracy of old information.
   - Discuss the plan with your senior resident or admitting attending physician.
2. Write down a brief plan. It is often helpful to first write the patient's "one-liner" ("52-year-old male with sigmoid diverticulitis") and brief plan on your team handout or census as an overarching guide. Refer back to this at the end to make sure your orders reflect each part of the broader plan.
3. Find a computer, ideally in an area with minimal distractions, to write your set of orders.
4. Move through the admission order set process. If available, it often helps to use the computer-guided workflow first and then double-check with the frameworks below.
5. Use the ADC VAANDIMLS system to ensure completeness of your orders:
   Admit: list the service, bed type (intensive care unit, floor, step-down), attending, resident/intern.

Diagnosis: list the diagnosis.

Condition/Code status: specify whether the patient is in good, fair, or poor (critically ill) condition. Specify code status.

Vitals: often obtained every 4 hours for typical floor patients but may vary based on a patient's condition or hospital policy.

Allergies: list the patient's allergies and what happens (eg, cefepime → anaphylaxis).

Activity: specify if the patient can ambulate, if he or she has any weight-bearing restrictions, needs bed rest, and so on. In general, if there is no reason to limit activity, choose the most liberal order (often "ambulate three times daily with nursing assistance").

Nursing orders: this is a broad category. List whether the patient needs any dressing changes or wound care. Think about all the tubes, lines, and drains a patient has and what care they will need. A nasogastric tube, for instance, should generally be ordered to low continuous wall suction with regular flushes. Consider DVT prophylaxis stockings or compression devices. Specify if the patient needs restraints. Specify times when you would like to be paged (for instance, with severe hypertension, fever, or changes in drain outputs). Set goals for respiratory care, such as the oxygen saturation to which nasal cannula oxygen should be titrated.

Diet: specify if the patient will be NPO or can have a diet. Consider if he or she needs consistency restrictions (eg, thickened liquids for aspiration precautions) or specific type (eg, diabetic diet).

IV fluids, Ins and Outs: write for any maintenance fluids or resuscitative fluid boluses. Typically, strict I's and O's are desired on surgical services.

Medications: order any necessary medications for the patient's presenting issue (on surgical services, this often includes pain medications, antibiotics, and antiemetics) and continue home medications or IV equivalents as appropriate. Pay special attention to any anticoagulants and when they should be restarted.

Labs: consider whether a full set of laboratory tests has been drawn yet, and what additional tests might be necessary now that the patient is being admitted. In addition, order any laboratory tests for the next morning.

Studies: order any necessary imaging. Consider if a chest x-ray is needed to confirm any new tube positions or as part of a preoperative workup.

Although very useful, remember that ADC VAANDIMLS does not cover everything. Be sure to also think about placing any consults you will need to place and initiating discharge planning (for instance, a patient could be anticipated to need physical therapy evaluation before discharge or a home wound vac system delivered).

6. Use a problem-based method to double-check your orders. For instance, a patient with diverticulitis could also have an acute kidney injury and may need particular fluid orders, holding of nephrotoxic home medications, and/or special laboratory tests.

 PEARLS

1. Use a framework such as ADC VAANDIMLS to think through admission orders.
2. Shortly after a patient's admission orders are placed and the patient has arrived on the floor, it is often mutually beneficial to discuss the patient with his or her nurse. This allows you to communicate directly about any unusual or complex orders, express any preferences about the order in which things are carried out (for instance, if you would like admission laboratory tests drawn before the patient goes down to radiology for an imaging study), and ensure no necessary orders were missed.
3. Patients need orders as soon as possible once they have arrived to the floor in order for their care plan to be put into place. If you are expecting a planned direct admission, you can often write basic orders in advance based on the plan that has been communicated to you. These can then be activated upon the patient's arrival, which allows for the plan to be initiated even if you are busy at the moment the patient first arrives.

Suggested Readings

1. Johnson CD, Zeiger RF, Das AK, Goldstein MK. Task analysis of writing hospital admission orders: evidence of a problem-based approach. *AMIA Annu Symp Proc.* 2006;2006:389-393.
2. Maxwell RW. *Maxwell Quick Medical Reference.* 6th ed. Minneapolis, MN: Maxwell Publishing Company; 2011.

30

POST-OP CHECK AND ORDERS

MEREDITH A. BAKER, MD | SYLVESTER A. PAULASIR, MD

POST-OP TO FLOOR/INTENSIVE CARE UNIT ORDERS

Patients admitted after surgery who came either from home or the emergency department (ED) need post-op orders that are very similar to admission orders (see previous chapter). Here we briefly discuss some orders that are more relevant to postoperative care and highlight a few important points to remember when placing them. Patients already admitted preoperatively typically need transfer orders (even if going back to same service and same room), which usually entails continuing the majority of existing orders, discontinuing orders that are no longer needed (eg, NPO order), and adding a few new orders (eg, wound care, pain medications, laboratory tests). Usually, if a patient is going/returning to another service, you are still expected to place post-op orders.

Communicating with the providers who will be taking care of the patient on the floor or in the intensive care unit (ICU) should also be routine practice. This should include what surgery was performed, if the procedure went as planned, and what the plan for the patient is. If admitting to your service, then communicate with the rest of your team however you usually do (and remember to update the list/census). If the patient is going/ returning to another service, page that service and speak to them directly. It is also generally advisable to speak with the postanesthesia care unit (PACU) nurse immediately after the orders are placed and clarify any questions he/ she may have. If the patient is being admitted to the ICU, you will most likely transport the patient from the operating room. Once in the ICU, place your post-op orders and talk to the ICU team about your specific plans for the patient.

As mentioned earlier, many "post-op" orders are similar to admission orders, including admitting information, vitals, monitoring, parameters to notify house officer, activity, diet, intravenous fluid, tubes/lines/drains (for example Foley to gravity, nasogastric tube [NGT] to continuous low wall suction, chest tube to water seal), venous thromboembolism prophylaxis, and consults (physical therapy, occupational therapy, Speech & Swallow, wound/ostomy registered nurse (RN), social work, registered dietician). A few things that are either different or more important postoperatively are as follows:

- Ins and Outs (I/O's): Obtaining accurate I/O's postoperatively gives the best measurement of fluid status, which influences the treatment plan for pulmonary and renal organ systems.
- Wound/Dressing Care: Most commonly, when the skin is closed and a dressing (eg, gauze and Tegaderm) is placed over the incision, you will want the dressing to remain on until post-op day (POD) 2 to allow for epithelialization.
- Laboratory Tests: Depending on the length and complexity of the operation, you may need to order immediate post-op laboratory tests such as complete blood count, basic metabolic panel, lactate, arterial blood gas, and coagulation panel. Also remember to order tests for the following morning if needed.
- Meds: Consider need for (*ABCDEFGHI*) *A*ntibiotics (ask attending about duration), *B*owel regimen, *C*rying (pain meds), *D*VT prophylaxis, *E*mesis (antiemetics), *F*ever (acetaminophen), *G*I prophylaxis (PPI or H2B, if home med or if needed based on risk [high stress, intubated, steroids, burns, etc.]), *H*ome meds,[1] and *I*nsulin.
- Pulmonary Care: Everyone: oxygen if needed (eg, wean to SaO_2 >93%), early ambulation, incentive spirometer (10x/hour), and analgesia. If the patient has obstructive sleep apnea, they may need continuous positive airway pressure. If intubated: ventilator settings, endotracheal suctioning, head of bed elevation to 30°, and chlorhexidine mouth washes.

POST-OP TO HOME ORDERS

For outpatient/day surgery, every hospital does postoperative orders a little differently. However, outpatient post-op orders should always include medication reconciliation ("med rec"), prescription(s), discharge order, and instructions.

- Med Rec: Go through the patient's home medications (list is typically confirmed by pre-op RN) and decide whether to continue, discontinue, resume, or modify them.
- Prescriptions: Scripts for nonnarcotic pain meds can be electronically sent to pharmacies, but a printed and signed paper prescription is required for narcotic pain meds. Remember to pick the prescription up from the printer, sign it, check that it has your correct DEA number (and NPI number for the first few months of residency), and hand it to the patient's nurse. Over-the-counter pain and "bowel regimen" meds are usually cheaper, but occasionally you will be asked to write/print/send in prescriptions for these as well.
- Discharge order: Usually done on the computer. If on paper, "d/c home from PACU when meets criteria" will usually suffice. Remember to specify if the patient must void before discharge or if you or another provider must evaluate the patient before discharge.
- Instructions: Should include (at minimum): activity (can vary from "if it hurts, don't do it!" to "no lifting more than 15 pounds for 6 weeks"), diet (usually resume previous), pain control (scheduled acetaminophen, ibuprofen if able, and narcotic pain meds PRN), wound/dressing (see previous text), bathing (usually okay to shower in 24 hours, no baths/swimming until *at least* follow-up appointment), follow-up information, and things to watch out for (call office or come to ED if occur or if other concerns).

You may ask your attending his/her preferences for orders and instructions. A few things that you should definitely ask include how many oxycodone tablets (if any!) to prescribe,[2] whether or not the patient can take ibuprofen (unless he/she just told Anesthesia that Toradol is okay, in which case you are safe to assume it is), when the patient can resume any meds (eg, warfarin) that were held pre-op, and, if relevant, whether the patient must void before they can go home (eg, inguinal hernia repair).

In general, we recommend dropping off the patient in the PACU, putting in orders, talking to the PACU nurse, and finally checking on the patient and the patient's wound/dressing before walking away from the PACU.

POST-OP CHECK

Typically done about 4 hours after the patient leaves the operating room (OR). However, if the patient is fully recovered from anesthesia (awake and alert), you can do the post-op check (POC) earlier. This involves a physical examination of the patient and documentation in the form of a "SOAP note." Make sure to state what surgery was performed. Other important points to include are as follows:

- Subjective: patient complaints, nursing concerns, pain control, nausea, PO intake.
- Objective: vitals, I/O's (OR and post-op), examination (including mental status, wounds/dressings, and drains), laboratory tests and imaging (post-op, if any).
- Assessment/Plan: assessment of how the patient is doing, plan including any changes based on assessment.

If you encounter a completely saturated dressing, change it (macerated skin cannot epithelialize). If the patient has an NGT, make sure it works. Most drains should be stripped. Any concerns you encounter on POC should be brought up to your Chief Resident so they can be addressed.

 PEARLS

1. When placing post-op orders, it is important to be thorough and not overlook anything. Having a system is the best way to accomplish this; this can include an established framework such as ADC VAANDIML.
2. Be sure to communicate any important orders to the PACU and floor nurses to ensure they are carried out and inquire any additional orders or questions they have. This can save you time.
3. If any concerns arise during your postoperative check, be sure to communicate them directly and clearly to your senior.

References

1. Maxwell RW. *Maxwell Quick Medical Reference.* 5th ed. Minneapolis, MN: Maxwell Publishing Company; 2006.
2. Stehr W, ed. *The Mont Reid Surgical Handbook.* 6th ed. Philadelphia, PA: Saunders; 2008.

31

DISCHARGE SUMMARIES

BRIAN C. GOH, MD, PhD | PRIYA S. GUPTA, MD, MPH

Discharge summaries are the primary method of communication in a patient's posthospitalization course—whether that be to a rehabilitation facility, skilled nursing facility, primary care physician (PCP), or readmission care team. The discharge summary is oftentimes the primary form of communication for the patient after discharge. As such, it is critically important that the discharge summary clearly and concisely encapsulates the patient's hospitalization with pertinent findings and data that will be necessary for the next phase of care. Handoffs and care team transitions are particularly vulnerable times for lapses in patient safety, and the discharge summary is the primary mechanism by which providers can relay important clinical information after hospitalization.

DISCHARGE REQUIREMENTS

In an effort to standardize the discharge summary, the Joint Commission has established requirements (Standard IM.6.10, EP 7) for all discharge summaries to include the following items:

1. Reason for hospitalization with a specific principal diagnosis
2. Significant findings

3. Procedures performed and treatment provided
4. Patient's discharge condition and disposition
5. Patient and family instructions
6. Attending physician's signature

In addition to these required domains, discharge summaries should also include other pertinent information such as the patient's complete reconciled medication list, diet, physical activity restrictions, instructions for visiting nursing if applicable, follow-up care, and any in-house testing that will be unavailable at the time of discharge. These results can be obtained by the discharge facility or by the patient's PCP for further longitudinal management. It is also important to highlight any incidental findings that were discovered during hospitalization; common findings that require long-term follow-up include pulmonary nodules, adrenal incidentalomas, or abdominal aortic aneurysms.

HOW TO WRITE YOUR DISCHARGE SUMMARY

Because there is no standardized method to the discharge summary, they come in many different styles and formats. Many providers opt to frame the brief hospital course as a narrative that details the patient's hospitalization. This approach oftentimes recounts a clear and coherent story but easily omits sometimes necessary detail. Other providers will outline the patient's hospitalization in a problem-based or systems-based format. This method is particularly useful for patients who have complicated, prolonged hospital stays, especially if the patient underwent intensive care unit (ICU) care. While more rigid than a narrative, the problem-based or system-based format is an excellent way to ensure that the summary is comprehensive and highlights all important aspects of the patient's hospitalization.

A timely discharge summary is critically important for continuity of care and to ensure accurate communication between the inpatient care team and those who will care for the patient after discharge. Oftentimes, when the patient is discharged to a rehabilitation facility, the receiving facility will require a completed discharge summary before admission to ensure accurate handoff and a seamless transition into posthospitalization care.

One of the most effective methods for ensuring a timely discharge is to anticipate upcoming discharges and prepare discharge paperwork accordingly. While logistically difficult, updating the patient's hospital course at regular intervals will greatly save time and effort when the patient's discharge approaches.

CONCLUSION

The discharge summary is a key component of the patient's longitudinal care and relays critical information to the patient's inpatient and outpatient health-care team. The summary details the events during the patient's admission and provides necessary information for the next phase of care, whether that be at a rehabilitation facility, in outpatient follow-up, or even readmission. Thus, it is important be comprehensive and concise in formulating a patient's discharge summary, to provide accurate continuity of care and ensure the highest level of patient safety.

 PEARLS

1. Following a chronological order can prove to be the easiest method for patients with a complicated hospital stay. Over time, you will hone your skills into a method that is fast and efficient.
2. Be sure to follow Joint Commission requirements. Luckily, with the advent of electronic medical record (EMR), this is usually kept track of for you.
3. Double check all information you have typed and ensure accuracy prior to final submission.

32

WRITING SCRIPTS

BRIAN C. GOH, MD, PhD | PRIYA S. GUPTA, MD, MPH

One of the many rites of passage as a new intern is the privilege of prescribing medications. This important skill is necessary for adequate patient discharge and a smooth transition after hospitalization. Before prescribing any medications, however, prescribers must select the appropriate drug therapy for each patient's situation. It is imperative to ensure that the patient does not have any allergies to the medication and/or class of medications you are prescribing. Additionally, it is equally as important to review the patient's current medications to ensure that there will not be any unforeseeable drug interactions. Apart from drug interactions, prescribers should also ensure that the medication is appropriate for the patient and their condition, e.g., avoiding nonsteroidal anti-inflammatory drugs (NSAIDs) in a patient with renal compromise. The prescriber should account for the patient as a whole—taking into account the patient's age, chronic diseases, and current medications before selecting a therapy.

PRECAUTIONS

All new prescriptions should include patient education regarding the medication's indications, intended use, and potential side effects, particularly warning signs. Special instructions on drug-specific avoidance of particular foods, alcohol, or over-the-counter medications should also be provided.

PROPER SCRIPT WRITING

As the advent of electronic medical record (EMR) systems becomes increasingly popular, so does the ability to electronically prescribe medications or print paper prescriptions directly from the EMR. If the option is available, many patients opt for the convenience of electronic prescriptions at the time of discharge so that they may pick up their prescriptions on the way home. Others prefer to have a paper prescription in hand so that they have the freedom to go to the pharmacy of their choosing.

All prescriptions should include:

- Two forms of patient identification such as the patient's name and date of birth
- Name and strength of the medication
- Directions for administration including route and indications for "as needed" medications
- Quantity to dispense and number of refills in both text and numerical format (eg, #10 ten)
- Date of prescription
- Duration of therapy
- Printed name and signature of the prescribing provider
- National Provider Identifier (NPI) number and Drug Enforcement Administration (DEA) number for controlled substances

Regulations regarding scheduled drug prescriptions, particularly opioid medications, vary from state to state, and you should become familiar of your state's rules and regulations. Quantity limits are often in place to ensure that the patient has adequate medication post hospitalization but not an excessive amount. Patients should follow up in specialty clinics or their primary care clinic for additional prescriptions or refills.

All prescriptions should be written legibly or printed with clear instructions, including relationships to meals and specific time of the day. The use of most abbreviations or shorthand should be strictly avoided to prevent any confusion or ambiguity. The National Coordinating Council on Medication Error Reporting and Prevention provides guidelines on which abbreviations are commonly mistaken and which abbreviations should be eliminated. All instructions should be written out using plain language, allowing the patient to understand the prescription and ask for any clarification. Patient understanding should be readily confirmed by having the patient repeat the instructions to the provider.

CONCLUSION

The capacity to prescribe medications is one of the most important aspects of being a physician and must be performed with great care and attention. Medication errors are common sources of adverse events and a significant contributor to patient harm. Providers must be diligent and thoughtful when prescribing medications to provide necessary patient care and ensure patient safety.

 PEARLS

1. Be sure to review allergies and all pertinent patient medications, their indications (if still in use) and their dose prior to prescribing a new medication.
2. Double check all new medications you write to ensure there are no errors in your script. Make sure you have included your NPI and DEA number, if applicable.
3. Medication name should be written without abbreviations. Route and dose can be written with appropriate abbreviations; such as, PO and mg.

33

BILLING AND CODING FOR RESIDENTS

STEPHANIE THERRIEN, BSc | WILLIAM R. DETERLING, BSBA

The purpose of this chapter is to expose you to an abbreviated version of medical coding and billing basics. The goal is not to turn you into a professional coder but instead to leave you with an understanding of the importance of timely, diligent, and detailed documentation and how doing so affects your practice and ultimately your patient. Topics to be discussed include: *What is coding and billing? Are coding and billing the same thing? What is an ICD10 code? What is a CPT code? Why do I need to know this?*

DEFINITIONS

Diagnosis and Procedural Codes: The diagnosis codes for professional billing are called International Classification of Diseases, Tenth Revision (ICD-10) and for inpatient hospital billing Diagnosis Related Group (DRG). For procedural billing, the codes utilized for professional billing are Current Procedural Terminology (CPT), Healthcare Common Procedure Coding System (HCPC) and for hospital billing International Classification of Diseases, 10th Revision, Procedure Coding System (ICD-10-PCS).

Medical Coder: an individual who is trained and certified in medical coding. Additional certification can be obtained through specialty certification.

Medical Coding: The act of medical coding is to take a symptom, diagnosis, procedure, or rendered service and translate it into an associated diagnosis and procedure code.

Medical Billing: Medical billers ensure that the services presented for reimbursement by the medical coder are billed properly to insurance and patients. At most institutions, the amount to be paid for a specific service is negotiated with an insurer and that amount is referred to as the "allowed amount" the insurer will pay.

Chargemaster, or Charge Description Master (CDM): A comprehensive listing of all billable services and items. This list captures each procedure, service, supply, drug, and diagnostic test with their associated charge. Each institution determines its own chargemaster charges and uses them to negotiate reimbursement rates with private insurers. It is essential that this list is managed and updated regularly to accurately reflect current pricing.[1]

HOW IT WORKS: IN LAYMAN'S TERMS

Whether you see a patient in clinic, or operate on them in the OR, you will generate a detailed note that outlines the conditions treated, how much time you spent, what you did, discussions you had, supplies you used, and diagnoses presented at the end of the visit or operative session. In doing this, you are providing your coding team with the information that they will utilize to generate or validate codes.

The process of medical coding is to review clinical documentation for diagnoses and services that can be assigned to an appropriate code. Medical coders are often responsible for auditing and appealing denied or unpaid claims in collaboration with the billing office or billing vendor. In large institutions, there are coders who specialize in certain specialties. Proper coding will reduce the incidence of claim denial, underpayment, and bundling of component procedure codes into one primary procedure code.

Once a code has been generated, the charge amount is retrieved from the professional and facility chargemaster. This is often done by using an item number that has been preassigned to one service. All billable items will then be sent to the billing team who will distribute a bill to the insurer or patient for payment.

E&M DOCUMENTATION STRUCTURE

As an example, documentation of an office visit; a problem focused history requires documentation of the chief complaint (CC) and a brief history of present illness (HPI), whereas a detailed history requires the documentation of a CC, an extended HPI, plus an extended review of systems (ROS), and pertinent past, family, and/or social history (PFSH).

Based on this documentation, the complexity of the patient's visit will be determined. This complexity is translated into three categories of CPT codes, new patient visit, established patient visit, and consults in the office or outpatient setting. These codes are commonly referred to as Evaluation and Management (E&M) codes.

99201-99205 New patient visits.

99211-99215 Established patient visits.

99241-99245 Office/Outpatient consults (code as office visit if code is not accepted by insurance)

For detailed professional visit (E&M) documentation guidelines the following link is provided:

https://www.cms.gov/Outreach-and-Education/Medicare-Learning-Network-MLN/MLNProducts/Downloads/eval-mgmt-serv-guide-ICN006764.pdf

To ensure that the proper codes are identified and accurate bills are generated, documentation of symptoms, conditions, time, and care provided must be contained in the note. It is important to know that insurance auditors take the view that if it is not documented it did not happen.

Example:

A medical weight management physician sees her patients monthly for monitoring. If she documents only that she discussed the plan of care, followed up on concerns, and wrote a prescription, she will be able to bill only a low complexity level.

If the same physician implemented the review of systems, documented changes, documented that she discussed the patient's active problem list that consists of CHF, DM2, Neuropathy, and so on, she can bill a higher level of complexity because of more comprehensive documentation, which may or may not have extended the length of time.

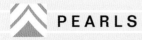

PEARLS

1. Understanding how to correctly document a chart has a direct impact on what codes are generated and, ultimately, what the level of reimbursement is received.
2. All providers must understand that the documentation must support the diagnosis and procedure codes submitted for payment. Selecting a complex CPT code that is not supported by documentation is considered overcoding.
3. Coding lower than what the documentation supports is undercoding. Both are viewed as inappropriate coding and can have different ramifications with the insurance carriers.

References

1. The role of the hospital chargemaster in revenue cycle management. In: LaPointe J, *RevCycleIntelligence*. Thinkstock; 2018. revcycleintelligence.com/features/the-role-of-the-hospital-chargemaster-in-revenue-cycle-management.
2. "AAPC." *AAPC – Advancing the Business of Healthcare.* AAPC Blog; 2018. www.aapc.com/resources/medical-coding/cpt.aspx.

34

HEALTH INSURANCE COMPANIES FOR RESIDENTS

STEPHANIE THERRIEN, BSc | WILLIAM DETERLING, BSBA

The purpose of this chapter is to touch upon economic aspects of the United States health care system basics and what you should know to best take care of patients. Topics to be covered include Health Maintenance Organization (HMO) versus Preferred Provider Organization (PPO) versus Point of Service (POS) (and other definitions), types of plans, differences between plans, and how those differences may affect the care you provide to your patient.

As a trainee, your interactions with insurance companies will be limited. Your interest in understanding their depths may not yet exist, but as you approach the completion of your training, the need to understand the general differences of plans and their financial ramifications will become very important.

WHY DO I CARE?

The cost of health care continues to rise. It stems from the implementation of new technology, expensive equipment, aging of a significant portion of the population ("*Baby Boomers*"), and, simply, more consumers needing coverage. No matter the cause, increased health costs affect everyone within the health,care system to one degree or another.

Quoted directly *from The Centers for Medicaid and Medicare National Health Expenditure Projections Forecast Summary* (2017-2026)[1]:

> *Under current law, national health spending is projected to grow at an average rate of 5.5% per year for 2017-2026 and to reach $5.7 trillion by 2026. While this projected average annual growth rate is more modest than that of 7.3% observed over the longer-term history prior to the recession (1990-2007), it is more rapid than has been experienced 2008-16 (4.2%).*
>
> *Health spending is projected to grow 1.0% point faster than Gross Domestic Product (GDP) per year over the 2017-26 period; as a result, the health share of GDP is expected to rise from 17.9% in 2016 to 19.7% by 2026.*
>
> *Among the major payers for health care, growth in spending for Medicare (7.4% per year) and Medicaid (5.8% per year) are both substantial contributors to the rate of national health expenditure growth for the projection period. Both trends reflect the impact of an aging population, but in different ways. For Medicare, projected enrollment growth is a primary driver; for Medicaid, it is an increasing projected share of aged and disabled enrollees.*[1]

When the costs for insurance companies and overall health care spending follow an upward trajectory, the trickle-down effect on consumers comes in the form of increased premiums, deductibles, and co-pays. Over time, these increases reduce what the average family has left over after each paycheck, or "available income." If the strain becomes significant enough, families or individuals may be forced to decide to subscribe to a less comprehensive, but financially sustainable, policy with a lower premium. This will in turn come with higher deductibles and higher co-pays to offset the loss of a higher premium. To avoid paying a deductible, high co-pay, or risk receiving a large medical bill, subscribers may choose to defer a necessary surgery, procedure, or office visit.[2] In your developing career, understanding the basics of insurance and having an idea how to work with them to provide services to your patients will make your life easier.

INSURANCE BASICS

Subscribers who are looking into the purchase of an insurance plan will find that there are two basic categories they can fall into, individual coverage or group coverage.[3]

Individual coverage is established when consumers obtain coverage for themselves or their family by contacting an insurer directly and receiving a policy that is paid for by the individual. An example of such would be someone who called an insurance agent or sought advice online, contacted a vendor (eg, Blue Cross Blue Shield) and received a policy of their choice. The premium for individual coverage is varied in both its cost and availability. Plan eligibility is often determined by the subscribers' past and current medical history. Individual plans do offer the most freedom of choice, as there is no employer restrictions as to the benefits the individual can purchase. However, premiums are typically high because the individual is not part of a shared risk pool, which is the advantage of a group policy.

Group coverage is established when a consumer is either an eligible employee of a participating employer or a student enrolled in a participating university. Unlike individual coverage, the cost of the premium is calculated based on the risk of the group to be insured. This is determined by the group's demographics, gender, and age, even geographic location. In group plans, the vendor and policy types are selected by the institutions. Variations of co-pays and annual deductibles are typically offered, which will affect employer and employee cost. Employers that offer health insurance as a benefit and The Affordable Care Act's Healthcare Exchange are examples of group coverage.

Allowed amount is the amount insurance will pay the provider, less any other provisions. The provider will bill insurance, insurance will pay the lesser of the provider charge or the insurance allowed amount. Therefore, it is important to ensure the provider charge is greater than the insurance allowed amount. One broadly accepted strategy to set provider charges is to take the Medicare allowed amounts and use a multiple of that amount. Typically, these multiples range from two to three times the Medicare allowed amount. Other considerations are the practice payor mix, which may influence the multiple selected.

Contractual adjustment is the difference between the provider charge and the insurance allowed amount. This is considered a contractual adjustment because the provider, when entering into an insurance contract, agrees to accept the insurance allowed amount as full payment. A contractual adjustment is a "write off" in which no payment will be made for that amount. It cannot be billed to the patient or secondary insurance.

HEALTH PLAN STRUCTURE

It is unlikely that by this point in your career, you have not heard the acronyms HMO, PPO, EPO, and so on. But what do they mean for you as a medical professional?

As a provider, even more so as a subspecialist, whether a patient is eligible to come see you for your services will depend entirely on the carrier and structure of his or her insurance plan. A failure to recognize or understand a patient's eligibility can result in unanticipated medical bills for the patient or nonreimbursed services for you and your institution.

The Breakdown: In general, plans that give a subscriber the most liberty in choosing where their care is to be managed are the most expensive. Such plans allow a subscriber to choose where they receive their care without any penalties (higher co-pay, etc.). If a subscriber is not enrolled in such a plan and chooses to go "*out of network*" to see a specialist, the institution and the subscriber will pay "outside utilization costs." In efforts to reduce these costs, plans with lower premiums may be offered to entice patients to stay within the network. Alternatively, an employer may put stipulations on where employees can and cannot go with the plan they selected.

OPTIONS

HMO

Stands for: Health Maintenance Organization.

Translation: HMO policy holders are expected to select a primary care physician (PCP) within an accepted organization and receive their care only through that organization. Patient's seeking care outside of that organization would need a referral for specialist care before services rendered for the policy to provide coverage.

What that means: If a patient visits a physician outside of his or her insurance network and does not have a referral in place, the visit may result in the patient being responsible for the claim payment. Some insurance plans place the referral burden on the provider, and if the referral is not in place, the provider will not get paid and there will be no patient balance.

PPO

Stands for: Preferred Provider Organization

Translation: Under this plan option, a primary care provider does not need to be delegated. Instead, subscribers are offered a network of physicians and specialists. Under this plan, a subscriber pays a higher premium for the ability to seek care out of network while still maintaining full coverage. Subscribers who frequent specialists outside of their plan's network (typically due to a specific condition) benefit most from this plan option.

What this means: When a PPO-covered patient comes in for a consult and their PCP is listed under a nonaffiliated institution, their claim will be covered, less any co-pay or deductible.

POS

Stands for: Point of Service Plans

Translation: Under a POS plan (a blend of HMO and PPO attributes), the subscriber must appoint a designated primary care provider. To visit any outside specialists, this appointed provider does not need a referral. There are higher patient costs for out-of-network care, such as deductibles, that would not be applied for in-network care.

What this means: A POS subscriber can seek care with an out-of-network provider; the patient would have the benefit of reduced patient balances but still have deductibles and or coinsurance applied. In network care would have the same benefits of a PPO plan with full coverage, less a co-pay.

Side note: It is important that patients coming in for a consult verify coverage for such. Their policy may have plan exclusions, preferred networks, or carve outs. Questions about such coverage should be directed to your billing office, or practice administrator, for confirmation.

When you enter the realm of surgical or procedural specialties, a referral may no longer be enough to cover services rendered, regardless of the plan structure. For both government and commercial insurances, there will be a list of covered services available on their website. Additional requirements and policy limitations will be available as well.

Preapprovals or prior authorizations are required by insurance companies to validate the medical necessity of the planed surgical intervention. Examples of services that require preapprovals or prior authorizations are bariatric surgery, deep brain stimulation, and exploratory gastrointestinal procedures. The patient's plan will dictate whether preauthorization is required. In most situations, front-line staff manage insurance requirements and ensure that the necessary authorizations are in place before surgery. For emergency surgery or surgical procedures that are not covered by the preauthorization, the hospital and surgeon have 48 business hours to contact the insurance for a retroactive authorization.

Now that we have outlined some of the most very basic, need-to-know insurance topics, lets cover some terminology that you should be comfortable with:

Source: The following definitions are taken directly from: MedicalCodingandBilling.org/health-insurance-guide.[3]

Premium: The amount a subscriber pays to his or her insurance company for health coverage each month or year.

Deductible: The amount of money a subscriber must pay out of pocket before payment is made. Typically, the lower the premium, the higher the deductible.

Coinsurance: The amount of money owed to a medical provider once the deductible has been paid. Coinsurance is usually a predetermined percentage of the total bill. If the policy's coinsurance is set at 15% and the allowed amount comes to $100, the policy holder owes $15 in coinsurance.

Co-pay: This type of insurance plan is like coinsurance but with one key exception: rather than waiting until the deductible has been paid out, the subscriber must make their copayment at the time of service. Most often, copayments are standardized by plan.

Out-of-pocket maximum: The amount of money paid for deductibles and coinsurance charges within a given year before the insurance company starts paying for all covered expenses.

In-network: This term refers to physicians and medical establishments that deliver patient services covered under the insurance plan. In-network providers are generally the cheapest option for policyholders. Insurance companies typically have negotiated lower rates with in-network providers.

Out-of-network: This term refers to physicians and medical establishments *not* covered under a subscriber's insurance plan. Services from out-of-network providers are usually more expensive than those rendered by in-network providers.

Preexisting condition: Any chronic disease, disability, or other condition listed at the time of application. In some cases, symptoms or ongoing treatments related to preexisting conditions cause premiums to be higher than usual.

Waiting period: Many employer-sponsored insurance plans mandate a period of 90 days before employees can enroll in their insurance plans.

Dual coverage: The act of maintaining a health plan with more than one insurer.

Coordination of benefits: This process is applied by individuals who have two or more existing policies to ensure that their beneficiaries do not receive more than the combined maximum payout for the plans.

Continuation of coverage: This is essentially an extension of insurance coverage offered to individuals no longer covered under a plan; it most often applies to former employees and retirees of companies that offer employee coverage.

Referral: An official notice from a qualified physician to an insurer that recommends specialist treatment for a current policy holder.

 PEARLS

1. It is important to understand the complex medical system you work in to better address any of your patient's concerns and questions.
2. This also includes covering yourself for services rendered and ensuring you receive what you have earned.
3. It is advised that, as you progress through your career, ask questions, speak to billing professionals, observe your frontline staff as they prepare prior authorizations. What you learn will greatly improve the payment for the care you provide in the future.

References

1. National Health Expenditure Data. *Centers for Medicare and Medicaid Services.* April 17, 2017. https://www.cms.gov, www.cms.gov/Research-Statistics-Data-and-Systems/Statistics-Trends-and Reports/NationalHealthExpendData/Downloads/ForecastSummary.pdf, https://www.rand.org/pubs/research_briefs/RB9605.html.
2. Buying Health Insurance. *Health Insurance FAQ's, Blue Cross Blue Shield.* 2018:2. https://www.bcbsm.com/index/health-insurance-help/faqs/topics/buying-insurance/difference-between-group-and-individual-coverage.html.
3. Understanding Health Insurance. *Everything You Need to Get Started in Medical Coding and Billing.* MedicalCodingandBilling.org; 2018. www.medicalbillingandcoding.org/health-insurance-guide/overview/.
4. Introduction to Health Care in the US. *The Khan Academy, The Brookings Institution/Khan Academy.* 2018. www.khanacademy.org/partner-content/brookings-institution/introduction-to-healthcare/v/introduction-to-health-care. All Khan Academy content is available for free at www.khanacademy.org.

35

PREPARING FOR THE OPERATING ROOM

ABRAHAM GELLER, MD | SIDHU P. GANGADHARAN, MD, MHCM

Preparation is paramount to success in surgical internship and residency. Perhaps nowhere is this truer than in the operating room (OR), and for good reason. The OR is not only where attending surgeons teach and evaluate residents, but it is also where good preparation can truly be the difference between life and death for a patient. How best to prepare for an operation will depend in part on the specific patient, his or her diagnosis, the operation to be performed, the attending surgeon's preferences, and your own fund of knowledge and skill level. Ultimately, preparing rigorously for the OR will allow you take the best care of the patient and propel your learning. We first present a quick guide and checklist to preparing appropriately and setting yourself up for success in the OR, followed by a more in-depth description of various aspects of preparation.

KNOW THE PATIENT

Understanding the patient's medical history and the reason for bringing him or her to the OR begins with a thorough review of the surgical history and physical as well as other providers' notes, laboratory tests, imaging, and pathology. This review can, and should, begin at least a day or two before the operation.

Key places to look include the attending surgeon's last clinic note, the patient's last discharge summary, and the operative reports from any prior operations, especially those related to the admission diagnosis. If the patient has undergone extensive workup by another medical specialty, notes from those encounters may contain valuable insight that could shape the plan for perioperative management.

Next, define a timeline for the disease being treated. When and how did the patient initially present? How was the workup initiated? Have objective diagnostic tests been done? What were the results? If a patient with gastroesophageal reflux disease is being considered for Nissen fundoplication, what were the results of his multichannel intraluminal impedance (pH monitoring) study and what was his DeMeester score? What treatments have already been tried? Did he get an adequate trial of proton pump inhibitors? Were they effective? When and why did the surgeon first get involved? A clear, logical path should begin to take form: *This 55-year-old man with obesity developed progressive postprandial heartburn, cough, and sour taste in the back of his throat over the last 12 months. An EGD was done that showed L.A. Grade A esophagitis but no Barrett's. Fluoroscopic swallowing study showed a moderately sized type I hiatal hernia and reflux to the level of the mid-esophagus. He underwent MII testing that showed a DeMeester score of 17, consistent with GERD. A 2-month trial of Prilosec has been effective, but the patient wishes to avoid long-term acid suppression. He is otherwise healthy and a good operative candidate, and desires definitive treatment. And that is why we're doing this operation.*

If the case you are preparing for is a cancer operation, what is the patient's TNM stage? What were her last tumor markers? Were they elevated before treatment? Review the patient's family history and results of any prior genetic studies. Did she receive neoadjuvant chemotherapy? When was her last dose? Did she tolerate neoadjuvant treatment well, or did she require dose reduction for poor tolerance? Neoadjuvant radiotherapy can induce (sometimes impressive) radiation fibrosis around the tumor bed and make for a challenging dissection. Importantly, it can interfere with the surgeon's ability to clearly define grossly negative margins. Being aware of these details before the start of the operation is essential.

Complete the picture by reviewing the patient's comorbidities and chronic conditions. If the patient has diabetes, is it managed with insulin or without? What and when was his last HbA1c? Thoroughly review the patient's list of home medications, and confirm *why* the patient is taking each medication. It goes without saying that the patient's past surgical history should be reviewed in great detail, including the date of every prior operation, why it was done, what approach was used, whether it was open or laparoscopic, and whether there were any complications. You should know about any incisions a patient might have; sometimes they do not report having had surgery until your examination detects an incision and you prompt their memory.

A focused but detailed physical examination is a critical component of the preoperative workup and should be confirmed the morning of the operation. Details of the physical examination should be noted insofar as they may affect the course of the operation. Does the patient have localized or diffuse tenderness at baseline? Does the patient have ascites or a fluid shift? The surgeon planning a midline laparotomy will want to know about any existing or previously repaired hernias. Local skin and soft tissue infections affecting the area of planned incision are among the few contraindications to surgical incisions, and their presence should be documented. Knowing whether a previous operation had been done open or minimally invasively may help you anticipate the extent of adhesions you might expect to encounter and thus alter your operative planning.

Always know the patient's most recent laboratory test results before the operation, particularly the hemoglobin/hematocrit and creatinine; having a baseline for comparison will be essential to the interpretation of these parameters postoperatively. Coagulopathy should not be a surprise to you, as it is detectable by history or laboratory testing or both. However, it is also essential to know about any antiplatelet or novel anticoagulant medications a patient is taking, as that may not impact routine laboratory values but would impact the risk of bleeding significantly.

As a surgeon, comfort and fluency interpreting various common imaging modalities is crucial. It is fine to read the radiologist's impression, but *always* review the images yourself. Sometimes subtle findings may go unreported in the official read, and failure to identify those findings preoperatively could affect how the operation goes—this could have real life-or-death ramifications for the patient. Equally important is using preoperative imaging to confirm the patient's anatomy, as these details, for example, a thick abdominal wall, replaced arterial or venous anatomy, or varices directly under the target incisions site, may significantly impact surgical planning.

Never underestimate the importance of a thorough social history. A patient's prior smoking history may speak to his propensity for healthy wound healing or risk of postoperative pneumonia. Alcoholic hallucinosis may easily be misdiagnosed as run-of-the-mill postoperative delirium if the patient's drinking habits are unknown, and it may progress to delirium tremens if not treated appropriately.

KNOW THE DISEASE

Familiarity with some basic principles of the patient's presenting diagnosis is critical to being an effective team member, both inside and outside of the OR. Develop the habit of thinking in terms of diseases rather than surgical operations. Advanced reading about the epidemiology, pathophysiology, and natural history of the disease shows the attending surgeon you are serious about learning what he or she has to teach you and may push him/her to allow you greater autonomy in the OR. Always keep in mind the top two or three differential diagnoses and how they can be differentiated from the patient's diagnosis. It is also important to become familiar with nonsurgical treatment alternatives for the disease, how effective they are, and how they compare with surgical management in terms of success rates, complication rates, and indications for first- versus Second-line treatment. How does the disease typically present, and how did it present in this patient? How is it diagnosed? What is the prognosis with and without surgery?

KNOW THE OPERATION

A working knowledge of the technical aspects of the operation should begin (but not end) with advanced reading of the steps to the operation in surgical texts or the primary literature. Recognize, however, that some surgeons have developed personalized, modified approaches that deviate from the textbook. Go beyond rote memorization of the steps of the operation; force yourself to consider the *rationale* behind each one (cognitive task analysis).

KNOW THE SURGEON

A critical element to active learning is understanding *why* the surgeon does things in this or that particular way. Develop a habit of being dissatisfied with not knowing the reason behind every move made during the operation. Efficient and purposeful movement is a tenant of good surgery, and every step of the operation has an underlying logic. This fact is not limited to the operation itself, but also applies to everything that happens in the OR before the skin incision: what instruments are chosen; how to position the patient; how to prep the skin, lay the drapes, and organize all the instruments, power cords, and tubing on the operative field. Some of these details may be discerned from the surgeon's operative reports from similar prior cases. Coresidents are another invaluable resource, and those who have operated with this attending surgeon before may have key insights into the surgeon's preferences and personal style. The attending surgeon will often explain why he or she likes to have the patient positioned in a particular way, or the instruments laid out on the field just so. Commit these details to memory. *After the case ends and you break scrub, take a minute or two to write them down.* Taking the initiative to put your knowledge and awareness to use in the next case by properly positioning the patient and organizing your instruments shows the attending surgeon you pay close attention to details. Surgeons notice these small details, and they may be more inclined to get you more involved in the next case. This sets off a positive feedback loop whereby good work leads to early advancement, which leads to opportunities for more good work, and so on.

Perhaps more important than knowing what your attending surgeon likes is knowing what he or she dislikes. Whether you agree with them or not, these preferences are often borne just as much out of objective evidence as they are personal negative experiences. Know how the surgeon likes to communicate. Some surgeons offer minimal verbal communication, whereas others will demand clear, closed-loop communication every time. Also pay attention to rationales given by different surgeons that seemingly contradict one another. This shows that many preferences are not necessarily evidence based. Paying attention to the diversity of approaches will allow you to choose the one that works best from your perspective.

As the case draws to a close, consider the plan for postoperative management. Is this patient on a well-defined pathway? If so, does the surgeon generally adhere to the generic pathway, or does she deviate in predictable ways? Does this particular patient have any reasons not to follow the pathway? If the patient is not on a pathway, it is important to know, in general terms, how the surgeon likes to manage these patients postoperatively. Does she like to advance diet more aggressively or more cautiously? Is she comfortable giving nonsteroidal anti-inflammatory drugs for pain control? How long does she like to hold off before restarting a patient's home anticoagulation? It may be surprising at first how much variation exists, even between surgeons within a single hospital. Take the opportunity to clarify any ambiguous details before the surgeon leaves you to close.

Lastly, constructive feedback is critical for self-improvement, and should be sought and incorporated early and often. However, asking for feedback can sometimes be tricky. Although we are generally led to believe that asking for feedback shows a desire to improve and is well received by our attendings, many people actually do not appreciate being unexpectedly put on the spot to come up with thoughtful, constructive feedback. Questions such as "What feedback can you give me?" are overwhelmingly broad and may actually be annoying when the attending is hurrying off to a full clinic. Good feedback should be S.T.A.T., that is, it should be specific, thoughtful, actionable, and timely. Help the surgeon give you STAT feedback by asking targeted, manageable questions: "What one area or skill would you most like to see me work on for next time?" "Which steps of the operation do I need to work on the most?" "What one thing can I work on to make the next case go even better?" After receiving feedback, briefly thank the surgeon for giving it: "Thank you. I'll be sure to work on that." "Thanks so much, that's good advice."

KNOW YOURSELF

Excellence in any field requires candid and critical self-reflection. Be honest with yourself about your strengths and weaknesses as a surgical resident. With time and dedication, most deficiencies in technique can be overcome. Although some technical skills may come more naturally, others may seem elusive even after many hours of dedicated practice. If you are sewing coronary arteries but you do not have the steadiest hands, there are still ways to train yourself to be capable of sewing coronary arteries, but it will require a willingness to work at it and an honest self-assessment of your weaknesses. You will need to figure out a solution that accommodates *your* weaknesses and plays to *your* strengths. It is important to enter an OR with the self-confidence that you have what it takes to make it through the operation successfully. Yet healthy self-doubt safeguards against errors of judgment and is conducive to a learning mindset. Strike a balance between having the self-confidence to execute the task in front of you and the self-doubt to take pause and be certain of every move before committing.

CHECKLIST

KEY POINTS

Thoroughly preparing in advance of every operation is essential for success during surgical internship, will benefit patients, and may lead to opportunities for early advancement in the OR.

Knowing about the patient entails a detailed knowledge of his/her history of present illness, workup and treatments to date, and all relevant past medical and surgical history and recent laboratory work.

Always personally review any recent relevant imaging the patient has had.

Take the time to read up on the patient's diagnosis, including its workup and nonsurgical treatments, and any major literature that has recently been published on the subject.

A working knowledge of the steps to the operation (beginning with a detailed understanding of the relevant anatomy) is essential to success in surgery.

Understanding the rationale behind each step of the operation makes it easier to commit to memory and greatly enhances learning.

Knowing what your attending surgeon likes and dislikes can help you avoid setbacks, shows you are detail oriented, and ultimately builds trust; this fosters a mutual working and learning relationship.

Constructive feedback and critical and specific self-reflection are essential to personal and professional growth.

Writing down impressions and observations after each case will help you to retain finer details and give you a leg up on the next case.

KNOW THE PATIENT

Do I know the patient's history?

What is my succinct but thorough one-liner on this patient?

Why is the patient getting this operation? What disease are we treating?

How has this patient been worked up for the disease we are treating?

How has the patient been treated for the disease up until now?

What are the patient's most recent relevant laboratory tests?

What are the most recent relevant images?

Does the patient have any comorbidities that may be relevant to the operation or perioperative period?

Does the patient have any chronic medical conditions? How are they managed? Are they well controlled?

What medications does this patient take at home? What is my plan for holding or resuming them perioperatively?

What allergies does this patient have?

What financial, psychosocial, and/or functional considerations may be relevant to discharge planning?

KNOW THE DISEASE

What are the epidemiology, pathophysiology, and natural history of the disease?

How is the disease worked up and diagnosed?

What are the top differential diagnoses and how are they distinguished?

What are the nonsurgical treatment options for this disease? Are they effective?

What are the indications for surgical versus medical management?

What is the prognosis?

KNOW THE OPERATION

What is the relevant anatomy encountered at each step?

What are the steps to the operation?

What is the rationale behind each step?

What is the rationale behind this particular *sequence* of steps?

What are the "danger points?" At each step of the operation, what are the important things that can go wrong?

KNOW THE ATTENDING SURGEON

How does the attending like to position the patient?

How does the attending like to organize instruments, tubing, and power cords on the operative field?

Where does the attending like to make the incision? Where does he or she place the trocars?

How does the attending like to communicate during an operation?

What are the attending's expectations of me during the operation?

What habits or practices does the attending dislike?

AFTER THE OPERATION

Clarify with the attending anything ambiguous about the post-op plan.

Find an appropriate moment to ask for feedback using specific, focused questions.

Write down any feedback the attending offers.

Record the steps of the operation.

Record how the attending likes the patient positioned and operative field organized and where the trocars/incision should be placed.

Reflect honestly on what you did well and what you did poorly, and develop a concrete plan for how to do better next time.

CONCLUSION

Ultimately, few operations are as perfectly straightforward as they "should be," and unforeseeable issues will inevitably arise. But chance favors the prepared mind, and the confidence that comes with being well prepared will maximize the likelihood of a successful operation and increase the learning potential of the experience.

 PEARLS

1. Thoroughly preparing in advance may lead to opportunities for early advancement in the OR. This includes a working knowledge of the steps to the operation (beginning with a detailed understanding of the relevant anatomy).
2. Knowing what your attending surgeon likes and dislikes can help you avoid setbacks, shows you are detail oriented, and ultimately builds trust; this fosters a mutual working and learning relationship.
3. Constructive feedback and specific self-reflection are essential to personal and professional growth.

36

SURGICAL CONSENT

JACQUELINE E. WADE, MD | LUCY C. MARTINEK, MD

INTRODUCTION

Informed consent is an established ethical and legal requirement for all surgical treatment. Surgical consent is not only a signature on a consent form but also an ongoing process of communication and shared decision-making that continues throughout preoperative, perioperative, and postoperative care.

Your job as a surgical trainee and representative of the surgical team is to appreciate the importance and nuances inherent in the process of obtaining informed consent and also to ensure the appropriate medical-legal documentation is efficiently collected. This chapter summarizes the key features involved in the consent process for the procedures and various treatments that are offered to patients.

COMPONENTS OF SURGICAL CONSENT

1. Attending surgeon who will be performing the procedure
2. The name of the procedure and possible associated procedures
3. Site or location of the procedure, along with the side it will be performed on (ie, left or right)

277

4. Purpose of the procedure
5. Alternatives to the treatment being consented for
6. Potential risks of not undergoing the procedure
7. Risks of the procedure
8. Benefits of the procedure

WHAT TO DO

Consent should be obtained before every surgery, procedure, initial blood product transfusion, or administration of medication which your institution has deemed to be potentially harmful requiring informed consent, for example, tPA for ischemic stroke.

Exceptions are emergent situations in which there are no available family members or health care professionals (HCPs) to consent on behalf of the patient and the patient's life is in immediate danger. In this case, consent is assumed owing to the urgent nature of the condition. Another exception occurs when the patient does not have the capacity to make a reasonable decision regarding his or her medical treatments and no HCPs are assigned or available. This situation will typically require two physicians to give consent on behalf of the patient in an emergent situation. If the condition is less life threatening, then a judge may become involved to assign a court-appointed guardian to consent for the patient.

Most people will agree that one of the most important parts of obtaining informed consent is to use simple terminology or layman's terms. Poor health literacy is very common in our society, and the majority of patients will not understand the consent if medical jargon is used. That is not to say medical terms should not appear on the final consent form, but the meanings of those terms should be described with the appropriate language. For example, the majority of patients will not know what an exploratory laparotomy is, but if you explain that it is an exploratory abdominal surgery via an incision at the middle of the abdomen, it would be more clear.

For non-English speaking patients, always obtain consent with the aid of an official medical translator. Avoid using family members or friends to translate the consent process, as they may not convey important information and details in order to achieve appropriate consent. Medical translators are often physically available in the hospital or via telephone systems that many institutions have established.

When obtaining consents over the phone, always have a witness speak to the person authorizing consent to confirm informed consent has been obtained by asking what procedure is being consented for and what the purpose of the treatment is. This witness should provide their signature and name on the consent form in addition to the primary consenter.

Finally, begin the discussion of the indications, alternatives, risks and benefits, recovery, and post-op care with your patients early. You do not want to hold up the operating room schedule because a patient has questions about the procedure and post-op care, which could have been answered earlier.

RISKS SPECIFIC TO COMMON SURGERIES LIKELY TO BE ENCOUNTERED DURING PGY-1 AND 2

Risks common to all surgical procedures include pain, bleeding, infection, allergic reaction, damage to surrounding tissues or structures, and death.

CENTRAL LINES

Pneumothorax, failure of implanted device (immediately or at a later date) requiring additional procedures, injury to blood vessels, embolism, arrhythmias.

CHEST TUBE PLACEMENT

Damage to nerves, injury to lung, need for additional procedures including additional tube placement and/or surgery, including thoracoscopy or thoracotomy.

LAPAROSCOPIC APPENDECTOMY WITH POSSIBLE CONVERSION TO OPEN

Resection of additional bowel, damage to bowel or nearby structures, placement of drains, difficulty with urination.

LAPAROSCOPIC CHOLECYSTECTOMY WITH POSSIBLE CONVERSION TO OPEN, POSSIBLE INTRAOPERATIVE CHOLANGIOGRAM, POSSIBLE COMMON DUCT EXPLORATION

Retained stones in bile ducts, injury to biliary ducts or vessels requiring additional surgery, injury to bowel.

INGUINAL HERNIA (LAPAROSCOPIC AND/OR OPEN)

Hematoma; seroma; mesh infection; difficulty urinating; injury to the spermatic cord resulting in loss of testicle or infertility (when applicable); injury to nerves causing prolonged pain or numbness in the groin, leg, and genital area; injury to bowel or bladder.

 PEARLS

1. Use simple terminology or layman's terms. The majority of patients will not understand the consent if medical jargon is used.
2. Be sure to include in your discussion the indications, alternatives, risks and benefits, recovery, and post-op care with your patients.
3. For non-English speaking patients, unless you are fluent in the patient's primary language, you must employ the aid of a translator (in person, or, remotely via phone/tablet) while obtaining surgical consent.

Suggested Readings

1. Childers R, Lipsett PA, Pawlik TM. Informed consent and the surgeon. *J Am Coll Surg.* 2009;208(4):627-634.
2. Angelos P. The evolution of informed consent for surgery using the best case/worst case framework. *JAMA Surg.* 2017;152(6):538-539.

37

PATIENT POSITIONING IN THE OPERATING ROOM

MOJDEH S. KAPPUS, MD | SOUHEIL W. ADRA, MD, FACS, FASMBS

Once your patient has entered the operating room, many steps must be taken to ensure the patient's safety. This includes confirming the patient's identity and the surgical procedure to be performed, positioning the patient and ensuring they are secured to the operating room table, taking measures to prevent infections and venous thromboembolism, initiating hemodynamic monitoring of the patient, and maintaining the sterility and counts of the operating tools and equipment. With the combined efforts of the anesthesiology team, surgical technician, circulating nurse, surgeon, and trainees this process may appear to occur in a quick and seamless fashion; however, these steps are critical and must be performed carefully.

As the anesthesiology team will be taking important steps to monitor the patient and obtain intravenous access and the surgical technician will be working to ensure that the sterile field remains sterile, the appropriate instruments are available, and that their counts are correct, it is important to listen carefully to the instructions of these medical providers to avoid errors or injury to the patient. While these medical professionals are at work, the surgeon and trainees will simultaneously begin the process of securing the patient to the operating room table with a safety belt, positioning and padding the patient, placing intermittent pneumatic compression devices on the patients extremities, and placing a Foley catheter when indicated, which usually occurs after the intubation of the patient.

INDICATIONS

PATIENT TRANSFER AND POSITIONING

Proper patient positioning allows the surgeon to have optimal exposure of the intended surgical field, it ensures that pressure points along the patient's body are appropriately padded to avoid injury, it allows for quick access by the anesthesiologist to the patient's airway and intravenous lines, and it ensures that the patient is securely fastened to the operating room table. The process of positioning the patient first begins with transferring the patient to the operating room table. This should be done in a manner that is safe for the patient and the surgical staff involved.

STEPS

PATIENT TRANSFER AND POSITIONING

1. *Supplies:*
   a. Hydraulic lift, roller board
   b. Padding (foam pads, gel pads, rolled sheets, blankets)
   c. Safety strap
   d. Draw sheet
2. *Preparation:* A draw sheet should be placed on the operating room table before the patient is transferred onto it. This will allow for the patient to be moved more easily after induction of general anesthesia.
3. *Transferring the patient:*
   a. Patients who are capable of transferring themselves from stretcher to operating room table without causing pain or significant bodily stress may be asked to do so. Before the patient begins transfer, ensure that his or her gown is unfastened in the back, the operating room table and

stretcher are locked and adjacent to each other without a gap or height difference between them, and there is a person standing at both sides of the patient.

b. If the patient is unable to transfer on his or her own, a roller board may be used to easily and ergonomically transfer the patient. The anesthesiology team member will direct the move and support the head of the patient. This is particularly important in a sedated or intubated patient with multiple monitors and intravenous lines. The anesthesia team member overseeing the move will loudly count and allow the move once the head of the patient is supported and all tubes and lines are protected. Once again, one person should stand at either side of the patient and both the operating room table and stretcher must be locked. With the lateral safety bar of the stretcher up and locked, the patient should be rolled toward the surgical staff member standing near the "stretcher side" of the patient. The other team member standing near the "operating room table side" of the patient will then place a roller board wrapped with a draw sheet under the patient's back. The patient will then be returned to supine position now overlying the roller board. The surgical staff standing on the "operating room table side" of the patient will pull the draw sheet, while the opposite side staff members will gently push the patient onto the operating room table. A fourth team member is usually needed to carry the patient's legs during the transfer. The patient is then rolled toward the "operating room table side" staff member while the opposite staff member removes the roller board. If a roller board is not available, a large piece of plastic, such as a large waste bag may be used.

c. A pneumatic air mattress is sometimes used as available in the morbidly obese patients, to prevent injuries to the staff moving the patient. Similar to the method by which the roller board is placed under the patient, a pneumatic device can be rolled behind the patient. Then with the patient rolled over to the operating room bedside, the pneumatic air mattress is unrolled. The multiple straps are then secured over the patient's trunk and lower extremities. Again, the anesthesiology team member clears the move before inflating the mattress. Great care must be taken in moving the mattress once inflated as it will move far too easily potentially overshooting and injuring the patient. Once the position is deemed appropriate by the anesthesiologist, the mattress is deflated and the straps undone before securing the patient to the table per routine.

d. A hydraulic lift may also be used to transfer the patient. Similar to the method by which the roller board is placed under the patient, a sling is unrolled under the patient as the patient is shifted from one side to the other. The sling is then attached to a hydraulic lift device, which can then be used to lift the patient off of the stretcher and then lower the patient on to the operating room table.

4. *Positioning for anesthesia:* If the patient will undergo a procedure without general anesthesia, then the patient will be positioned for surgery immediately (as detailed later). More often, the patient will be placed in supine position for induction of general anesthesia and to secure the airway. Someone must stand at each side of the patient lying in the supine position, until they have been secured to the table with a safety strap. At this point, the surgical staff may step away from the patient to remove the stretcher from the operating room. Safety straps may differ at various institutions but generally may be secured by wrapping the strap around the operating room table rails and over the upper thighs of the patient and securing it in place. The strap should fit snugly against the patient but with room for two fingerbreadths underneath. The strap should not be so tight so as to cause discomfort to the patient. A blanket should be placed over the patient's body before the safety strap is placed for modesty and comfort. Foam padding under the strap may also be used. Of note, the patient may be positioned on a wedge or a ramp made of blankets to facilitate intubation position if a difficult airway is anticipated, especially in morbidly obese patients. This wedge is usually removed after the airway is secured, under the supervision of anesthesiology who will secure the airway and support the head. A pillow may be placed under the knees to gently flex them, which may be helpful in patients with back pain.

5. *Placement of intermittent pneumatic compressions devices:* Patients undergoing surgical procedures are at increased risk of venous thromboembolism. This risk is augmented by numerous surgical and patient-specific factors. The majority of adult patients and some pediatric patients will require placement of intermittent pneumatic compression devices (IPC). IPC devices used on the calves augment the velocity of blood flow in the femoral veins and stimulate the release of endogenous fibrinolytic factors to prevent venous thromboembolism.

6. *Placement of Foley catheter:* Placement of a Foley catheter may be indicated for a select group of patients depending on the type of surgical procedure they are undergoing, duration of surgery, need for intraoperative monitoring of urine output or in patients anticipated to receive large-volume infusions or diuretics (Centers for Medicare & Medicaid Services guidelines). Foley catheters should not be placed in patients who do not meet appropriate indications, as this may predispose them to the development of catheter-associated urinary tract infections. If the catheter is needed only for the procedure, it should be removed at the end of the procedure if possible.

7. *Positioning for surgery:* After induction of general anesthesia and securing the airway, the patient may be repositioned depending on the surgical procedure to be performed. This should be initiated only after checking with the anesthesia team, as they need to guide this team effort while supporting the head and protecting the airway and lines. Care should be taken to protect pressure points with padding to prevent injury to the patient. The patient may be propped up on their side using rolled sheets, padding or a "beanbag." Various types of stirrups and footboards may also be employed to secure the lower extremities for a patient being placed in steep reverse Trendelenburg or lithotomy position, respectively. Either or both of the upper extremities may be tucked at the side of the patient using the draw sheet and foam padding to protect the patient from neurovascular injury. The most commonly used patient positioning techniques are listed in Figure 37.1.

PLACEMENT OF INTERMITTENT PNEUMATIC COMPRESSIONS DEVICES

1. Supplies
   a. Intermittent pneumatic compression machine
   b. Connection tubing
   c. Intermittent pneumatic compression calf wrap
2. Inform the patient that you will be placing an intermittent pneumatic compression device to help prevent the formation of deep venous thrombosis (DVT) during surgery. Inform the patient that they should not feel any pain from the IPC and may liken it to a "leg massage." IPC should be initiated as soon as possible even before induction of anesthesia.
3. Examine the patient's calves for any open wounds or injuries. Ask the patient if they have a history of recent DVT in the lower extremities. An acute DVT or open wound are contraindications to placement of an IPC on the affected extremity; contralateral leg placement of IPC should be performed.
4. Gently lift the patient's calf, and slide the wrapping underneath.
5. Lower the patient's calf down over the wrapping and secure the wrap around the calf just above the medial malleolus inferiorly and below the tibial tuberosity superiorly. Secure the wrap with Velcro attachments. The wrap should fit snuggly against the patient but with room for two finger-breadths underneath. The wrap should not be so tight so as to cause pain to the patient.
6. Once both calves have been individually wrapped, connection tubing may be used to connect the leg wrap to the IPC machine.

Position	Description	Pressure Points
Supine	The patient lies on their back, facing upward.	Occiput, scapula, thoracic spine, sacrum, coccyx, calcaneus,. 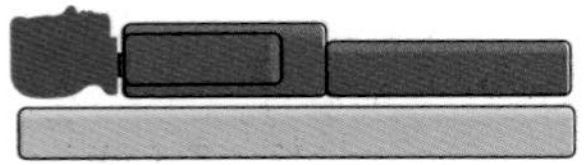
Prone	The patient lies facing downward.	Facial structures, chest, iliac crest, breasts, genitalia, knees, feet. *Place a rolled blanket under the shoulders to prevent cervical hyperextension and decrease chest compression. 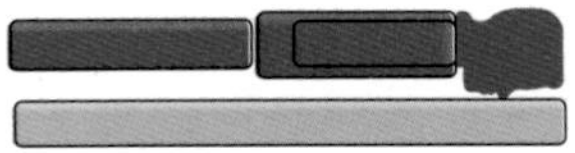
Jackknife	Prone position with patient and operating room table flexed at the waist.	Facial structures, chest, iliac crest, breasts, genitalia, knees, feet. 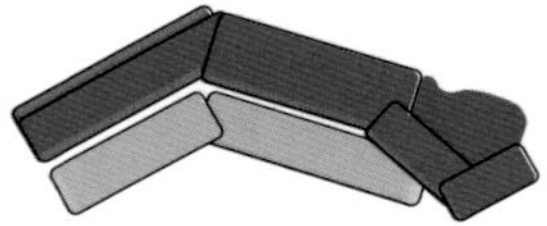
Lateral	The patient lies to one side with lower leg flexed at hip and upper leg straight with padding between.	Lateral bony prominences *Place an axillary roll under the dependent axilla to prevent compression and injury of the brachial plexus 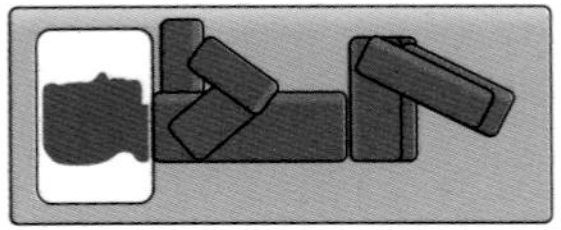
Lithotomy	Supine position with legs suspended in stirrups at an even height with minimal rotation of the hips, and 90 degree flexion at the knee	Hips, knees, common peroneal nerve, arthritic or artificial joints *Ensure that the stirrups are not so far elevated that the patient's lower extremity weight is being suspended from the knees 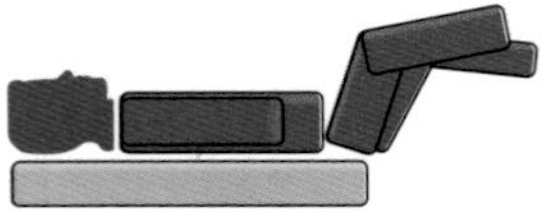

FIGURE 37.1 Commonly used patient positioning techniques (Courtesy of Safa Lohrasbi, DO).

7. Ensure that the IPC machine is plugged into a power outlet and is turned on.
8. You may check to ensure that the IPC machine is working by gently placing your hands over the leg wraps to ensure that they are inflating bilaterally.

COMPLICATIONS

Improper patient positioning and padding may result in neurologic injuries, especially to the extremities. Lithotomy position may result in temporary or permanent injury to the common peroneal, sciatic, or femoral nerve. Hyperextension of the arms may result in ulnar nerve or brachial plexus injuries.

 PEARLS

1. Before performing any procedure in the operating room, introduce yourself to the circulating nurse, surgical technician, anesthesiologist, and surgeon, and inform them of the procedure you wish to perform.
2. Always inform the patient of the steps you are taking (eg, safety strap placement, IPC placement) before you proceed. Make sure to the turn the intermittent pneumatic compression device on after you have finished attaching it before the patient is induced for anesthesia.
3. Always ensure the patient is secured to the operating room table before leaving the patient's bedside to prevent fall injuries to the patient.

Suggested Readings

1. Gould MK, Garcia DA, Wren SM, et al. Prevention of VTE in nonorthopedic surgical patients. Antithrombotic therapy and prevention of thrombosis. In: 9th ed. American college of chest physicians evidence-based clinical practice guidelines. *Chest.* 2012:141(2);e227S-E277S.
2. Ramanathan R, Duane TM. Urinary tract infections in surgical patients. *Surg Clin.* 2014:94(6);135101368.

38

AIRWAY MANAGEMENT AND INTUBATION

BIJAN J. TEJA, MD, MBA | CINDY M. KU, MD | STEPHANIE B. JONES, MD

Although the first thing that usually comes to mind when people think about emergency airway situations is intubation or cricothyroidotomy, perhaps the skill that is most commonly lifesaving is the ability to bag mask ventilate. Particularly in community hospitals, where a person with airway expertise is sometimes not immediately available, patients in the recovery area or other locations who have become hypoxic or hypercarbic have been resuscitated by surgical residents using bag mask ventilation. Most patients can be successfully bag masked for as long as needed until help arrives. It is therefore critical for you to develop the ability to mask ventilate early in your training.

You may also be asked to perform intubations, particularly during your critical care rotations. As you become more senior, you may have the opportunity to perform emergency cricothyroidotomies when intubation, bag mask ventilation, and placement of a laryngeal mask airway (often used as a rescue device) all fail. Surgical airways are discussed in more detail in the cricothyroidotomy chapter.

INDICATIONS

The most common indications for intubation are:

- Hypoxia
- Hypercarbia (if severe enough to cause altered mental status)
- Inability to protect the airway (rule of thumb: Glasgow coma score ≤8, although this is certainly not a definitive rule)
- To perform procedures
- Hemodynamic instability is sometimes cited; however, just because a patient is on pressors does not mean he or she needs to be intubated

STEPS

FOR BAG MASK VENTILATION IN AN EMERGENCY SITUATION

1. Call for help.
2. Connect the bag mask to an oxygen source, and turn the oxygen flow up to 10 to 15 L/min.
3. Obtain a tight seal with the mask. Lift the angle of the jaw with your third, fourth, and fifth fingers in an E shape while holding the mask with your thumb and index finger in a C shape (Figures 38.1 and 38.2).
4. Squeeze the bag with your other hand.
5. Look for fogging of the mask and chest rise (and improvement in oxygenation if the indication for bag mask ventilation was hypoxia).
6. If you do not have a good seal, reposition or use two hands to bag mask while someone else squeezes the bag (two-hand mask technique)

   Predictors of difficult mask ventilation: Presence of a beard, body mass index>26 kg/m², lack of teeth, age >55 years, history of snoring.

FOR INTUBATION

If nonemergent, perform an airway evaluation, including Mallampati classification (Figure 38.3), dental assessment (prominent, loose, or chipped teeth), mouth opening, and neck range of motion at the very least. You should also check prior intubation notes to find out if the patient had a difficult airway in the past. Finally, you can check mandibular protrusion, thyromental distance, and hyomental distance.

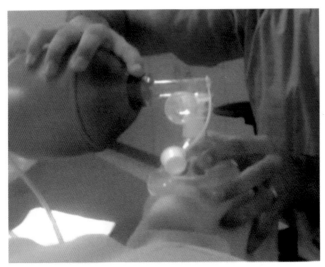

FIGURE 38.1 One-hand bag mask ventilation: The third, fourth, and fifth fingers lift the angle of the jaw into the mask, and the thumb and index finger hold the mask over the mouth and nose to create a good seal.

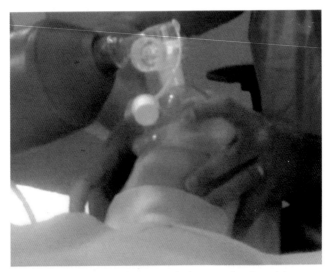

FIGURE 38.2 Two-hand mask ventilation: used when one-hand mask is unsuccessful and a second operator is available to squeeze the bag. For the second hand (right hand), the thumb and part of the palm can be used to push the mask down and obtain a tight seal, while most of the force is used to lift the angle of the jaw into the mask (this allows the soft tissue of the mouth to be pulled up and away from the airway, assisting with ventilation).

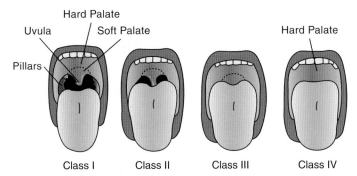

FIGURE 38.3 Mallampati classification for predicting difficult intubation. (Reprinted with permission from Diepenbrock N. Quick Reference to Critical Care. 4th ed. Philadelphia: Lippincott Williams & Wilkins; 2012.)

Predictors of difficult intubation: High Mallampati score, short neck, receding mandible, prominent maxillary incisors, history of difficult intubation.

Steps for Intubation

Options for placing an endotracheal tube include standard direct laryngoscopy and video laryngoscopy and fiberoptic intubation for more difficult cases. An overview of direct laryngoscopy technique with a Macintosh (Mac) blade is provided:

1. Prepare your equipment (commonly used mnemonic: SOAP-M):
    a. Suction at the head of the bed in case the patient vomits
    b. Oxygen source for bag mask at 10 to 15 L/min
    c. Airway equipment (including backup equipment such as videolaryngoscope if needed)
    d. Pharmacy: ie, drugs for intubation (see later text)
    e. Monitors, including turning the sound on the monitor so you can hear if desaturation occurs, and checking the blood pressure (BP)—if it is low, ideally start a vasopressor infusion or give a bolus BEFORE you push drugs to prevent cardiac arrest (most drugs for intubation cause decreased cardiac output and decreased afterload). Also, set the BP measure frequently if no arterial line
2. Adjust bed height so that the patient's face is at the level of your xiphoid cartilage.

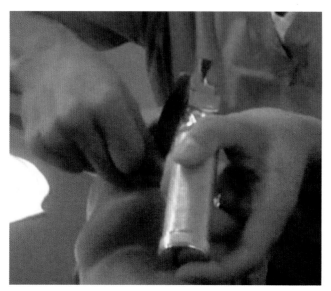

FIGURE 38.4 Opening the mouth using counter pressure of the right thumb on the mandibular teeth and right index finger on the maxillary teeth and insertion of laryngoscope with the left hand.

3. Extend head (assuming no c-spine pathology) once induced. This often opens the mouth.
4. If mouth does not open adequately with head extension, manually open it using counter pressure of the right thumb on the mandibular teeth and right index finger on the maxillary teeth (Figure 38.4).
5. Insert the blade with your left hand just right of midline (Figure 38.5). You may need to roll the lip away with your left index finger to prevent bruising if it gets caught under the blade with insertion.
6. Deflect the tongue to the left as you advance the blade toward the epiglottis. Your blade should advance to the base of the tongue, just shy of the epiglottis, to allow you to bring the epiglottis up and expose the vocal cords.
7. Lift along the axis of the handle to bring the laryngeal structures into view (Figure 38.5). Do NOT use the blade as a lever (pull the handle up with a rigid wrist, rather than rotating the blade with the patient's teeth as a fulcrum—rocking the blade on the patient's teeth can cause injury).
8. Hold the endotracheal tube in your right hand like a pencil. Advance it gently along the right side of the mouth to avoid obscuring your view (Figure 38.6).

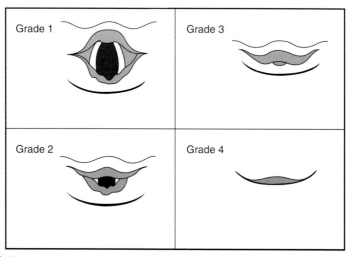

FIGURE 38.5 Cormack and Lehane classification to describe the quality of the view on laryngoscopy. (Reprinted with permission from Wolfson, AB. Cloutier RL, Hendey GW, Ling LJ, Schaider JJ, Rosen CL. Harwood-Nuss' Clinical Practice of Emergency Medicine, 6th ed. Philadelphia: Wolters Kluwer Health, 2014. Fig 1.1.)

9. Once the proximal end of the balloon cuff is 1 to 2 cm past the vocal cords, remove the laryngoscope.
10. Inflate the cuff with the minimum volume required to prevent a leak of positive pressure, usually ~25 cm H_2O (overinflation can cause mucosal ischemia of the tracheal wall).
11. Check for correct placement using end-tidal CO_2 (either color change monitor or quantitative waveform monitor).

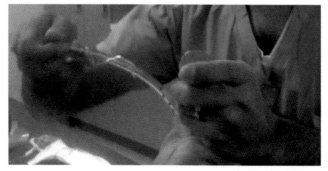

FIGURE 38.6 Insertion of endotracheal tube gently with the right hand.

COMMONLY USED MEDICATIONS FOR INTUBATION

Propofol: Most popular agent. Facilitates binding of gamma-aminobutyric acid (GABA) to its receptor, among other effects. Very rapid onset. Single dose effect terminates within minutes because of rapid redistribution. Disadvantage is hypotension due to drop in systemic vascular resistance (SVR), preload, and contractility. Safe in chronic kidney disease and cirrhosis. Often avoided in patients with severe coronary artery disease or cardiac valvular disease due to hypotension. If you use this medication to intubate a patient in the intensive care unit (ICU), be sure to have phenylephrine boluses ready to counteract hypotension.

Etomidate: Mimics GABA. Advantage over propofol is that cardiac output, contractility, and SVR are well maintained. Disadvantage in critically ill patients is adrenal suppression, but this is usually only an issue when this medication was used as an infusion in the ICU.

Ketamine: N-methyl-D-aspartate antagonist. Advantage is preserved respiratory drive. Your patient will often continue to breathe spontaneously with this drug, and blood pressure will not usually drop as significantly, which make it a popular choice for intubation in the critically ill at many centers. Large boluses avoided in patients with cardiac disease because of increases in systolic blood pressure, heart rate, and cardiac output. Also causes disturbing dreams and delirium; risk of this reduced by co-administration of low doses of benzodiazepines (1-2 mg of midazolam, for example).

Fast-acting opioids are also sometimes used as adjuncts.

COMMONLY USED NEUROMUSCULAR BLOCKING AGENTS (TO OPTIMIZE INTUBATING CONDITIONS)

Succinylcholine: Consists of two joined acetylcholine (ACh) molecules, which depolarize the muscle by binding the ACh receptor. Rapid onset (30-60 seconds) and rapid metabolism by serum pseudocholinesterase (duration <10 minutes). Raises serum potassium by 0.5 in healthy patients. Contraindicated in patients with hyperkalemia, burn injuries, massive trauma, many neurologic disorders, and myopathies and children/adolescents (risk of undiagnosed myopathy), because of risk of life-threatening potassium elevation in these patients.

Rocuronium: Nondepolarizing agent; ACh receptor antagonist that prevents muscle depolarization. Rapid onset (dose dependent, 1-3 minutes), duration 20 to 35 minutes, or longer in patients with renal failure.

PEARLS

1. Make sure you know how to bag mask ventilate. It is often life saving until help arrives.
2. If you do not have a good view with laryngoscopy, do not try to intubate blindly or force an endotracheal tube past resistance. This creates swelling and will make subsequent attempts more difficult.
3. If an intubation is urgent but not emergent, try to let the family know beforehand that their loved one is being intubated. You can mention to the family that it may be some time before they will be able to speak with their loved one again. You will be happy you gave their family a chance to speak with them before the endotracheal tube was placed.

Suggested Reading

1. Jones D. *Pocket Surgery*. 2nd ed. Philadelphia: Lippincott Williams & Wilkins; October 2017.
2. Airway management. In: Butterworth IV JF, Mackey DC, Wasnick JD, eds. *Morgan & Mikhail's Clinical Anesthesiology*. 6th ed. New York, NY: McGraw-Hill. http://accessmedicine.mhmedical.com/content.aspx?bookid=2444&sectionid=193559024. Accessed July 29, 2019.

39

SURGICAL PREPPING AND DRAPING

DEBRA J. SAVAGE, MSN, RN, CNOR | KORTNEY ROBINSON, MD, MPH

INTRODUCTION

Prepping and draping is fundamental to positive outcomes in surgical procedures. Across different specialties, the way in which prepping and draping
are completed varies. However, the primary purpose behind prepping and
draping is to reduce postoperative infections. Surgical prepping decreases the
amount of transient bacteria and resident microorganisms on the patient's
skin and therefore decreases the risk of a surgical site infection. Transient
bacteria are limited to the exposed areas of the skin and are easily removed
by mechanical cleansing. Resident microorganisms inhabit deep structures of
the dermis and the hair follicles. Resident bacteria require chemical agents to
eliminate them and prevent their regrowth for a period of time. The goal of
the surgical skin prep is to remove soil and transient microorganisms of the
skin and reduce the resident bacteria count below pathological levels. Prep
must be completed in a time-efficient manner with the least possible tissue
irritation.[1]

BASIC SUPPLIES

- Surgical scrub
- Clippers
- Sterile gloves
- Prep solution
- Time and patience
- Towels and drapes

TIMELINE OF PREPPING

NIGHT BEFORE SURGERY

- For elective cases, the Centers for Disease Control and Prevention recommends that the patient bathe the night before surgery.[2] Often the patient is given a solution with chlorhexidine gluconate to use in the shower or bath the night before surgery while utilizing clean towels and wearing clean garments.

MORNING OF SURGERY

- For elective cases, the patient should repeat/complete a shower with the surgical scrub as earlier.[1]

HAIR REMOVAL

- Remove hair only when necessary (ie, if it will interfere with the procedure). If possible, complete this in the preoperative area and not in the operating room (OR) itself.
- Use clippers only (not razors).
  - Exceptions (urology and neurosurgery where clippers are not safe or will not get the hair short enough).

PREPPING

- Begin at the site of the incision, use friction and scrub in a back and forth or circular motion depending on antimicrobial used. Proceed circumferentially outward. For example, do not drag microbes from the groin area to the umbilical region for a laparotomy.

■ Choose a prep based on surgery, site, patient allergies, and surgeon preference.
■ See details of prep agents in the following text.

ANTIMICROBIAL PROPERTIES OF SURGICAL PREP AGENTS

■ **Broad spectrum:** kills a wide range of microorganisms
■ **High log reduction capability:** has the ability to decrease microbial colonies by a log of 1 (a 10-fold reductionism colonies), a log of 2 (a 100-fold reduction), a log of 3 (a 1000-fold reduction), and so on
■ **Persistency:** maintains its effectiveness over a long period of time
■ **Nonirritating:** causes the least amount of tissue irritation
■ **Nontoxic:** is safe for use on the skin and other superficial tissues
■ **Fast acting:** acts rapidly and is totally effective with the first application

MOST COMMONLY USED ANTIMICROBIAL AGENTS AND PREPPING PROCEDURES

POVIDONE-IODINE

■ Pros: Can be used on open wounds and mucous membranes (ie, urogenital tract).
■ Cons: Povidone-iodine (commonly known as betadine) kills when it dries; therefore, you must wait till the area is dry! Persistence is not high.
■ With povidone-iodine preps, begin at the incision site and use friction and scrub in a circular motion, moving away from the site in all directions. This directs any contaminants away from the critical area.
■ For a two-stage prep, one starts with a soap. After scrubbing the area, lay a towel over the area to soak up the excess, pat dry, and then remove the towel by grasping the edge furthest away from you and removing it toward you. Then paint the area using the povidone-iodine paint sticks using an outward circular motion, starting at the incision site.
■ One-stage prep: paint only, prep as earlier.

CHLORHEXIDINE GLUCONATE (WITH OR WITHOUT ALCOHOL)

- Pros: Chlorhexidine gluconate (CHG)-containing products continue to kill bacteria for ~48 hours after it dries (high persistence). It also has a high log reduction.
- Cons: CHG can trigger allergic reactions and should not be used on open wounds or mucous membranes, above the neck, in the ear, or in the eye. It can cause corneal damage and is toxic to the auditory ear canal.
- These products are most often prepackaged with an ampule of solution in the "stick" of the applicator. They can also be packaged in a single-use bottle for scrub only (without alcohol). When using the premixed CHG with ETOH solution (contained in glass ampule inside the applicator), crush the ampule using a squeezing motion then allow gravity to work (the pad will become saturated with the solution). Once the pad is wet, paint the patient using the pad while holding the handle of the applicator. First scrub the incision site for about 30 seconds and then the rest of the surgical area. You may prep the area in any direction.

ALCOHOLS

Alcohols are often used in combination with another chemical (ie, iodine povacrylex and alcohol or 2% CHG and alcohol).

- Pros: Provide the quickest reduction in bacterial counts.
- Cons: Must dry a minimum of 3 minutes; 1 hour if used on hair. This is owing to fire risk.[1] Have no persistent chemical effect unless used in combination with CHG.
- When alcohol-based skin preps are utilized, minimizing fire risk is the responsibility of the team.
  - Clip hair at surgical site before applying prep.
  - Prevent pooling, soaking into linens or patient's hair.
  - Use sterile towels to absorb drips and excess solution.
  - Remove saturated materials before draping the patient.
- *Follow manufacturer guidelines for drying time.*

ST-37

- Pros: Less irritating.
- Cons: Not as effective as the previously described products.

- ST-37 is an antiseptic that is used when the patient is allergic to the other prep solutions.
- Start prepping with your incision site and work your way out.

SALINE

- Pros: Not irritating.
- Cons: Least effective.
- Saline is used as a last resort only when it is impossible to use one of the more effective prep solutions.
- Start prepping with the incision site and work your way out.

PREPPING PROCEDURE

DETERMINE THE AREA TO BE PREPPED AND THEN EXPOSE THAT AREA

- The prep area should extend at least 6 to 8 inches in all directions beyond the planned incision site.
- The size of the prepped area needs to be large enough to accommodate extensions of the incision, additional incisions, and all potential drain sites. Think of the laparoscopic appendectomy (midline and left-sided incisions) that may require conversion to open (right-sided incision).
- The prepped site also needs to be large enough to avoid wound contamination by inadvertent drape movements during the procedure.
- Utilize towels or absorbent material to prevent dripping.

PERFORMING SKIN PREPS FOR EXTREMITIES WITH TOURNIQUET USAGE

- Seal off the tourniquet with an impervious drape.
- Begin at the incision site and scrub away from the incision site circumferentially.
- Hand and foot preps begin at incision site, including the fingers or toes, and moving up the extremity.
- It is more effective (measured by bacterial counts) to clean the foot before beginning the antiseptic skin preparation for surgery, than with prep alone.[1]

SURGICAL HAND SCRUB

- While the prep is drying, complete your surgical hand scrub (please see Chapter 41 on Scrubbing, Gloving, and Gowning).

DRAPING

RATIONALE AND PROCESS BEHIND DRAPING

- Draping provides a barrier between the sterile field and the surrounding area.
- The sterile field consists of the patient, the operating room bed, the instrument table, the mayo stand, and any other equipment necessary for the surgical procedure (ie, microscope, C-arm).
- Drapes provide a barrier to prevent migration of microorganisms.
- Drapes are resistant to tearing, puncturing, or abrasion.
- Drapes are antistatic, nonallergenic, dull, and nonglaring to minimize distortions under OR lights.

DRAPE CHARACTERISTICS

- Most facilities utilize disposable drapes because of their characteristics such as softness, lint free, light weight, compact, moisture resistant, nonirritating, and static free. They also have the ability to retard "strike through," which can prevent contamination.
- Drapes include towels, fenestrated sheets, nonfenestrated sheets, and plastic drapes.
- There are several types of drapes:
  - **Laparotomy sheet or universal drape**—used for abdominal area
  - **Thyroid sheet**—used for the neck area
  - **Breast sheet**—used for chest or breast areas
  - **Extremity sheet**—covering the patient's extremity (arm or leg), which may also cover arm boards, arm table, or other equipment that is utilized in the surgical procedure
  - **Laparoscopy sheet with leggings (including perineal opening)**— utilized for laparoscopic gynecologic, urological, or colorectal cases
  - **Split sheet**—can be used for extremities or difficult draping situations where other drapes do not conform to the surgical area
  - **Half sheets, table covers, plastic drape, and various equipment drapes**—used to drape tables, arm boards, C-arms, x-ray machines, microscopes, and robotic equipment and to prevent contamination of the surgical areas if needed.

DRAPING PROCEDURE

The draping process is a team effort; your scrub nurse or surgical technologist will assist with the draping by organizing the drapes in the order of use, handling of drapes to prevent contamination, and assisting the team with the draping procedure.

- Drape from the operative site to the periphery starting with towels (1-5 depending on area to be draped).
- Drape from the sterile area to the unsterile area by draping the closest area first.
- When draping the opposite side, the scrubbed person should walk around the OR bed to drape or hand-off of the drape to the sterile team member.
- Remove plastic strips to expose the sticky area and carefully place those down on the sterile field where you want them.
- Follow pictorial directions on the drapes (arrows or sticklike figures).
- When draping and passing the sterile drape to a nonsterile person to secure to the IV pole (ie, anesthesia or circulating nurse), one should cuff the drape over their gloved hand to prevent contamination of sterile gloved hand.

 PEARLS

1. Prep wide enough to accommodate extension of surgical incisions or conversion to open procedure. Place towels or other absorbable material on the sides of the patient to collect spillage. Remove these before draping. If prep pools under a patient, it can give the patient a chemical burn and/or be a fire hazard.
2. It is always a good idea to follow manufacturers' guidelines for details on prepping with various preps.
3. The sterile area of the surgical team goes from 2 inches below the neck to the waist, so falling above or below that is no longer considered sterile (this is true even for your hands)!

References

1. AORN. Association of perioperative Registered Nurses. *Facility Reference Center.* Denver, CO: AORN, Inc. 2018. Available at https://aornguidelines.org/glance/filter?gboscontainerid=162. Accessed July 22, 2018.
2. Berríos-Torres SI, Umscheid CA, Bratzler DW, et al. Centers for disease control and prevention guideline for the prevention of surgical site infection, 2017. *JAMA Surgery.* 2017;152(8):784. doi:10.1001/jamasurg.2017.0904.

40

SCRUBBING, GOWNING, AND GLOVING

KIRSTEN DANSEY, MD | HEIDEE ALBANO, BSN, RN, CNOR

SURGICAL SCRUBBING

The next step after the patient has been positioned and prepped is scrubbing. A couple of key things to keep in mind before scrubbing:

- Wear the proper attire that covers all your hair, including beard and mustache.
- Give your gloves to the tech before scrubbing.
- Leave jewelry, beepers, and cell phones on the counter before scrubbing.

There are sinks outside of the operating room where there is usually an alcohol-based scrub, which does not require water, or scrub brushes with chlorhexidine gluconate or povidone iodine. More traditional surgeons will often scrub their hands with the aqueous-based scrubs for the first operation of the day. With the aqueous based scrubs, you should open the packet before you wet your hands, as it becomes difficult to open with wet hands. Follow these steps:

1. Open the sponge/scrub packet.
2. Use the plastic nail cleaner to clean under your nails.
3. Wet the brush and use the side with the bristles to clean your nails again.
4. Use the sponge side to clean every portion of your hand. You start with fingers, making sure to clean between each digit (add in each side of the finger should be scrubbed), move to the palm then to the dorsum of the hand, then divide your forearm into four sections. Scrub each section, and then repeat with the other hand. You should scrub for at least 3 minutes.
5. When rinsing take care not to touch anything inadvertently, and if you do, then rescrub. Let water rinse down from your fingers to the elbows.

When using the alcohol-based hand antiseptic, follow the specific directions given on the box. Before doing so, make sure to use freestanding plastic nail cleaners to clean under your nails before starting to scrub with the alcohol solution.

1. Spray the alcohol onto your palm, then use the other hand to clean the nails.
2. Let the solution spray onto your palm and distribute over your hand, between your fingers, and forearms.
3. Let dry.

GOWNING

You will then go into the operating room where the scrub tech will ask you, "Wet or dry?" Usually the aqueous-based solutions will need you to dry your hands, do not let the towel touch your scrubs. You will usually have to bend at the hips slightly with your arms out. Use the towel to dry your hands. If you used the alcohol-based solution, then you need to let it dry before you start gowning.

The scrub tech will usually open the gown and you will walk into the gown with your arms pointing forward aimed into the arm holes. Make sure your arms come out such that the gown cuffs do not rise beyond your wrists. Keeping your arms in the sterile area, do not let your hands fall at your side and prepare to receive your gloves from the scrub technician.

While you are doing the above, the circulating nurse will Velcro-secure and tie your gown behind you. You will then be gloved (see next section).

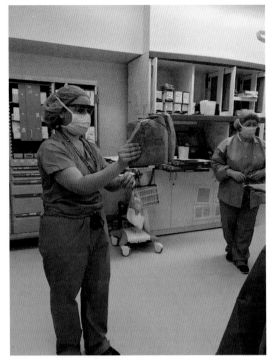

Gowning 1 - Accepting gown

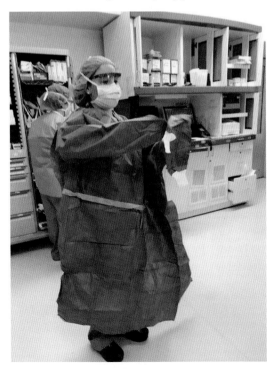

Gowning 2 - Insert arms to gown

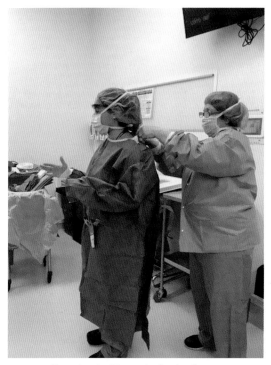

Gowning 3 - Nurse ties back of gown

After you are gloved, there is a final waistbelt that you will need assistance with. Hold the two ties in each hand, release the left tie from the paper tab, continuing to hold the paper tab with the right hand. Hand off the paper tab to the scrub tech. Spin to the left. Release the remaining tie off the cardboard tab, and tie the two ends together.

GLOVING

The surgical scrub will help you glove. They usually start with the right hand, and you insert your hand into the open glove then repeat with the left. If you need to glove yourself then you will put the side where your thumb is on your forearm. Open the glove with the white cloth cuff of the surgical gown and flip the glove onto the hand. The scrubs will not let you glove and gown yourself until you are comfortable doing so.

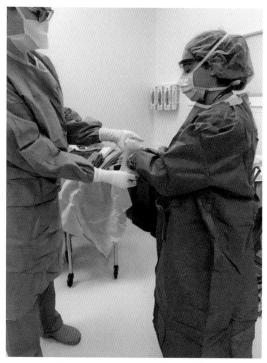

Gloving 4 - Insert hand into glove

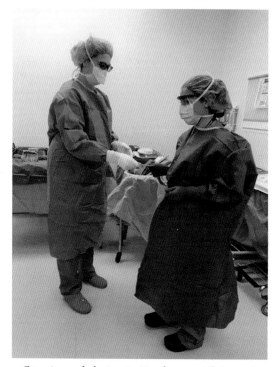

Gowning and gloving 5 - Hands paper tab to scrub

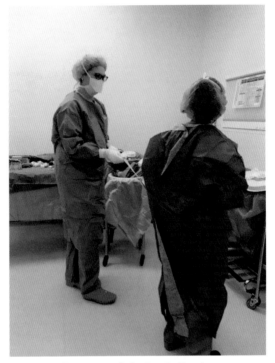

Gowning and gloving 6 - Turning

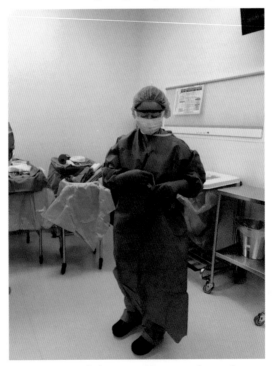

Gowning and gloving 7 - Tie two ends together

PEARLS

1. Be sure to trim your nails every day and keep them clean. If you believe you have broken your sterility, speak up and rescrub or manage as appropriate.
2. If you feel a sneeze coming on be sure to face forward and sneeze, do not turn your head! Simply step back from the operating table.
3. Be vigilant during the procedure should you come in contact with a non-sterile area, and keep your hands at all times above your waist. Do not cross your arms under your armpits.

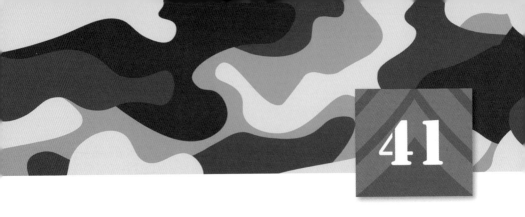

41

STERILE TECHNIQUE

STEPHANIE THERRIEN, BSc | JEFFREY R. KEANE, JR., BSN, RN, CNOR

Sterile technique is defined by the Association of Perioperative Registered Nurses as the use of specific actions and activities to prevent contamination and maintain sterility of identified areas during operative procedures by microorganisms that can cause an infection. With more than 27 million surgical procedures performed in the United States each year,[1] surgical site infection (SSI) was the third most frequently reported nosocomial infection.[2] SSIs can lead to longer hospital stays, which can incur greater expenses.

The exact processes and techniques that encompass sterile technique are numerous and complex. It is designed and used to protect the patient from SSIs by preventing or minimizing postoperative infection through the creation of an environment that is free from microbial or environmental contamination.[3] Such an environment is achieved by using sterile fields, sterilized equipment, and active vigilance of the operative field by every member of the operative team.

If a sterile field is breached, the patient becomes at risk of developing an SSI. The Centers for Disease Control and Prevention define an SSI as "an infection at the site of surgery within 30 days of an operation or within 1 year of an operation if a foreign body is implanted as part of the surgery."[2] Contamination of the surgical site with an organism is the precursor for an SSI. The most common organisms involved in SSIs are *Staphylococcus aureus,* coagulase-negative staphylococci, *Enterococcus* species, and *Escherichia coli.*[4] For most SSIs, the source of pathogens is the endogenous flora of the patient's skin and mucous membranes.[5] Exogenous sources of SSI pathogens include surgical personnel, the operating room environment, and all tools, instruments, and materials brought into the sterile field during a procedure.[2]

THE TEAM

Surgeon: the primary surgeon for the procedure, typically the attending surgeon.

First assistant: another physician, usually a resident or an advanced practice clinician (such as a nurse practitioner or physician assistant).

Circulating nurse: a registered nurse who is qualified by training and experience in operating room nursing. This individual is responsible and accountable for all activities that occur during surgical procedures and is responsible for monitoring the patient during the procedure.

Certified Surgical Technologist (CST): the "scrub" who prepares the sterile field by setting up surgical instruments, supplies, and solutions. During the operation, the CST will pass instruments and manage the sterile field. He or she will also assist the circulating nurse in performing *counts* to prevent retention of surgical items.

Operating room attendants: paraprofessionals who are responsible for providing support services when required in an operating room.

Sterilization technicians: health care professionals who specialize in the sterilization of reusable medical supplies, instruments, and equipment. They pay special attention to cleaning, testing, assembling, packaging, and sterilizing these equipment and instruments.

STEPS: ESTABLISHING A STERILE FIELD/ASEPTIC TECHNIQUE

1. The field should be in a location with minimal traffic where it does not have to be moved.[3]
2. Cover surfaces and/or operative fields with sterile drapes.[3]
   a. If the drape does not cover the surface entirely, a 1-inch margin around the drape is considered not to be sterile.
   b. Any part of the drape that is not under direct supervision of the surgical team is considered not to be sterile.

   c. When a scrubbed assistant opens a sterile drape, it is opened first toward the sterile individual.

3. All objects used in a sterile field must be sterile.
   a. Check packages for sterility by assessing package integrity, dryness, and expiration date before use.
   b. Wet, torn, previously open, or dropped instruments and supplies cannot be entered into the sterile field and should be considered nonsterile and discarded.
   c. Any sterile object that meets a nonsterile object becomes nonsterile. If a sterile item becomes compromised, all surfaces and objects involved are also considered to be contaminated.
   d. Any item that has passed its expiration date is considered nonsterile.
   e. Reusable medical devices shall be reprocessed according to the manufacturer's directions for use.
   f. Once a patient has entered the operating room where sterile supplies have been opened, those supplies are to be discarded if the operation is canceled, whether or not they have been used.

STEPS: DISPENSING STERILE SUPPLIES

1. To reduce potential contamination, sterile fields should be opened as close as possible to the surgical start time.[3]
2. Sterile supplies should undergo minimal handling.[3]
3. Before entering an item into the sterile field, it should be inspected for sterility using the methods described earlier.[3]
4. When entering an item into the sterile field, the method of transfer should maintain item sterility by[3]:
   a. Never shaking an item from its package
   b. Never flipping an item on to the sterile field

STEPS: MAINTAINING A STERILE FIELD

1. Circulating operating room (OR) staff should neither touch nor reach over sterile items/sterile fields.[3,6]
   a. If a staff member needs to open a sterile pack, they should do so in such a way that the wrap is opened away from themselves to prevent contamination.
2. Scrubbed assistants should not touch or reach over unsterile items/areas.[3,6]

3. Sterile personnel should stay within the sterile field.[3,6]
   a. If sterile personnel change positions during the procedure, they should do so in such a way that they never turn their back to the sterile field.
4. Sterile supplies should not at any point be left unattended.[3,6]

PEARLS

1. Movement around the sterile field must not compromise or contaminate the sterile field; this means: Keep OR traffic to a minimum, tie loose hair back. If you are not scrubbed, do not laugh, talk, or lean over a sterile field.
2. Before using a sterile item, check chemical indicators (can be either inside or outside of the package), package integrity, and whether there is an expiration date.
3. If the sterility of an item is doubted, it is to be considered not sterile.

References

1. Graves EJ, Gillum BS. Detailed diagnoses and procedures, National hospital discharge survey, 1994. *Vital Health Stat.* 1997;13:1-145.
2. Chan D, Downing D, Keough C, et al. *Joint Practice Guideline for Sterile Technique during Vascular and Interventional Radiology Procedures.* December 2012. Available at https://www.jvir.org/article/S1051-0443(12)00742-7/pdf.
3. Meara G, Reive R. *Surgical Aseptic Technique and Sterile Field.* January 2013. Available at https://www.albertahealthservices.ca/assets/wf/eph/wf-eh-surgical-aseptic-technique-sterile-field.pdf.
4. Schaberg DR, Culver DH, Gaynes RP. Major trends in the microbial etiology of nosocomial infection. *Am J Med.* 1991;91:72S-75S.
5. Altemeier WA, Culbertson WR, Hummel RP. Surgical considerations of endogenous infections—sources, types, and methods of control. *Surg Clin North Am.* 1968;48:227-240.
6. Carson J, ACORN, The Royal Children's Hospital Melbourne. *Aseptic Technique in the Perioperative Unit.* 2012-2013. Available at https://www.rch.org.au/surgery/local_procedures/Aseptic_Technique_in_the_Perioperative_Unit/.

42

SURGICAL INSTRUMENTS

AMY R. EVENSON, MD, MPH | COURTNEY BARROWS, MD

An understanding of the identification and use of surgical tools will aid in the efficient and safe performance of operative procedures. This chapter aims to depict common instruments used in open surgical procedures and describes their uses. Many of these instruments are available in laparoscopic formats as well. Please note that significant regional and institutional variability occurs in the names and specific uses of instruments. Similarly, individual surgeon preference for particular instruments in particular circumstances may differ from these descriptions. A system to record and remember the preferences of specific staff is advised and will serve to aid trainees in determining their own preferences over time.

SCALPEL BLADES

Scalpel blades are available in numerous sizes and shapes. Scalpel blades frequently used in general surgery procedures are depicted in Figure 42.1. A 10-blade is used to open large, straight incisions. A 15-blade allows for more precision in curved incisions and is often also used for laparoscopic port

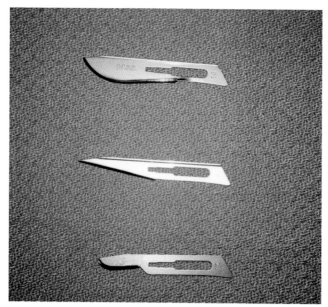

FIGURE 42.1 Common scalpel blades. From top, 10-blade, 11-blade, 15-blade.

incisions. For both the 10- and 15-blade the "belly" or rounded portion of the blade is used for skin contact. An 11-blade is pointed at the tip and is often used for stab-type incisions (drain placement, for example) or creating arteriotomies or venotomies in vascular surgery.

FORCEPS

Forceps are used to grasp or manipulate tissues, ties, vessel loops, or umbilical tapes. The choice of forceps depends on the target tissue and depth of field. The tips of forceps may be toothed or smooth. Toothed forceps concentrate the force generated by the user on a smaller area of tissue and are typically used when tension may be applied, such as during wound closure. Smooth forceps distribute the pressure more evenly but may lead to significant crush injury when too much force is applied. Additionally, smooth forceps are preferred during vascular anastomoses to avoid injury to the vascular intima. Forceps are available in various lengths to suit the depth of field of the procedure.

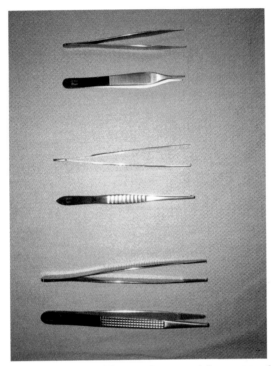

FIGURE 42.2 Common toothed forceps. From top, Adson, rat-toothed, Bonney.

Toothed forceps frequently used in general surgery are depicted in Figure 42.2. Adson forceps are short, toothed forceps typically used to manipulate skin during opening and closure of incisions. Rat-toothed forceps are slightly heavier, longer forceps that are often used on fascia. Bonney forceps are the heaviest-toothed forceps in common use and are also often employed during fascial closure. Ferris Smith forceps are similar to Bonney but have a wider grip area. Neurotoothed forceps are preferred by some surgeons during manipulation of the bowel for resection and anastomoses.

Smooth forceps frequently used in general surgery are depicted in Figure 42.3. Despite being referred to as smooth, many forceps in this class have ribbing at the tips. Debakey forceps are widely used in general and vascular surgery. They are used during dissection of structures to provide tension. They may be used to pass ties, umbilical tapes, or vessel loops. Gerald forceps are finer at the tips than Debakey and are often used during vascular surgery. Dressing forceps are typically longer and have wider tips. They are

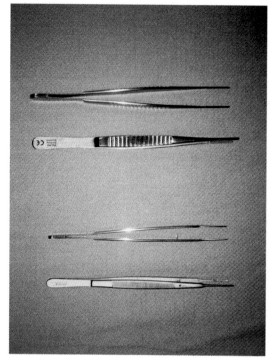

FIGURE 42.3 Common smooth forceps. From top, Debakey, Gerald.

used to manipulate dressings as the smooth tips will not catch the fabric as toothed forceps would. Some forceps in this category may also have varieties with teeth.

SCISSORS

Scissors may be straight or curved and come in many lengths. There are many special types of tips used for specific purposes. Scissors commonly used in general and vascular surgery are seen in Figure 42.4. Metzenbaum ("Metz") scissors are frequently used to cut tissue or fine suture. They may also be used in blunt dissection. Metzenbaum scissors have a long shank-to-blade ratio. Mayo scissors are heavier and often used to cut heavy fascia, suture, mesh, or dressings. Potts scissors have sharply angled blades that are used to cut arteriotomies and venotomies (Figure 42.5). Tenotomy or iris scissors have very fine blades and allow precise cuts in limited spaces (Figure 42.6).

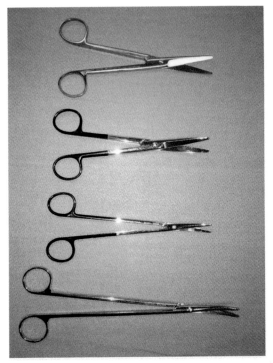

FIGURE 42.4 Common scissors. From top, straight Mayo, curved Mayo, straight Metzembaum, curved Metzembaum.

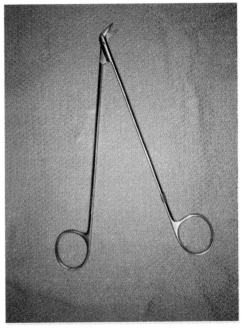

FIGURE 42.5 Potts scissors.

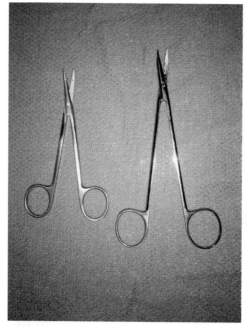

FIGURE 42.6 Left, iris scissors. Right, tenotomy scissors.

CLAMPS AND CLIP APPLIERS

Clamps are among the most widely used and versatile instruments available to surgeons for dissection, securing sutures or ties, and manipulating tissues. Clamps have finger rings and ratchets to securely hold tissue, ties, or suture. Clamps come in a wide range of tip configurations, lengths, and weights. Snaps or hemostats may be straight or curved (Figures 42.7 and 42.8). A very fine snap may be called a mosquito or Jake. Heavier or longer clamps are often called Kelly or curved-6's, where the number refers to the length of the instrument in inches. Right-angled clamps are used for dissection, passing ties, and clamping tissues or blood vessels (Figure 42.9). Tonsil or Schnidt clamps have a long shank-to-tip ratio and are used for passing ties or drains and grasping tissue. Allis clamps are used to grasp tissue with sharp teeth. Babcock clamps have a flat surface and are considered atraumatic (Figure 42.10). Kocher clamps have grooves and teeth and are used to securely grasp heavy tissue such as fascia (Figure 42.11). Ring forceps may be used to grasp tissue but are

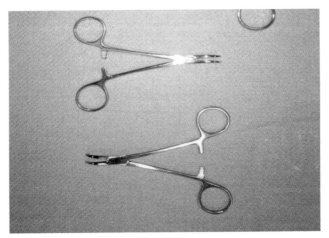

FIGURE 42.7 Clamps. Curved snaps.

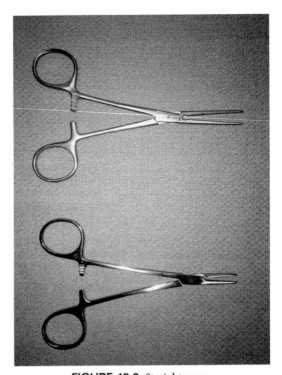

FIGURE 42.8 Straight snaps.

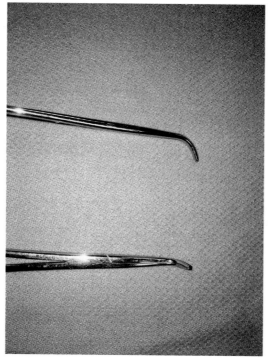

FIGURE 42.9 Right-angle tip detail.

commonly used to hold gauze sponges (also known as a sponge stick) to provide retraction and exposure in deep field or control bleeding with pressure (Figure 42.12).

Towel clamps may be sharp (or perforating) or smooth (or nonperforating, Edna) (Figure 42.13). Some surgeons prefer to secure drapes to the patient's skin using perforating towel clamps, whereas others use skin staples or adhesive dressings to prevent movement of the drapes.

Clip appliers are used to place metal clips on blood vessels. Clips and clip appliers are available in several sizes. These instruments may be single use and reloadable or automatic with multiple preloaded clips (Figure 42.14).

NEEDLE DRIVERS

Instruments used for suturing are broadly classified as finger-ring types and double-spring types. Finger-ring types are available in many lengths and with different tip weights and configurations for use in various settings

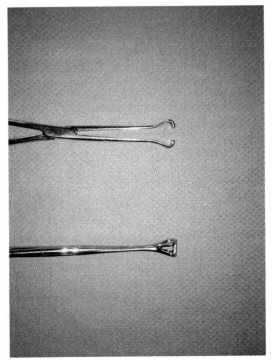

FIGURE 42.10 Babcock detail.

(Figure 42.15). Castro-Viejo drivers are the most commonly used double-spring needle drivers and have fine tips for use with small needles used in vascular surgery (Figure 42.16).

RETRACTORS

Retractors are used to provide exposure of the operative field. Retractors range from simple, handheld devices to elaborate, multipiece systems. Figure 42.17 demonstrates various handheld retractors. Richardson and lady finger retractors have a single blade attached to the handle at a right angle (Figure 42.17A). Deaver retractors have a curved blade typically used to retract the abdominal wall. A sweetheart retractor has a wider tip than blade and can provide additional exposure at the depth of the field of exposure (Figure 42.17B). A bladder blade is relatively shallow and has a curved lip at its sides (Figure 42.18). Army-Navy retractors have a blade at each end of the retractor, each of a different length, whereas Senn retractors have a blade at one end and a rake

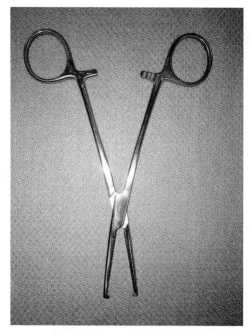

FIGURE 42.11 Kocher clamp.

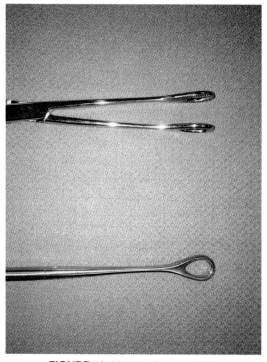

FIGURE 42.12 Ring forceps detail.

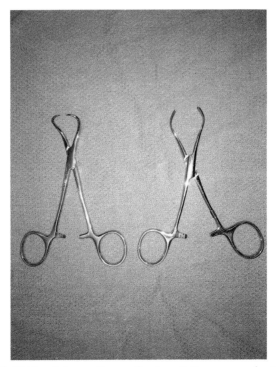

FIGURE 42.13 Towel clamps. Top, perforating. Bottom, nonperforating (Edna).

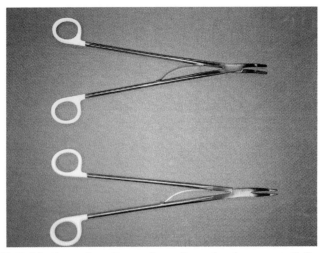

FIGURE 42.14 Clip appliers. Top, medium clip applier; bottom, small clip applier.

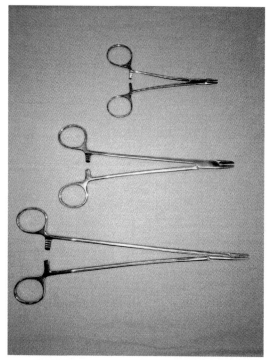

FIGURE 42.15 Finger-ring needle drivers.

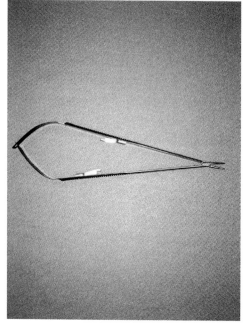

FIGURE 42.16 Double-spring needle driver (Castro-Viejo).

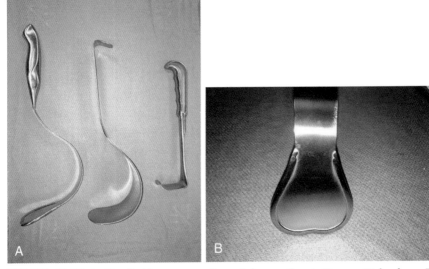

FIGURE 42.17 A, Handheld retractors. From left, sweetheart, Deaver, Richardson. B, Sweetheart detail.

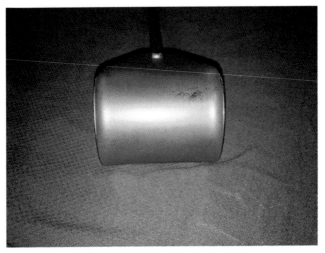

FIGURE 42.18 Bladder blade detail.

at the other (Figure 42.19). Ribbon retractors are flat, malleable retractors that may be bent to provide customized exposure (Figure 42.20). The choice of retractor depends on the depth and width of the exposure required. Handheld retractors offer infinite configurations but require ongoing management of the

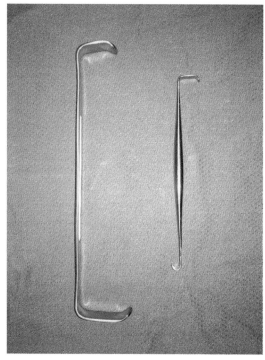

FIGURE 42.19 Double-bladed handheld retractors. Left, Army-Navy retractor. Right, Senn retractor.

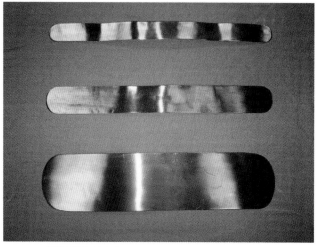

FIGURE 42.20 Ribbon or malleable retractors.

instrument by a surgical assistant. Fatigue and inability to see the exposure provided are limitations of this approach, especially for long procedures or deep operative fields.

Self-retaining retractors may be placed in the field and their position maintained without further manipulation by the surgical team. Figure 42.21 shows common self-retaining retractors. The individual blades on these retractors may be sharp or blunt. Self-retaining retractors are available in a number of lengths and depths. Balfour retractors consist of two blades mounted on a crossbar that may be opened to various distances (Figure 42.22A). Balfour retractors may allow the placement of an additional blade on the crossbars of the device (Figure 42.22B). Sternal retractors may use a crank mechanism to increase the width of the exposure (Figure 42.23).

Mechanical retracting systems allow reliable exposure of a large field. These systems are more elaborate and require more time to set up. They may be very flexible in configurations, allowing a broad use in general and

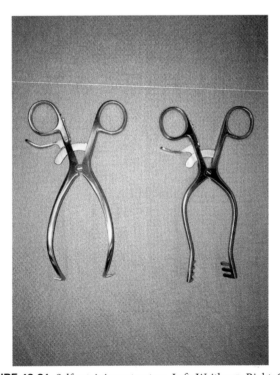

FIGURE 42.21 Self-retaining retractors. Left: Weitlaner. Right: Gelpi.

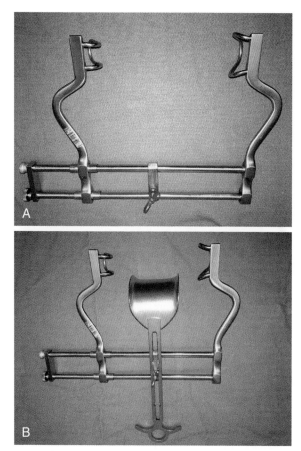

FIGURE 42.22 A, Balfour retractor. B, Balfour retractor with additional bladder blade.

vascular surgery. The commonly used Bookwalter is depicted in Figure 42.24A-C). Most mechanical retraction systems use one or more posts attached to the operating table to provide a secure base for retraction coupled with a crossbar, ring, or assortment of limbs to suspend blades into the operative field. Additional mechanical retraction systems include the Thompson, iron intern, and Omni systems. Various systems offer specific advantages and disadvantages; the choice of mechanical retracting system is beyond the scope of this chapter and is typically made after significant experience with several systems throughout residency and/or fellowship training.

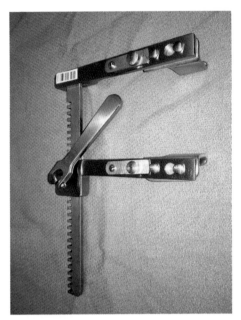

FIGURE 42.23 Sternal retractor.

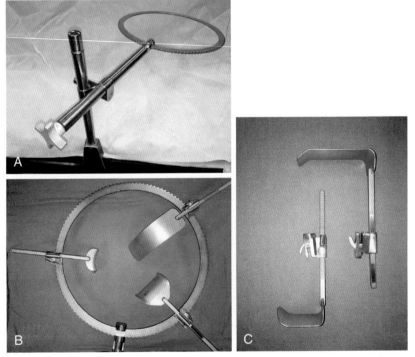

FIGURE 42.24 A, Bookwalter retractor post, bar, and ring. B, Bookwalter ring with retractors. C, Bookwalter right-angled retractors and ratchets.

PEARLS

1. It is imperative to become familiar with surgical tools and their specific uses. Many of these instruments are available in laparoscopic formats as well.
2. Please note there may be significant regional and institutional variability occurring with regards to the instruments name.
3. Similarly, individual surgeon preference for particular instruments in particular circumstances may differ from these descriptions. A system to record and remember the preferences of specific staff is advised and will serve to aid trainees in determining their own preferences over time.

43

NEEDLES AND SUTURES

SAYURI P. JINADASA, MD, MPH | ALOK GUPTA, MD

There are varying types and sizes of sutures. Their use depends on the type of tissue being repaired and the time duration intended for the suture to stay in place.

SUTURE SIZE

Sutures are sized in the United States following the United States Pharmacopeia (USP) method. This takes into account knot security, tensile strength, and suture diameter. Gauge varies from #12-0 to #4, going from the thinnest to the thickest diameter. For example, #2, #1, 0, 00, and 000 are a list of suture sizes in decreasing diameter. To simplify the vernacular, 00000 is colloquially referred to as "5-0." This is an easy way to remember that, for example, 7-0 is smaller than 2-0. Table 43.1 lists common suture sizes used in cases listed from the largest to smallest diameter.

TABLE 43-1 Common Suture Sizes and Uses Listed in Order of Smallest to Largest Diameter Gauge

USP Standard	Common Uses
6-0	Common for use in vascular graft sewing
5-0 4-0	Used for larger vessel repair or skin closure
3-0 2-0	Skin closure when there is a lot of tension, closure of muscle layers, or repair of bowel
0 1	Used for closing of abdominal fascia, various orthopedic procedures

Reprinted with permission from Jinadasa SP, Gupta A. Surgical bootcamp: wound closure. In: Jones DB, ed. *Pocket Surgery*. Wolters Kluwer; 2018.

SUTURE MATERIAL

There are four main classifications of suture material, including physical characteristics, handling characteristics, biocompatibility, and biodegradation.

- Physical: size (diameter), number of filaments, tensile strength, coefficient of friction
- Handling: pliability, packaging memory, knot slippage, tissue drag
- Biocompatibility: degree of inflammatory reaction and propensity for wound infection, allergic reactions
- Biodegradation: tensile breaking strength and mass loss, biocompatibility of degradation properties

The two most practical properties of suture material are whether or not they are absorbable and whether they are monofilament or multifilament.

ABSORBABLE VERSUS NONABSORBABLE

Absorbable suture materials are those that are naturally degraded and absorbed by the body over time by way of hydrolysis (synthetic sutures) and enzymatic degradation (natural sutures).

- Used for suturing internal tissue or in patients who cannot return for suture removal
- Dissolution time depends on suture type, size, and type of tissue
- Examples: surgical gut suture, Vicryl, Monocryl, polydioxanone suture (PDS)

Nonabsorbable sutures are made of materials not readily broken down by the body.

- Used when a suture may be removed after a certain period of time (eg, nylon sutures to close a superficial laceration) or when they can or need to be left permanently (eg, vessel repair or bowel anastomosis)
- Fibroblasts encapsulate or wall off nonabsorbable sutures
- Provoke less of an immune response and cause less scarring than absorbable sutures; therefore, they are used where cosmetic outcome is important
- Examples: silk, nylon, stainless steel, polyester, prolene

MONOFILAMENT VERSUS MULTIFILAMENT

Monofilament sutures are composed of a single smooth strand.

- Cause less drag through tissue and therefore are less traumatic
- More likely to slip and therefore approximately 5 to 7 knots are required when tying
- Crush and crimp easily, creating weak spots that lessen tensile strength

Multifilament sutures consist of multiple fibers braided or twisted together.

- Provide increased tensile strength and pliability
- Increased drag and trauma on the tissues
- Less likely to slip and therefore require only 3 to 4 knots when tying
- Can be coated with different materials that can decrease drag and make it easier to slide knots into place (this may compromise knot security)

SYNTHETIC VERSUS NATURAL

Monocryl: absorbable, synthetic, monofilament; ideal for subcuticular closures.

Nylon: nonabsorbable, available as monofilament or multifilament, synthetic; because of its elasticity, particularly well suited for retention and skin closure.

- Monofilament nylon sutures have memory (a tendency to return to their straight state); therefore, more throws are required for knot security compared with braided nylon sutures

PDS: absorbable, monofilament, synthetic; ideal for secure fascial closures.

Prolene: nonabsorbable, monofilament, synthetic; used in general soft tissue approximation and/or ligation.

- Causes minimal tissue reaction and does not adhere to tissue

Silk: nonabsorbable, multifilament, natural; used for bowel anastomoses and vessel ligation.

Stainless steel: nonabsorbable, available as monofilament or multifilament, synthetic, nonabsorbable; often used for sternal closure.

- Disadvantages associated with handling: possible cutting, pulling, or tearing of patient's tissue or injury to surgeon

Surgical gut (catgut): absorbable, monofilament, natural; indicated in general soft tissue approximation and/or ligation.

- Plain: consists of purified collagen derived from animal intestines; breaks down enzymatically, and tensile strength is maintained for 7 to 10 days; completely absorbed within 70 days
- Chromic: plain gut treated with chromium salts that result in prolonging tensile strength to 10 to 21 days and absorption time to over 90 days

Vicryl: absorbable, multifilament, synthetic; used in general soft tissue approximation and/or ligation.

DISSOLUTION TIME

The dissolution time of suture material depends on:

- type of material
- blood supply to the tissue
- structure of the tissue
- degree of fluid accumulation on the suture material

Table 43.2 shows the dissolution time for several commonly used sutures.

TABLE 43-2 Dissolution Time of Sutures

Suture	# Days
Monocryl	90-120
PDS	180-210
Plain gut	70
Chromic gut	90
Vicryl	55-70

Reprinted with permission from Jinadasa SP, Gupta A. Surgical bootcamp: wound closure. In: Jones DB, ed. *Pocket Surgery*. Wolters Kluwer; 2018.
PDS, polydioxanone suture.

MISCELLANEOUS

Pledgeted suture: suture supported by a small, flat, nonabsorbent pad (pledget) so that the suture will not tear through tissue; used routinely in valve replacement operations.

The strength of a knotted suture decreases by approximately 50% owing to the stresses from bending and twisting that are introduced into the suture when knotting.

NEEDLE ANATOMY

Figure 43.1 shows the components of a needle.

Point: sharpened part of the needle that first penetrates the tissue.

- Determines ease of penetration and the initial size and shape of the hole made in tissue
- **Blunt tip:** sharp enough to penetrate fascia and muscle but not skin; also, can be used to suture friable tissue such as kidney or liver
  - minimizes risk of needle stick injury

Diameter: gauge or thickness of the needle wire; select based on the tissue to be sutured; finer diameter for softer tissue (eg, bowel) and wider diameter for tougher tissue.

Body: portion that is grasped by the needle holder.

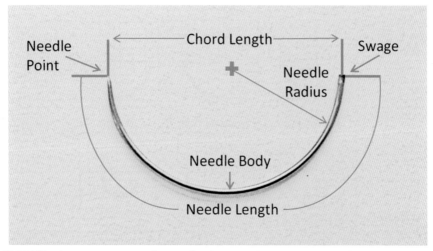

FIGURE 43.1 Components of a needle. (Reprinted with permission from Jinadasa SP, Gupta A. Surgical bootcamp: wound closure. In: Jones DB, ed. *Pocket Surgery*. Wolters Kluwer; 2018.)

NEEDLE CURVATURE

- The curvature of the needle body comes in a variety of different shapes and sizes that give the needle different characteristics
- Classified by the fraction of a circle the needle takes up

  Figure 43.2 shows several basic needle shapes.

TAPERED VERSUS CUTTING

Tapered: body of tapered needles are round in cross section that taper to a point; they separate tissue fibers rather than cut them.

- Most atraumatic needle type, therefore used in tissue that can be easily penetrated, for example, deep fascia closure, bowel, vessels, nerves, tendons
- Not used on skin because of difficulty to penetrate tissue

  Cutting: body of cutting needles are triangular in cross section; cut rather than separate tissue and therefore make it much easier to penetrate tough tissue.

- Used in areas of tough, fibrous, or dense tissue and for suturing skin

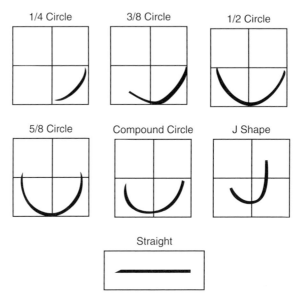

FIGURE 43.2 Basic needle shapes. (Reprinted with permission from Jinadasa SP, Gupta A. Surgical bootcamp: wound closure. In: Jones DB, ed. *Pocket Surgery*. Wolters Kluwer; 2018.)

- **Conventional cutting needle:** apex cutting edge is on the inside of the needle curvature
- **Reverse cutting needle:** apex cutting edge is on the outside of the needle curvature
  - Has improved strength and increased resistance to bending

  Figure 43.3 demonstrates the geometry of tapered and cutting needles. Table 43.3 shows multiple commonly utilized needle codes and their uses.

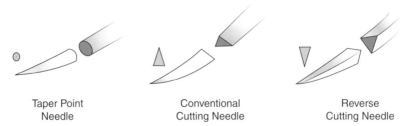

FIGURE 43.3 Needle point geometry. (Reprinted with permission from Jinadasa SP, Gupta A. Surgical bootcamp: wound closure. In: Jones DB, ed. *Pocket Surgery*. Wolters Kluwer; 2018.)

TABLE 43-3 Common Needle Codes and Meanings

Code[a]	Meaning	Common Uses
BV	Blood Vessel	Blood vessels
CT	Circle Taper	Closure of deep tissue layers
SH	Small Half (Circle)	Bowel closure; closure of tissue layers after breast surgery
UR	Urology	Laparoscopic port site closure

Reprinted with permission from Jinadasa SP, Gupta A. Surgical bootcamp: wound closure. In: Jones DB, ed. *Pocket Surgery*. Wolters Kluwer; 2018.
[a]Subtypes of needle shapes are classified by numbers from larger to smaller size.

WHICH NEEDLE TO USE?

- Depends on procedure, tissue type, exposure, and accessibility to tissue being sutured and surgeon preference
- Goal is to minimize trauma to tissue
  - Should be as slim as possible without compromising strength
  - Stable in grasp of needle holder
  - Able to carry suture material through tissue
  - Sharp enough to penetrate tissue with minimal resistance
  - Rigid enough to resist bending but able to resist breaking
- Care should be taken to match the size of the needle to the size of the tissue bite required

Figure 43.4 shows a needle suture package with a guide to how to determine what the key components of the suture and needle are.

MISCELLANEOUS

Eyed needles: manufactured separately from suture thread.

- requires rethreading
- reuse leads to loss of sharpness
- more than a single strand is pulled through tissue; therefore, more trauma and a larger gap is created than is filled by sutures
- Advantage: any needle and suture combination can be achieved

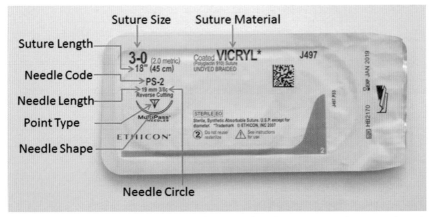

FIGURE 43.4 Suture packaging guide. (Reprinted with permission from Jinadasa SP, Gupta A. Surgical bootcamp: wound closure. In: Jones DB, ed. *Pocket Surgery*. Wolters Kluwer; 2018.)

"**Pop-offs**": Needles designed to come off of the suture with a sharp straight tug; commonly used for interrupted sutures, where each suture is passed only once and then tied; risk of needle-stick injury while tying is minimized.

SUTURING TECHNIQUE

NEEDLE HOLDER

- Needle holder should be selected to match the size and strength of the needle being used
- If too large, can result in damage to needle and distortion of needle curvature
- Needles should be grasped at approximately two-thirds of the needle length from the point
- The needle and holder should be roughly perpendicular
- The needle tip should enter the target tissue at a 90° angle
- When applying force to achieve passage of the needle through tissue, it should be applied in a direction following the curvature of the needle
- If placement of the needle in tissue needs to be readjusted, the needle should be removed and reinserted

SUTURE REMOVAL TIMING

Different parts of the body heal at different speeds. Common time to remove sutures will vary:

- Face: 3 to 4 days
- Scalp: 5 days
- Trunk: 7 to 10 days
- Limbs: 7 to 10 days
- Foot: 10 to 14 days

 PEARLS

1. Each needle type and curvature has its unique circumstance where it is best used. Over time you will become familiar with their various uses in dealing with different types of tissue.
2. Selection of absorbable versus nonabsorbable is related to the type of forces applied to the area under repair and how long you wish to provide support for the healing process.
3. Keeping a written record of when your attendings use particular types of sutures and needles will help you learn this important topic.

ACKNOWLEDGMENT

This chapter originally appeared in *Pocket Surgery*, by Daniel B. Jones.

44

BASIC TECHNICAL SKILLS

BLAINE T. PHILLIPS, MD, MPH | DANIEL B. JONES, MD, MS

Suturing is an essential skill set for any resident required to care for wounds or lacerations. Surgical residents who find themselves in the operating room are also required to demonstrate proficiency when suturing within the body through both open and minimally invasive techniques (see chapter on Fundamentals of Laparoscopic Surgery).

In general, primary closure is indicated when a clean wound or uncontaminated laceration extends beyond the dermis and is treated in a timely manner. Some contaminated wounds and lacerations may also be closed by primary intention. The decision to use sutures for primary closure, as opposed to staples or adhesives (tissue glue or surgical tape strips), depends on the anatomic location and characteristics of the wound or laceration, the health of the patient, and the availability of supplies. Secondary closure is recommended when there is a high risk of infection, when there is extensive tissue loss (eg, from traumatic lacerations or burns) or if the wound or laceration was unable to heal by primary intention (eg, due to dehiscence or the development of an infection).[1] Tertiary closure is often appropriate when there is a delay in treatment, when initial debridement is required, or when there is a high risk of infection from an animal bite. It is also indicated for patients with impaired wound healing and for wounds or lacerations that are either dirty or infected. Some contaminated wounds and lacerations may also require delayed primary closure.

This chapter will describe proper needle driver technique and provide step-by-step instructions for performing vertical mattress, horizontal mattress, simple interrupted, and running subcuticular sutures. The indications for these different suture types will also be provided since this can vary depending on the anatomic location of the wound and its characteristics. A brief overview on how to avoid and manage needlestick injuries will also be offered.

NEEDLE DRIVER HANDLING

Although there are numerous different types of needle drivers, the vast majority of them have the same component parts. These include the ring handles, ratchet locking mechanism, shanks, joint or fulcrum, and jaws (Figure 44.1). Each type of a needle driver has its own unique set of properties and should be utilized based on the type of procedure being performed, the level of dexterity required, the anatomic location where sutures are indicated, and the size of the needle being used (Table 44.1).

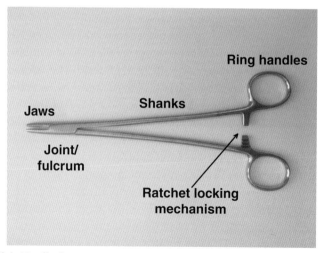

FIGURE 44.1 Needle driver components. The vast majority of needle drivers are made up of the same component parts: jaws, joint or fulcrum, shanks, ratchet locking mechanism, and ring handles. The jaws can either be smooth or cross-serrated. Smooth jaws are beneficial when small needles are being used, and cross-serrated jaws are useful when firm needle traction is required. Gold-plated ring handles indicate that the jaws of the needle driver contain tungsten carbide inserts. These inserts enhance jaw longevity and grip strength as tungsten carbide is harder and more durable than stainless steel.

TABLE 44-1 Various Types of Needle Drivers

Type of Needle Driver	Unique Properties	Indication	Instrument Size[a]	Needle Size
Mayo-Hegar	Wide range of available sizes	Most commonly used needle driver	5″-12″	Medium to large
Olsen-Hegar	Scissors located between jaws and fulcrum	Plastic surgery	4.75″-7″	Medium
Heaney	Curved jaws	Gynecology	8.25″-13.75″	Small to medium
Castroviejo	Spring handle with serrated shanks instead of ring handles Available with or without spring and latch locking mechanism Available with curved or straight jaws	Microsurgery	3.5″-8.5″	Fine

[a]Ranges provided may not include all available sizes.

When handling needle drivers, there are several different grips that one can adopt. Each grip has its own set of advantages and disadvantages. Needle drivers should be handled in a manner that maximizes their design and intended purpose. The grip you use will depend on the level of dexterity or strength required for the specific task at hand (eg, microvascular surgery versus large incisional hernia repair under tension), your hand size, your level of training, and what is most comfortable for you. It should be noted, however, that each attending surgeon with whom you work will likely have a preference on the grip you use.

In order of *increasing* precision and control and *decreasing* needle motion with release of the ratchet locking mechanism and strength in suture placement, needle driver grips include the palm grip, thenar eminence grip, tripod grip, and pencil grip. The palm grip utilizes the wrist and arm for rotational strength and is characterized by placement of the proximal end of the needle driver within the palm of your right hand without placement of any digits through the ring handles (Figure 44.2). Meanwhile, the thenar eminence grip is nearly identical to the palm grip, except the tip of the fourth digit is placed through the lower ring handle and the posterior aspect of the fifth digit presses against the lower ring handle (Figure 44.3). The placement of the third digit is also modestly different in that it holds the needle driver at a more proximal location by wrapping around and applying pressure over the intersection of the lower shank and ring handle. These small changes in hand placement

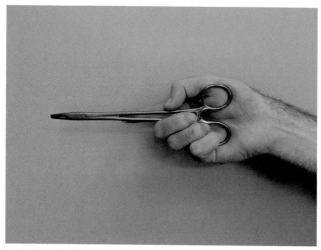

FIGURE 44.2 Palm grip. The palm grip holds the proximal end of the needle driver in the palm of the right hand without placing any digits through the ring handles. Needle driver control is achieved when the tips of the third to fifth digits stabilize the lower ring handle, the lower shank (and sometimes the upper shank), and the ratchet locking mechanism against the hypothenar eminence as the thenar eminence and first digit simultaneously stabilize the upper ring handle and its associated shank against the third or fourth digit pressing the ratchet locking mechanism in the opposite direction. The second digit rests distally over the shanks to provide further control and precision. When using the palm grip, the ratchet locking mechanism is unlocked when the thenar eminence pushes in the opposite direction of the hold provided by the third to fifth digits. As the needle driver is unlocked, the first digit prevents the upper shank from flipping open in an uncontrolled manner. The first digit is also used to lock the ratchet locking mechanism and to open and close the jaws after the ratchet locking mechanism has been unlocked. The basic mechanics associated with manipulating the ratchet locking mechanism via the palm grip are different when the needle driver is placed in the left hand.

for the thenar eminence grip prevent the arm from being utilized as a source of rotational strength when compared to the palm grip. Instead, the thenar eminence grip only uses the wrist for rotational strength. The tripod grip employs the wrist for rotational strength and is similar to the thenar eminence grip with regard to hand placement, except the tip of the first digit is placed through the upper ring handle (Figure 44.4). Finally, the pencil grip acquires rotational strength solely from the digits and adopts a hand confirmation that resembles proper penmanship (Figure 44.5). The pencil grip is primarily used when manipulating Castroviejo needle drivers, which do not have ring handles, during microsurgical procedures (Figure 44.6). As highlighted through this discussion, needle driver mechanics while suturing are largely dependent

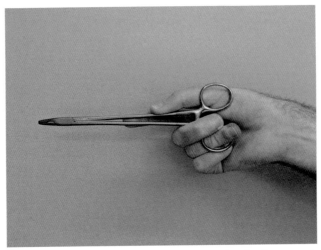

FIGURE 44.3 Thenar eminence grip. Hand placement for the thenar eminence grip is nearly identical to that of the palm grip, except the tip of the fourth digit is placed through the lower ring handle and the posterior aspect of the fifth digit presses against the lower ring handle. The placement of the third digit is also modestly different in that it holds the needle driver at a more proximal location by wrapping around and applying pressure over the intersection of the lower shank and ring handle. When using the thenar eminence grip, the ratchet locking mechanism is unlocked when the thenar eminence pushes in the opposite direction of the hold provided by the third and fourth digits. As the needle driver is unlocked, the first digit prevents the upper shank from flipping open in an uncontrolled manner. The first digit is also used to lock the ratchet locking mechanism and to open and close the jaws after the ratchet locking mechanism has been unlocked. The basic mechanics associated with manipulating the ratchet locking mechanism via the thenar eminence grip are different when the needle driver is placed in the left hand.

upon the grip being utilized. It is worth noting that your mechanics and overall performance with any of these techniques will be enhanced by stabilizing the most distal part of your arm that is not being used to generate movement as this will increase your control and comfort while simultaneously decreasing your fatigue.

The needle should be loaded at the very tip of the jaws of the needle driver and approximately one-half to two-thirds along the needle body from the needle point (or one-half to one-third along the needle body from the needle swage) (Figure 44.7). Loading the needle away from the tip and deeper into the jaws should be avoided as this can both flatten and weaken the needle. Needles should also be loaded by locking only one or two ratchets from the ratchet locking mechanism in order to avoid damaging and warping the needle with

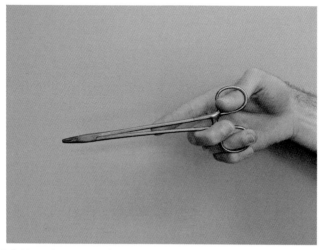

FIGURE 44.4 **Tripod grip.** Hand placement for the tripod grip is essentially identical to that of the thenar eminence grip, except the tip of the first digit is placed through the upper ring handle. When using the tripod grip, the ratchet locking mechanism is unlocked when the first digit pushes in the opposite direction of the hold provided by the third and fourth digits. The basic mechanics associated with manipulating the ratchet locking mechanism via the tripod grip are different when the needle driver is placed in the left hand.

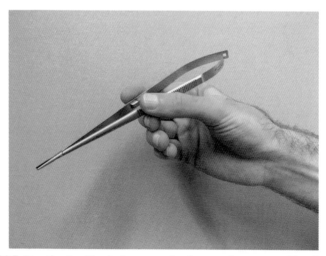

FIGURE 44.5 **Pencil grip.** Hand placement for the pencil grip resembles that of proper penmanship and requires placement of the first and second digits on opposite shanks while the third to fifth digits rest comfortable behind the needle driver. When using the pencil grip, the ratchet locking mechanism is unlocked when the first and second digit push in opposite directions. The basic mechanics associated with manipulating the locking mechanism via the pencil grip are essentially the same when the needle driver is placed in the left hand.

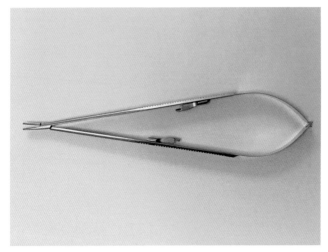

FIGURE 44.6 Castroviejo needle driver. The Castroviejo needle driver does not have ring handles and allows for excellent precision and control. It is primarily used in microsurgery.

unnecessary pressure at the jaws. The needle is typically loaded at a perpendicular angle with respect to the needle driver. This allows for enhanced maneuverability. Occasionally, however, loading the needle at a slightly more obtuse angle can be beneficial. When this is indicated, the needle should be loaded closer toward midway point of the needle body.

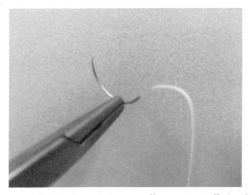

FIGURE 44.7 Suture needle loading. Suture needles are typically loaded at the very tip of the jaws and perpendicular to the needle driver and secured one-half to two-thirds along its body from the needle point. Occasionally, a slightly obtuse angle is preferred when loading the needle.

BASIC SUTURING TECHNIQUES

Although there are certainly differences with each of the suturing techniques described in the following four subsections, there are common concepts that apply to all of these methods as well. For example, needles should always enter and exit at an angle perpendicular to the tissue surface. This includes the skin and the surfaces of the wound within the wound cavity itself. In other words, bites should have approximately the same radius when traversing the wound. You should also be sure to capitalize on the great utility of your tissue forceps in providing the necessary tension to help guide your needle through tissue. However, always be gentle when manipulating the dermis and epidermis with your forceps and resist the temptation to use them to pull your needle when exiting through tissue. Instead, use your needle driver and try to grasp the needle as far away from the point as possible to avoid dulling the needle. Knots should be tied securely in order to avoid slippage and air knots, but too much tension can cause the suture to break or tear through the tissue (see chapter on Knot Tying). It is even possible for excessive tension to result in poor wound healing or strangulation that leads to tissue ischemia or necrosis. You should also be sure to maintain horizontal tension on your suture along the length of the wound after the first loop is placed and after making the final throw. These concepts on knot tying apply to both hand and instrument ties.

VERTICAL MATTRESS SUTURE

Vertical mattress sutures utilize interrupted stitches composed of both large and small bites within the same vertical plane. The large bites focus tension deeper within the wound and serve to bring the wound together and evert the wound edges. The small bites are placed after the deep bites and function to approximate the wound edges while under less tension. Vertical mattress sutures are indicated for wounds that require closure under tension and wound edge eversion, such as those on concave body surfaces like the posterior neck.[2] There is also a running version of this suture.

Steps (Figure 44.8 A-H)

1. Use small-toothed forceps (eg, Adson forceps) to load the needle driver in the forehand configuration.
2. Near the apex of the wound, elevate and stabilize the skin with small-toothed forceps (continue to use forceps appropriately throughout) and pass the needle perpendicularly through the skin approximately 0.5 cm away from the edge of the wound.

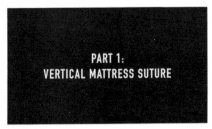

FIGURE 44.8A Vertical mattress suture.

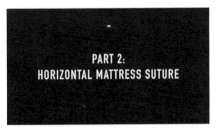

FIGURE 44.9A Horizontal mattress suture.

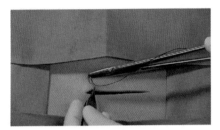

FIGURE 44.8B Pass needle through skin 0.5cm away from wound edge.

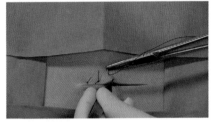

FIGURE 44.9B Pass needle through skin 0.5cm away from wound edge.

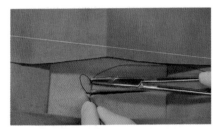

FIGURE 44.8C Take equal bites.

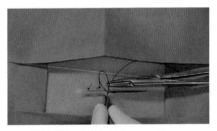

FIGURE 44.9C Take equal bites.

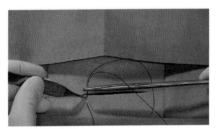

FIGURE 44.8D Pass needle back through skin in the same vertical plane 0.2cm away from wound edge.

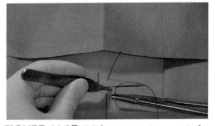

FIGURE 44.9D Make mirror image stitch through skin in the same horizontal plane 0.5cm away from previous stitch.

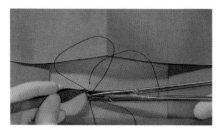

FIGURE 44.8E Take equal bites.

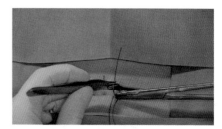

FIGURE 44.9E Take equal bites

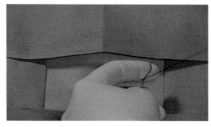

FIGURE 44.8F Tie surgical knot.

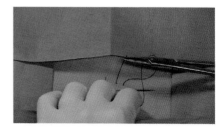

FIGURE 44.9F Tie surgical knot.

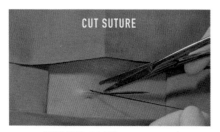

FIGURE 44.8G Cut suture.

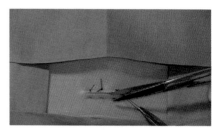

FIGURE 44.9G Cut suture.

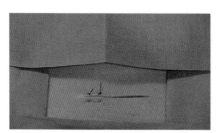

FIGURE 44.8H Repeat as necessary.

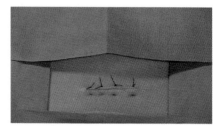

FIGURE 44.9H Repeat as necessary.

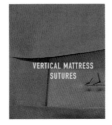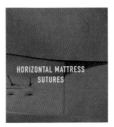

FIGURE 44.10 Finished product with vertical mattress sutures on the left and horizontal mattress sutures on the right.

3. Take an equal bite through the other side of the wound, exiting perpendicularly through the skin approximately 0.5 cm away from the wound edge.
4. Use small-toothed forceps to load the needle driver in the backhand configuration.
5. In the opposite direction, pass the needle perpendicularly through the skin approximately 0.2 cm away from the edge of the wound within the same vertical plane as your first two original bites.
6. Take an equal bite through the other side of the wound, exiting perpendicularly through the skin approximately 0.2 cm away from the wound edge.
7. Tie a surgical knot and cut the suture with suture scissors so that 0.4 cm tails remain.
8. Repeat as necessary sequentially along the wound with subsequent stitches placed approximately 0.4 cm apart from one another.

HORIZONTAL MATTRESS SUTURE

Horizontal mattress sutures utilize interrupted stitches composed of equally placed bites within the same horizontal plane. This suture distributes tension along the length of the wound edge and also serves to evert the wound edges. Horizontal mattress sutures are indicated for patients with fragile skin or for wounds that require closure under tension and wound edge eversion.[2] There is also a running version of this suture.

Steps (Figure 44.8 9 A-H)

1. Use small-toothed forceps (eg, Adson forceps) to load the needle driver in the forehand configuration.
2. Near the apex of the wound, elevate and stabilize the skin with small-toothed forceps (continue to use forceps appropriately throughout) and pass the needle perpendicularly through the skin approximately 0.5 cm away from the edge of the wound.

3. Take an equal bite through the other side of the wound, exiting perpendicularly through the skin approximately 0.5 cm away from the wound edge.
4. Use small-toothed forceps to load the needle driver in the backhand configuration.
5. In the opposite direction, pass the needle perpendicularly through the skin along the same horizontal plane and approximately 0.5 cm from the previous stitch.
6. Take an equal bite through the other side of the wound, exiting perpendicularly through the skin along the same horizontal plane and approximately 0.5 cm from where the suture originally entered the skin.
7. Tie a surgical knot and cut the suture with suture scissors so that 0.4 cm tails remain.
8. Repeat as necessary sequentially along the wound with subsequent stitches placed approximately 0.4 cm apart from one another.

SIMPLE INTERRUPTED SUTURE

Simple interrupted sutures utilize single interrupted stitches. This suture allows for accurate skin approximation while minimizing the risk of wound dehiscence due to suture compromise. Simple interrupted sutures are indicated for uncomplicated wounds and lacerations under moderate tension. It is one of the most commonly used suturing techniques.[3]

Steps (Figure 44.11 A-F)

1. Use small-toothed forceps (eg, Adson forceps) to load the needle driver in the forehand configuration.
2. Near the apex of the wound, elevate and stabilize the skin with small-toothed forceps (continue to use forceps appropriately throughout) and pass the needle perpendicularly through the skin approximately 0.5 cm away from the edge of the wound.
3. Take an equal bite through the other side of the wound, exiting perpendicularly through the skin approximately 0.5 cm away from the wound edge.
4. Tie a surgical knot and cut the suture with suture scissors so that 0.4 cm tails remain.
5. Repeat as necessary sequentially along the wound with subsequent stitches placed approximately 0.5 cm apart from one another.

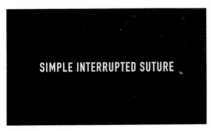

FIGURE 44.11A Simple interrupted suture.

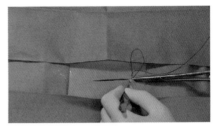

FIGURE 44.11D Take equal bites on each side of the wound.

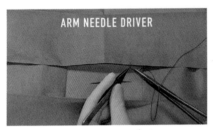

FIGURE 44.11B Arm the needle driver

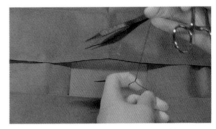

FIGURE 44.11E Tie a surgical knot.

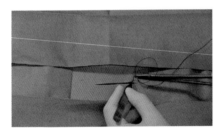

FIGURE 44.11C Pass the needle perpendicularly through the skin and have it exit perpendicularly through the edge of the wound.

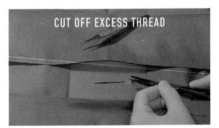

FIGURE 44.11F Cut excess suture and leave 0.5 cm tails. Repeat as neccessary along the length of the wound

RUNNING SUBCUTICULAR SUTURE

Running subcuticular sutures predominantly utilize continuous stitches of variable size just below the dermal-epidermal junction. Bites parallel to the skin surface are slightly smaller at the apices of the wound to allow for enhanced skin approximation. Perpendicular bites are typically required to anchor and bury the suture at both ends. Running subcuticular sutures are indicated for clean wounds with easily approximated edges under low tension, such as straight surgical wounds made during surgery.[3] This type of suture allows for improved cosmesis.

Steps

1. Use small-toothed forceps (eg, Adson forceps) to load the needle driver in the forehand configuration.
2. Make an anchoring stitch with a buried knot approximately 1 cm from the apex of the wound.*
   a. Elevate and stabilize the skin with small-toothed forceps (continue to use forceps appropriately throughout) and make a deep to superficial bite in which the needle exits perpendicularly through the deeper part of the dermis. This bite only needs to be on one side of the wound.
   b. Make a surgical knot with an instrument tie and cut the blind end of the suture to a length short enough that it can be buried within the incision. Typically, a length of 0.3 cm is adequate.
3. Pass the needle from deep within the dermis and have it exit perpendicularly just below the dermal-epidermal junction directly at the apex of the wound.
4. Use small-toothed forceps to load the needle driver in the forehand configuration.
5. Pass the needle parallel to the plane of the skin just below the dermal-epidermal junction on one side of the wound and lightly pull the suture tight with your nondominant hand.
6. Use small-toothed forceps to load the needle driver in the backhand configuration.
7. Along the contralateral side of the incision, find a location in the skin a few millimeters back from where the suture just exited on the ipsilateral side of the wound and pass the needle parallel to the plane of the skin just below the dermal-epidermal junction on this side of the wound. Lightly pull the suture tight with your nondominant hand.

---

*Anchoring can be achieved at both ends through other approaches. One such option includes pulling both ends of the suture to the appropriate tension, applying liquid adhesive to these ends, and then covering them with adhesive strips. Through this technique, surgical knots are not required for anchoring. Another option includes making an anchoring stitch with a buried knot that incorporates *both* sides of the wound when beginning your running subcuticular suture. Alternatively, one can also make an anchoring stitch with a buried knot that incorporates both sides of the wound when finishing your running subcuticular suture. However, instead of using a two-handed technique to tie the looped end of the previous stitch to the end of the suture connected to the needle, an instrument tie is utilized. Both of these techniques that incorporate buried knots require the blind or looped ends to be cut with suture scissors to a length short enough that they remain buried.

8. Continue steps 4 through 7 until the end of the wound is reached. It is often advised that these bites are made slightly smaller in length toward the apices of the wound and can be slightly larger in the middle. Your last bite should exit just below the dermal-epidermal junction at the opposite apex of the wound.

9. Make an anchoring stitch with a buried knot at the opposite apex of the wound.*
   a. Pass the needle from deep within the dermis and have it exit perpendicularly just below the dermal-epidermal junction directly at the apex of the wound. However, DO NOT pull the suture tight.
   b. Instead, make a buried knot by using a two-handed technique to tie the looped end of the previous stitch to the end of the suture connected to the needle.

10. Bury the end of the remaining suture by taking a deep bite from within the apex of the wound that exits perpendicularly through the skin approximately 1 cm away.

11. Use suture scissors to cut the suture just above the level of the epidermis so that the suture easily disappears down into the skin.

NEEDLESTICK INJURIES

Although this manual has a separate chapter on needlestick and sharp injuries and the necessary precautions to take if one occurs (see chapter on Needlesticks and Occupational Exposure), this discussion on basic technical skills would be incomplete without briefly reviewing preventative strategies for suture needlesticks. In general, you should always complete the necessary occupational hazard training at your institution to help prevent injury and infection, plan for safe needle handling (eg, wearing gloves) and proper disposal *prior* to using suture needles, and quickly dispose of used suture needles in appropriate sharp disposal containers.[4] These recommendations apply to suture needle use in the emergency department, on the wards, and within the operating room.

---

*Anchoring can be achieved at both ends through other approaches. One such option includes pulling both ends of the suture to the appropriate tension, applying liquid adhesive to these ends, and then covering them with adhesive strips. Through this technique, surgical knots are not required for anchoring. Another option includes making an anchoring stitch with a buried knot that incorporates *both* sides of the wound when beginning your running subcuticular suture. Alternatively, one can also make an anchoring stitch with a buried knot that incorporates both sides of the wound when finishing your running subcuticular suture. However, instead of using a two-handed technique to tie the looped end of the previous stitch to the end of the suture connected to the needle, an instrument tie is utilized. Both of these techniques that incorporate buried knots require the blind or looped ends to be cut with suture scissors to a length short enough that they remain buried.

In the operating room specifically, however, there are several effective strategies that can either help prevent needlestick injuries from taking place or can help decrease the risk of transmission of blood-borne pathogens when they do occur. First and foremost, never hesitate to tell your attending when you have been stuck by a needle or sharp. Although you may not want to disrupt the procedure or may have silently convinced yourself that the integrity of your skin was not compromised, you should still always report this immediately and follow the proper protocols. Double gloving is also an effective method to decrease skin perforations and, thereby, exposure to infectious agents.[5] Finally, suture needles should never be left unattended on the surgical field. When you are done with your suture, always make sure to safeguard your suture needle in the proper fashion before returning it to the scrub nurse or surgical technologist (Figure 44.12). This can be accomplished by arming the needle driver with the swage end of the needle loaded distally within the jaws and the needle point placed either directly over and touching the fulcrum or within the jaws itself. Once the suture needle is locked in this position, the needle driver and suture needle may be safely returned to the scrub nurse or surgical technologist through effective communication and with the ring handles presented to him or her. Unfortunately, this latter technique is infrequently taught to surgical trainees. Please note that, even with these safeguards, needlestick injuries may still occur.

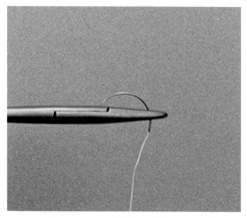

FIGURE 44.12 **Proper needle return technique.** Proper needle return technique in the operating room requires the needle driver to be locked with the jaws clasping the body of the needle near the swage and the needle point either positioned directly over and touching the fulcrum or within the jaws itself. The needle driver should then be handed back to the scrub nurse or surgical technologist with the ring handles presented toward him or her. Always remember to say, "Needle back," as you return the loaded needle driver.

CONCLUSION

The importance of practice cannot be understated. Since it is challenging to simulate the experience of suturing on human skin, a slight learning curve is acceptable when *first* implementing this skill set on patients. However, the basic mechanics of handling a needle driver, manipulating soft tissue with small-toothed forceps, and suturing with different techniques should be mastered prior to performing these skills on patients. Therefore, we encourage you to practice suturing outside of the operating room whenever you get the chance. Improvement in performance in these basic technical skills is almost solely dependent on one's desire to practice, and your senior residents and attendings will notice if you make this investment. In the end, you should aim to improve your economy of movement so that every action you take has purpose.

 PEARLS

1. The importance of small-toothed tissue forceps cannot be understated. Surgeons-in-training are typically so focused on their needle drivers that they tend to ignore the great utility provided by their tissue forceps when first suturing. Remember to use your tissue forceps to *gently* manipulate the dermis and epidermis as you guide your suture needle through the skin. Fine-toothed Adson forceps are the most commonly used forceps and are ideal when working with percutaneous and dermal wounds and lacerations. Be sure to practice using forceps to reload needles, as this will decrease your risk of needlestick injuries and possible viral exposure, and avoid using your forceps to pull needles to prevent blunting on your needle.
2. You should always load your needle driver at the tip of the jaws and secure your needle a distance of one-half to two-thirds from needle point in either a perpendicular or slightly obtuse angle.
3. The palm grip does not place any digits through the ring handles of the needle driver. This may seem uncomfortable at first for the surgical novice. Therefore, we recommend that you place tape over the ring handles of your needle driver and practice locking and unlocking the ratchet locking mechanism in an efficient and controlled manner while holding the needle driver with the palm grip.

4. Avoid bending and breaking needles by selecting needle drivers that are appropriately sized for the specific needle being used. You can also avoid deforming needles by loading them at the tip of the jaws of your needle driver and by suturing along the curve of the needle.

5. Occasionally a layer of deep dermal sutures will be required before placing epidermal sutures for deeper wounds and lacerations. This is known as two-layer suturing and helps prevent seroma and hematoma formation and their associated risks of infection.

6. Exercising proper technique when manipulating your needle driver will enhance your control and precision while minimizing your fatigue.

7. Once mastery of these basic technical skills has been completed with your right hand, you should start practicing them with your left hand.

8. Master your suturing technique at home by using suture practice kits. Never practice your suturing skills on a patient without prior training.

References

1. Hollander JE, Singer AJ. Laceration management. *Ann Emerg Med*. 1999;34(3):356-367.
2. Zuber TJ. The mattress sutures: vertical, horizontal, and corner stitch. *Am Fam Physician*. 2002;66(12):2231-2236.
3. Forsch RT, Little SH, Williams C. Laceration repair: a practical approach. *Am Fam Physician*. 2017;95(10):628-636.
4. NIOSH Alert. *Preventing Needlestick Injuries in Health Care Settings*. U.S. Department of Health and Human Services, Public Health Service, Centers for Disease Control and Prevention, National Institute for Occupational Safety and Health, DHHS (NIOSH) Publication No. 2000-108; 1999.
5. Mischke C, Verbeek JH, Saarto A, Lavoie MC, Pahwa M, Ijaz S. Gloves, extra gloves or special types of gloves for preventing percutaneous exposure injuries in healthcare personnel. *Cochrane Database Syst Rev*. 2014;(3):CD009573. doi:10.1002/14651858.CD009573.pub2.

Suggested Readings

1. ACS/ASE Medical Student Simulation-Based Surgical Skills Curriculum. https://www.facs.org/education/program/simulation-based.
2. Don't stick me, but don't take all day. *J Am Med Assoc*. 1990;264(9):1191.

45

KNOT TYING

MOHAMAD RASSOUL ABU-NUWAR, MD | EMILIE B. D. FITZPATRICK, MD | DANIEL B. JONES, MD, MS

Surgical knots are used to approximate tissues to heal by primary intention or to tie off tubular structures, such as ducts and blood vessels. The ability to form a secure knot is absolutely paramount to the success of any operation. Failure of a surgical knot can result in disastrous consequences (ie, intraoperative or postoperative hemorrhage, evisceration, dehiscence) and most often occurs as a result of a knot untying due to slippage.

Surgical knot tying is often the first technical skill to be required of surgical novices. It begins by training to create the proper hand movements and manipulation of the suture material to create a secure knot. The main techniques include the one-handed tie (OHT), two-handed tie (THT) and instrument tie (IT).

There are three distinct basic knots to be mastered: the slip knot, square knot, and surgeon's knot. These motions should be practiced until they become automatic. Merely learning only how to perform these throws is not sufficient to master the formation of a secure knot. Equally important is the understanding and ability to maintain the correct orientation and tension between the threads as each throw is cinched down. This is often confusing at first but is absolutely essential to master. Students often learn they must alternative the direction of pull as they cinch each throw but may not understand why this is so crucial.

MECHANICS

The mechanical performance of a suture is the most important aspect when selecting the thread and type of knot to be used. While beyond the scope of this chapter, we will focus on the mechanical parameters that impact choice of knots to ensure knots do not fail by knot slippage or knot breakage.

Knot slippage is resisted by frictional forces of the knots. The coefficient of friction is a reflection of suture size and type of thread used, monofilament threads having significantly lower coefficients than multifilament. The coefficient of friction directly impacts the thread's ability to hold down a knot with minimal added tension. Due to this, threads with higher friction rates (vicryl) can be secured confidently with as few as four to six throws while monofilament threads (polydioxanone [PDS]) generally need eight throws. Friction forces gradually increase with each additional throw until maximum security is obtained and the knot will fail by breakage and not slippage. It is therefore paramount to use the proper number of throws as too many only leave behind foreign material that may cause problems (stitch sinus).

The coefficient of friction along with the type of knot also impacts what is known as knot rundown force. As the name implies, this is the sheering force needed to cinch a knot down upon itself. The drawback being that higher rundown forces ultimately wear down the suture material and result in knot breakage. The highest rundown force is encountered in surgeon's knots (2:1), followed by square knots, and lastly slip knots that are cinched through slipping and effectively exert no rundown force. IT would hold to logic that when using suture material with a high coefficient of friction, throwing knots with a lower knot rundown force is ideal.

Knots may also fail when they slip above the ears of the cut thread; it is generally advocated to cut "ears" 3 mm in length. Mechanical trauma to the thread, such as grasping the thread with the needle driver, weakens the sutures integrity and promotes knot failure.

GENERAL PRINCIPLES

A basic understanding of the physics and topology of knots is usually not directly (or correctly) taught but is a necessary element in order to obtain mastery of knot tying in a wide variety of situations and circumstances. Beginners should not be allowed to tie knots that are merely "passable" but should be pushed to perfect their technique at the earliest stages of development.

1. Given the material being used, the simplest knots are always preferred (no show boating).
2. Knot and knot "ears" should be left as short as possible to avoid a foreign body reaction.
3. When pushing knots, friction between the ("sawing") must be avoided so to not weaken the suture material integrity.
4. When handling the suture material, care should be taken to not damage the material by aggressive manipulation with the needle driver or forceps.
5. The finer the material, the less force needed to be exerted by the surgeon as this may only cut the thread and the surrounding tissue.
6. Attention to not performing knots too tight that may otherwise produce tissue strangulation where it is not desired.
7. After passing the first throw, tension needs to be maintained in the appropriate direction so as to avoid the knot becoming loose.
8. A properly tied knot does not need extra ties, this only adds volume but does not decrease the rate of knot slippage.

BASIC KNOTS

Half hitch: The half hitch is the basic building block of most knots used in surgery, whether tying one-handed, two-handed, or using instruments. It is used in performing both the square and slip knot.

A half hitch is formed by crossing the two ends of the thread to form a closed loop, the working end is placed on top and is then passed through the loop. There are two configurations of the half hitch, determined by which of the two threads is passed over the other. Each throw of the thread forms one half hitch.

The two configurations correspond to the two "throws" to be mastered and are referred to as "alternating throws." Secure knots are created by forming a series of multiple half hitches, with an emphasis on alternating between the two throws and applying the correct amount of tension (Figures 45.1-45.4).

Square knot: A critical principle to understand here is what constitutes a true "square knot." A common misperception is that a square knot is formed simply by forming alternating throws. While this is a requirement, it alone is

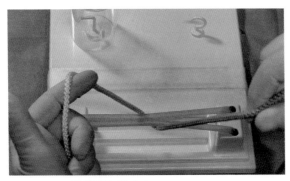

FIGURE 45.1 Starting position.

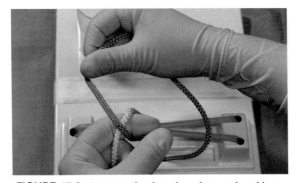

FIGURE 45.2 Crossing the threads to form a closed loop.

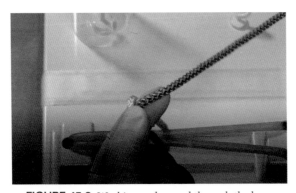

FIGURE 45.3 Working end passed through the loop.

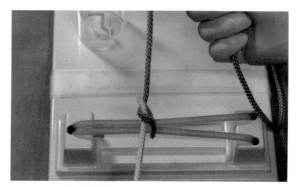

FIGURE 45.4 Knot cinched down.

not sufficient for adequately tying square knots. Confusion is only perpetuated as the term "square" is often used to connote alternating throws. In fact, a true "square knot" requires in addition to alternating throw that each throw is cinched down in a flat orientation. This second point is the defining difference from a slip knot.

To lay down a flat knot, equal tension must be maintained on both threads as it is tightened. The direction of pull is in a horizontal plane and must be in line with the orientation of the knot (Figure 45.5). The ends of the thread will lie in a direction parallel to the standing thread. If the two throws are reliably alternated, the axis of the knot, or direction of pull, should remain constant.

In contrast, repeating the same throw multiple times results in a "granny knot" configuration, this is not a secure knot (Figure 45.6). Repeating the same throw also results in the twisting of the knot's orientation, with the ends of the threads projecting at right angles to the standing parts.

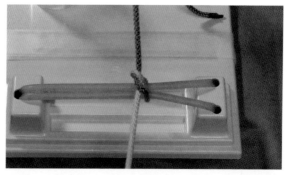

FIGURE 45.5 Hitch cinched down with both hands in a horizontal fashion to form the square knot.

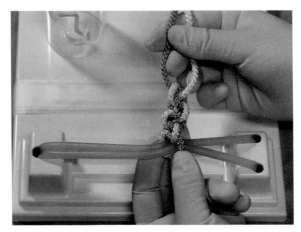

FIGURE 45.6 Multiple square knots in succession.

Slip knot: The critical difference between a square knot and a slip knot is the relative tension that is maintained on the two threads as each half hitch is cinched down. As described above, square knots require equal tension to be maintained on both threads, in a horizontal plane, and in parallel to the orientation of the standing threads.

When tying slip knots, tension is maintained preferentially on one end of the thread, which is held upright or as a "post." Each throw is formed by manipulating the other "free" end of the suture and cinching it down around the "post" (Figure 45.7). Slip knots are useful when in confined area (deep in a hole), where cinching throws in a horizontal plane is not feasible.

Slip knots can be a very useful tool when used deliberately and correctly, but the assumption that a series of slip knots will always form a secure knot is

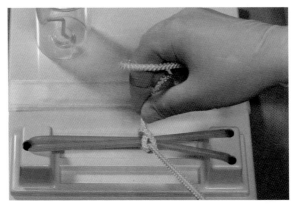

FIGURE 45.7 Post with the knot cinched down in a vertical fashion.

false. A good example is the setting of fascial closure, where a large diameter monofilament is often used and is under tension. The first throw of a slip knot will not hold in place on its own. Once a second (or third) half hitch is added, the friction between the bends of the thread increases enough to hold the knot down tight. The benefit of throwing the first two throws as slip knots is that it allows you to control the tension, prevent tying an air knot, and gives you tactile feedback to notice if your knot has slipped which can then be corrected. Once you are satisfied that the knot is well seated, the remaining throws should be cinched down flat to form a series of square knots (Figure 45.8).

A square or granny knot can be converted into a slip knot by pulling up on one of the two threads. This is useful for salvaging an air knot.

Surgeon's knot: The surgeon's knot is an all-time favorite. It has the greatest knot pushdown friction as well as the propensity to hold its position once placed. It is a great tie to utilize especially in tying off tubular structures. Care should be used when doing this with a multifilament braided tie as it can wear down the suture material if improperly handled or placed with too much friction. Using a monofilament suture with this knot plays to its advantages, such as when closing skin under tension using nylon.

When forming a surgeon's knot, the first throw is formed as a double-throw (Figure 45.9). The tail end of the suture is passed around the working end twice. This prevents slippage of the initial knot while the next throw is formed and cinched down (Figure 45.10). If the first double-throw is cinched down flat and still does not hold sufficient tension to maintain skin approximation, it can be converted to a higher friction "clove hitch" by pulling up on the working end to form a post (Figures 45.11 and 45.12).

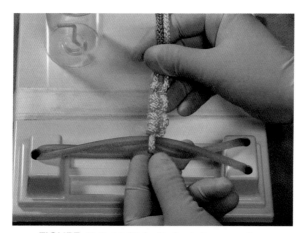

FIGURE 45.8 Multiple slip knots in succession.

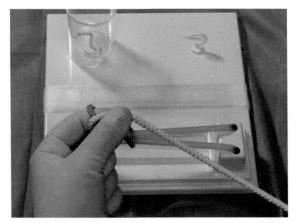

FIGURE 45.9 Closed loop and passing first throw.

ONE-HANDED VERSUS TWO-HANDED TIES

Looking at this from another perspective, all throws initially formed are hitches; it depends on how they are placed that will determine if they are a square or slip knot. Generally, the two-handed technique is associated with tying flat knots (square), while one-handed is used to form sequential hitches on a post (slip).

It is true that the hand movements associated with tying two-handed provide an easier set up for lying down throws flat, while one-handed throws are

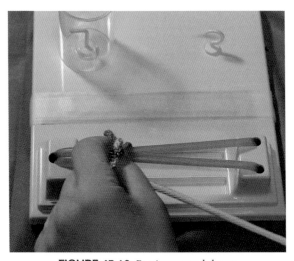

FIGURE 45.10 Passing second throw.

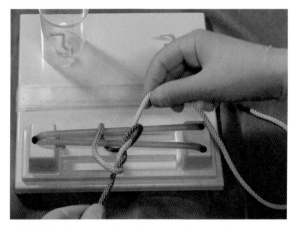

FIGURE 45.11 Cinching down the knot in a flat manner.

set up to naturally be cinched on a post. However, depending on the tension discipline of the thrower, it is just as plausible to convert an intended square/flat knot tied with two hands into a series of hitches on a post. This takes time and practice, while developing a "feel" for the material, its friction, and the underlying tension.

If tying delicate structure (end of anastomosis, small vessel), it is best to use THT to perform a surgeon's or square knot. The benefit comes due to the lack of tension placed on the native tissue when erecting your "post" as a laxity of tension on the post can lead to forming an air knot.

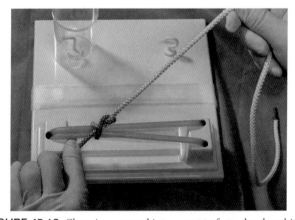

FIGURE 45.12 Changing one end into a post to form the clove hitch.

In a THT, both hands are active participants. It starts by crossing both ends of the thread to form a closed loop. Once the loop has been formed, the index finger and thumb of one hand pass through the loop while the other hand hands off the end of the thread. It is then pulled through completing the knot. The knot is pulled and tightened down in a horizontal plan with attention that the knot is properly laid out before the final cinch.

Alternatively, in an OHT, all the manipulation is done by a single active hand. The other hand passively works by maintaining tension on the "post." This is where it should become clear that while knots may be called by some as OHTs or THTs, in the end it all comes full circle back to our three basic ties.

INSTRUMENT TIE

The instrument tie, a cornerstone in the armamentarium of the surgeon, is particularly useful due to its ability to make use of short suture material that would be insufficient for hand ties. Additionally, it provides the ideal scenario to form perfect square knots rapidly and with maximum economy of motion. The long end of the suture is wrapped twice around the instruments tip, which is then opened to grasp the short tail, after which the knot is cinched down. Following the initial knot, remaining knots are done with a single wrap around the instrument tip (Figure 45.13). Attention must be paid to make sure alternating hitches are thrown and that they are laid down in the proper orientation and tension.

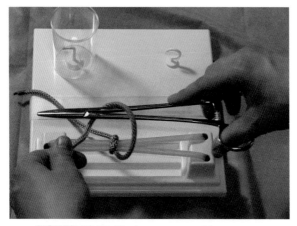

FIGURE 45.13 Single wrap around instrument.

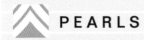 **PEARLS**

1. Instrument tying offers many advantages including, thread conservation, speed, and an improved economy of motion.
2. Practice different types of ties until you are comfortable with all of them, so that you can demonstrate your skill level and speed in front of your attending while maintaining a secure tie.
3. Ask questions in the operating room (OR). At times your surgeon will prefer a certain knot over another, it is important to understand the reasoning behind this.

46

SURGICAL DICTATION

SEEMA P. ANANDALWAR, MD, MPH | SYLVESTER A. PAULASIR, MD

An operative report is an important document in a patient's medical record that summarizes the procedure(s) performed and the important steps of the case. This document has two important functions: (1) to provide information regarding the events of the operating room and (2) to give an accurate description of the different components of the operation for continuity of care to all future providers. According to the Joint Commission on the Accreditation of Healthcare Organizations (JCAHO), a report must be written or dictated immediately after an operation or high-risk procedure, either by a fully transcribed operative note or a brief progress note in order to ensure a proper hand-off of care. Prior to transferring care, there must be documentation of, at minimum, the following components: name of the primary surgeon, procedures performed, description of findings, estimated blood loss, specimens removed, and postoperative diagnosis. A thorough and complete operative note, however, typically contains the following sections:

Patient's name/medical record number (MRN)
Date
Primary surgeon/assistants
Preoperative diagnosis
Postoperative diagnosis
Procedure(s) performed

Indications
Description of procedure
Findings
Anesthesia
Estimated blood loss
Specimen
Complications
Disposition

Operative reports are usually dictated by the primary surgeon or assistants in the case via a hospital dictation system, transcribed and sent to the surgeon for final editing, and then submitted into the medical record. A more detailed explanation of each section is outlined below and a sample operative report is included at the end of this chapter. Finally, the best way to learn the components of an operative report is to read as many operative reports as possible.

PATIENT'S NAME/MEDICAL RECORD NUMBER

This is important for ensuring that the operative note gets placed into the right medical chart. It is important to not only say the patient's name, but to also spell it out to make sure it is transcribed correctly. In addition, the medical record number (MRN) will help further in identifying the correct patient within the medical record system.

DATE

This should be the date of the operation, regardless of when the operative report is dictated. It is very important that this date is accurate because all calculations of postoperative days will be based off of this date.

PRIMARY SURGEON/ASSISTANTS

The primary surgeon of record should be the attending surgeon or the surgeon responsible for the care of the patient. Assistants include any fellow, resident, or medical student who is assisting and taking part in the case. Only people who were scrubbed in for at least portions of the case should be listed here. Observers, scrub techs, or scrub nurses should not be listed under this section.

PREOPERATIVE DIAGNOSIS

The preoperative diagnosis is the presumed diagnosis that prompted the operative intervention prior to starting the case (ie, appendicitis). This typically is a diagnosis that indicates the reason for going to the operating room.

POSTOPERATIVE DIAGNOSIS

The postoperative diagnosis is the determined diagnosis after the case is completed. For example, if a patient was presumed to have appendicitis prior to starting the case and during the case the appendix appears normal but the right ovary is torsed, the preoperative diagnosis would be appendicitis and the postoperative diagnosis would be ovarian torsion.

PROCEDURE(S) PERFORMED

This includes any and all procedures performed in a succinct but informative fashion. This should include all relevant information for appropriate continuity of care. For example, an appropriate "procedures performed" is: Exploratory laparoscopy with lysis of adhesions and small bowel resection.

INDICATIONS

This section is a brief "history of present illness" (HPI) related to the patient's surgical illness and any events justifying the need for operative intervention. This may include imaging, abnormal labs, portions of the hospital course, short descriptions of previous procedures, and/or a description of the symptoms leading to the presumed diagnosis.

DESCRIPTION OF THE PROCEDURE

This is the most detailed portion of the operative report. This section should explain all of the important events in the case in chronologic order. This portion should be detailed enough that the reader should be able to visualize the surgery, understand why things were done the way they were, and any findings noted during the procedure.

The beginning of this section should begin with the patient entering the room, state that he/she was "prepped and draped in the usual sterile fashion," and always include that a time-out was completed. Once these steps are stated, the description of the actual procedure can begin. This typically starts with the location and size of the first incision, and then a step-wise detailed description of the entire procedure, including a rationale for each important decision. For example, if a bowel resection was performed for ischemic bowel, prior to a description of the resection, details of how the bowel looked and the reasons for nonviability necessitating a resection should be included. This portion of the operative note should end with how the incisions were closed, including the type of sutures, what dressings were used, any drains left in the surgical site, and if the patient was successfully extubated.

FINDINGS

This is a short (only a few words) description of what was found during the surgery (ie, inflamed appendix).

ANESTHESIA

This section indicates the type of anesthesia used. This is sometimes abbreviated to common shorthand versions (ie, general endotracheal anesthesia = GETA).

ESTIMATED BLOOD LOSS

This section states the amount of blood that the surgeon estimates was lost during the case. This is helpful particularly during the immediate postoperative care of the patient.

SPECIMEN

This section should indicate any specimen that was sent to pathology. This indicates to future providers which items are to be followed-up as they continue to care for the patient.

COMPLICATIONS

This section outlines any complications that may have happened during the operation. Examples of complications include pneumothorax during line placement and cardiac arrest necessitating chest compressions, among others. This is an important aspect of the transition of care to ensure that future providers understand major events that occurred during the procedure.

DISPOSITION

The disposition includes where the patient is expected to go immediately following surgery (ie, postanesthesia care unit [PACU], intensive care unit [ICU], etc).

SAMPLE OPERATIVE REPORT

Patient's name/MRN: John Doe/00000001
Date: 08/01/2018
Primary Surgeon/Assistants: Dr Jane Smith
Preoperative diagnosis: Acute uncomplicated appendicitis
Postoperative diagnosis: Acute uncomplicated appendicitis
Procedure(s) performed: Laparoscopic appendectomy
Indications: This is a 25 year-old female presenting with 1 day of right lower quadrant abdominal pain, WBC of 13, and CT scan revealing an 8 mm appendix with wall thickening, enhancing fat, and surrounding free fluid. These findings were highly suspicious for acute appendicitis. All risks and benefits were explained to the patient and the decision was made to take the patient to the operating room for a laparoscopic appendectomy.
Description of procedure: The patient was brought into the operating room and placed in supine position. General endotracheal anesthesia was induced. The abdomen was prepped and draped in the usual sterile fashion. A successful time-out was completed. An open Hassan technique was used to enter the peritoneal cavity. An infraumbilical incision was made and carried down to the fascia which was divided to expose the peritoneal cavity. A trocar and laparoscope were inserted into the abdomen under direct visualization. Next, a left lower quadrant and supra pubic port were inserted under direct visualization. Care was taken to avoid injury to the inferior mesenteric artery and

the bladder during trocar insertion. The abdomen was thoroughly explored with the laparoscope to ensure that there were no intra-abdominal injuries during trocar insertion. The patient was placed in Trendelenburg and left side down and attention was directed toward the right lower quadrant. The appendix was identified and noted to be acutely hyperemic without gross signs of perforation. A window was created between the base of the appendix and cecum. Linear cutting stapler was used to divide the appendix from the cecum. The mesoappendix was then divided using a vascular load stapler. The base of the cecum was found to be intact and healthy. The appendix was placed in a sterile endoscopic bag and removed through the periumbilical port site. The specimen was sent to pathology. Purulent fluid was suctioned out of the RLQ and pelvis. Staple lines were inspected and found to be intact and hemostatic. All ports were removed under direct visualization. The fascia of the umbilical port was closed in a figure-of-eight fashion with 0-vicryl sutures. The skin was closed using 4-0 monocryl in a subcuticular fashion. The abdominal wall was cleaned and dried, steri-strips were placed and incisions were dressed with gauze and Tegaderm. No drains were left. The patient was successfully extubated at the end of the case.

Findings: Inflamed appendix, no signs of perforation
Anesthesia: GETA
Estimated blood loss: 5 cc
Specimen: Appendix
Complications: None
Disposition: PACU

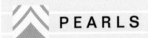

PEARLS

1. Be sure to clearly identify the patient and yourself during your dictation. Well-done dictations are crucial. They ensure appropriate continuation of care and can be valuable even many years down the line.
2. Practice makes perfection! As with all aspects of your career, continuous practice will ensure a fluidity and speed in your work and will ensure you do not miss any key and relevant points.

47

NEEDLESTICKS AND OCCUPATIONAL EXPOSURE

JANE CHENG, MD, FACC, FHRS | SARAH MABEN, MD

In the healthcare profession, exposures and injuries can frequently occur. It is important to take the necessary precautions to prevent these from occurring, but it is also important to recognize when an exposure or injury occurs and how to proceed.

FACTS ABOUT OCCUPATIONAL INFECTION

All health care providers who perform invasive procedures with sharp instruments are at risk for injury; however, the operating room (OR) setting presents the greatest risk. Surgeons-in-training have the greatest risk of exposure to blood-borne pathogens, given their frequent encounters with use of sharp instruments. Learning new technical skill sets also increases the propensity for injury. Virtually all surgical residents (99%) have a needlestick injury by their final year of training. Furthermore, many of these injuries are not reported to an employee health service. Not reporting these incidences puts surgeon-in-training at risk for exposure to human immunodeficiency virus (HIV), hepatitis B (HBV), and hepatitis C virus (HCV) exposures.

PREVENTING NEEDLESTICKS AND TRANSMISSION OF DISEASES

While healthcare workers are at increased risk for a needlestick, taking precautions can help prevent and decrease risk of exposure. Improvements have been made in instruments and tools to help increase safety; these include safety scalpels and blunt-tip suture needles.

While working in the healthcare setting, especially with sharps and/or during a procedure, one should keep in mind that all patients are potential exposures. As such, one should use up to five points of personal protective equipment to prevent blood/body fluid contact, including cap, eye shield, mask, gown, and gloves. All healthcare workers should also have appropriate vaccinations.

Education and training of healthcare professionals is also important such as double-gloving, the neutral (safe) passing zone, and appropriate use of blunt-tip needle (not sharp like hypodermic needles), which makes these needles less prone to cause injury.

Preventing percutaneous injuries also includes the following:

- Eliminating unnecessary needle use
- Using devices with safety features
- Developing safe work practices for handling needles and other sharp devices
- Safely disposing of sharps and blood-contaminated materials

SAFETY IN THE OR.

- When using needle or sharps in the OR, make sure you hand back needles that are protected by the instrument.
- Do not reach for instruments on the scrub tech stand unless it was well communicated.
- Do not place loaded needle drivers down on tables, or operating field.
- Always communicate where sharps are.
- Clearly communicate and say "needle back," "needle down," "knife back," or "knife down" when passing instruments.

WHAT TO DO IF YOU ARE STUCK WITH A NEEDLE

Timely reporting of occupational exposures to employee health services is required to ensure that appropriate surveillance, precautions, and treatment measures are taken. Failure to report exposures precludes interventions that could benefit the injured party, placing healthcare workers at unnecessary risk.

If you experienced a needlestick or sharps injury or were exposed to the blood or other body fluid of a patient during the course of your work, you should follow these steps:

- Wash needlesticks and cuts immediately with soap and water. Do not wait until you are finished with the case.
- Flush splashes to the nose, mouth, or skin with water.
- Irrigate eyes with clean water, saline, or sterile irrigants.
- Report the incident to your supervisor.
- Immediately seek medical treatment (often occupational health during daytime, and emergency room during nights/weekends).

WHAT BASELINE TESTING SHOULD BE PERFORMED AFTER EXPOSURE?

Source patient:

- HIV antigen/antibody (Ag/Ab) or HIV Ab (rapid HIV testing preferred if accessible)
- HCV Ab or HCV RNA (HCV viral load) (CDC prefers HCV RNA)
- HBV surface Ag

POST-EXPOSURE MANAGEMENT OF HEPATITIS B VIRUS

Individual with known response to HBV.

- Baseline testing is not necessary

Individuals who have been vaccinated against HBV, but vaccine response is unknown.

- Anti-HBs should be checked.
- If the exposed person has been vaccinated and is a known responder to the vaccine, then no postexposure prophylaxis is necessary.

- If test for anti-HBs is inadequate, then hepatitis B immunoglobulin (HBIG) should be administered along with vaccine booster.

  Individuals who are unvaccinated.

- HBIG should be administered and hepatitis B vaccine series should be given.

  Follow-up HBV testing.

- Perform follow-up anti-HBs testing in those who receive hepatitis B vaccine after exposure.
- Test for anti-HBs 1 to 2 months after final dose of vaccine.

POSTEXPOSURE MANAGEMENT OF HEPATITIS C VIRUS

The risk of transmission of HCV with needlestick is 1.8% (ranges from 0% to 7%). If personnel are exposed to an HCV-positive source, then the source should test for anti-HCV and ALT. If the source patient is not infected, then baseline testing is not necessary. Post exposure prophylaxis is not recommended after exposure. The following algorithm (Figures 47.1) should be followed for those exposed to HCV positive or unknown sources.

POST EXPOSURE MANAGEMENT OF HUMAN IMMUNODEFICIENCY VIRUS

What is the risk of HIV transmission?

Postexposure prophylaxis (PEP) is generally recommended when an exposure to an HIV-positive person has occurred. After exposure, the exposed area should be immediately cleaned as described above. Initiation of short term antiretroviral therapy should be initiated within 36 to 72 hours after exposure to reduce the risk of acquisition of HIV infection following exposure. Triple-therapy is now the preferred regimen, including three drugs from at least two drug classes—typically two nucleoside reverse transcriptase inhibitors with a non–nucleoside reverse transcriptase inhibitor, a boosted protease inhibitor, or an integrase inhibitor, for the regimen should be continued for 28 days or until the source patient's labs are negative for HIV, at which time prophylaxis can be stopped. Side effects of antiretroviral can be severe, but are generally self-limited.

Recommended HBV PEP

Vaccination and antibody response status of exposed healthcare personnel*	Treatment		
	Source HBsAg† positive	Source HBsAg† negative	Source unknown or not available for testing
Unvaccinated	HBIG§ x 1 and initiate hepatitis B vaccine series	Initiate hepatitis B vaccine series	Initiate hepatitis B vaccine series
Previously vaccinated			
Known responder¶	No treatment	No treatment	No treatment
Known nonresponder**	HBIG x 1 and initiate revaccination or HBIG x 2††	No treatment	If known high risk source, treat as if source were HBsAg positive
Antibody response unknown	Test exposed person for anti-HBs§§ 1. If adequate,¶ no treatment is necessary 2. If inadequate,** HBIG x 1 and vaccine booster	No treatment	Test exposed person for anti-HBs§§ 1. If adequate, no treatment is necessary 2. If inadequate, administer vaccine booster

* Persons who have previously been infected with HBV are immune to reinfection and do not require postexposure prophylaxis
† Hepatitis B surface antigen
§ Hepatitis B immune globulin; dose is 0.06 mL/kg intramuscularly
¶ A responder is a person with adequate levels of serum antibody to HBsAg (i.e., anti-HBs ≥10 mIU/mL)
** A nonresponder is a person with inadequate response to vaccination (i.e., serum anti-HBS <10 mIU/mL)
†† The option of giving one dose of HBIG and reinitiating the vaccine series is preferred for nonresponders who have not completed a second 3-dose vaccine series; for persons who previously completed a second vaccine series but failed to respond, two doses of HBIG are preferred
§§ Antibody to HBsAg

FIGURE 47.1 Algorithm after exposure. (Used with permission from: CDC. https://www.cdc.gov/hai/pdfs/hiv/occupational_exposure_HIV_08_11x17.pdf.)

TABLE 47-1 Risk of Transmission

Route of Exposure	Risk of Exposure When Source Person is HIV Positive	Factors Increasing Risk
Percutaneous	~1/435 episodes (0.23%)	Hollow bore needles, visibly bloody devices, deep injury, and device used in an artery/vein
Mucous membrane	~1/1000 episodes (0.09%)	Large volume
Cutaneous	<1/1000 episodes (0.09%)	Must involve nonintact skin integrity

HIV, human immunodeficiency virus.
From HIV/AIDS. Available at https://www.cdc.gov/hiv/risk/estimates/riskbehaviors.html

Gastrointestinal side effects (nausea, vomiting, gastrointestinal [GI] upset, and diarrhea) are most common. Headache, fatigue, and insomnia are other side effects. Antiemetic and antidiarrheal medications can be prescribed to help with adherence.

If the source patient is HIV positive, the full 28-day course of triple therapy should be completed and the exposed individual should undergo HIV testing at 6 weeks, 3 months, and 6 months (Table 47.1).

 PEARLS

1. Prevent percutaneous injuries by eliminating unnecessary needle use, developing safe work practices for handling needles and other sharp devices, and safely disposing of sharps and blood-contaminated materials.
2. Be sure to review patient comorbidities. Always know when to be exceptionally vigilant with patients known to be disease carriers.
3. Whenever a workplace injury occurs, immediately tend to the event and be sure to report the incident to your supervisor and occupational health. Timely attention is critical.

Suggested Reading

1. Günthard HF, Saag MS, Benson CA, et al. Antiretroviral drugs for treatment and prevention of HIV infection in adults: 2016 recommendations of the International Antiviral Society-USA Panel. *JAMA.* 2016;316(2):191-210.

48

FIRE PREVENTION IN THE OPERATING ROOM

DANIEL O. KENT, MD | CHARLOTTE L. GUGLIELMI, MA, BSN, RN, CNOR

Performing surgery can be an immensely rewarding and enjoyable experience. There are few things as satisfying as completing a successful operation while protecting the patient from harm. Advances in technology, years of experience, and data analysis have allowed surgeons to treat a wider variety of conditions with much greater safety than ever before. As such, it can be easy to overlook how dangerous of an environment the operating room actually is; there are very few places where exist such a high concentration of potentially dangerous equipment, instruments, hazardous materials, explosive gases, and infectious bodily fluids within such close contact to both patients and staff. To maintain a high degree of safety in the setting of so many hazards, it is very important to be aware of the risks within the operating room environment and manage them appropriately. One area of paramount importance is the prevention of fires.

Although operating room fires are relatively rare in incidence in the modern era (approximately 200-650 fires reported per year in the United States, or roughly one in 65,000 operations[1,2]), the risk is ever present in the operating environment. In fact, the Emergency Care Research Institute (ECRI) recently named surgical fires as one of the top 10 health technology hazards.[3] Flammable materials, supplemental oxygen, and energy devices are ubiquitous in nearly all environments where surgery is carried out, from the operating room to the bedside to the clinic office. The low number of actual fires is a result of coordinated, rigorous fire prevention techniques that have been employed throughout hospitals and surgery centers nationwide. However, there still are approximately 20 to 30 episodes of major disfigurement or disability as a result of operating room fires per year and 1 to 3 deaths from these injuries.[2,4] In addition, as new devices and techniques are constantly being invented and employed in the operating room, the effort to prevent fires is ever ongoing.

Of fires that occur in the operative field, approximately two-thirds of them occur on the upper body above the xiphoid process. 40% to 45% of fires occur on the head, neck, or upper chest, and around 20% within the airway itself.[5] It is thought that the higher concentration of oxidizing gases (supplemental O_2 or nitrous oxide given for anesthesia), more potential fuel sources (hair, drapes, skin crevices where chemical preparations can pool), and more delicate anatomic structures contribute to this increased risk. Certain operations have been identified as "high risk" for fires due to the anatomic location and materials used during the surgery, such as oropharyngeal surgery, facial surgery, endoscopic laser surgery, cutaneous surgery, tracheal surgery, and burr hole surgery.[6] Awareness of the potential fire risk based on the location of the planned operation is an important step in preventing fires in the operating room.

WHAT CAUSES FIRES?

Fire is the process by which a material undergoes rapid oxidation by an oxidizing agent, resulting in the production of light, heat, and oxidation byproducts. To produce fire, three "ingredients" are necessary: a fuel source, an ignition source, and an oxidizing agent.[1] These three ingredients are often referred to as the "triangle of fire"[7] or "fire triad."[8] With these three ingredients together, a chain reaction ensues and the fire continues until all of the available fuel or oxidizer is consumed. We will now explore these three ingredients in the context of the operating room environment and how they interact with each other to potentially produce a fire.

A *fuel source* can be thought of as anything that can burn. In the operating room, and specifically the operating field, there are many fuel sources present. Since the primary goal of fire prevention in the operating room is to prevent injury or harm, it is important to consider the potential fuel sources associated with the people in the operating room. The human body itself is combustible, with different tissues having variable rates of combustion. Hair, especially if saturated with chemicals such as alcohol, can easily catch fire. Gastrointestinal gases, such as hydrogen, methane, and hydrogen sulfide, may be present in certain operations (such as repair of a hollow viscus perforation) and may cause an explosion if the hazard is not managed appropriately. Anything covering the body, such as linens, gowns, drapes, dressings, adhesives, shoe covers, head covers, clothing, and scrubs, are all potential fuel sources.[8] Medications or chemicals used in the operating room, such as certain flammable anesthetic gases (although rarely used nowadays), alcohol-based skin preparations, and preserving agents are potentially flammable. Lastly, various surgical materials, such as towels, sponges, plastics, cables, can all potentially catch fire.[9]

An *ignition source* is anything that provides the activation energy to induce the rapid oxidation of a fuel, resulting in fire. The operating room is filled with equipment that can serve as potential ignition sources, and the surgeon as well as the operating room staff should be familiar with proper setup and use of such devices. Common equipment used in the operating room that may function as an ignition source include electrodessication devices (eg, radiofrequency and harmonic energy), electrocautery, coagulators (argon beam), thermal equipment (warming devices), lasers, lighting equipment (fiber optic lights and cables for endoscopy and laparoscopy), monitors, and defibrillators.[8] Statistically, the most common ignition sources of in the operating room have been identified to be electrosurgical equipment (68%) and lasers (13%).[7,9] However, any electrical equipment can produce a spark, even at the wall outlet. The specifics of these devices are beyond the scope of this chapter, and you should learn about these how these tools are used in surgery as well as how to operate them properly and safely.

An *oxidizing agent* is a chemical that rapidly reacts with the fuel source to produce fire. The most common oxidizers in the operating room are oxygen (delivered as supplemental O_2), and nitrous oxide, both of which are delivered to the airway by the anesthesiologist.[8] These gases are at highest concentration above the xiphoid process, within the airway, and can sometimes accumulate under the drapes depending on the technique used for draping the patient.[2] Environments with oxygen concentrations above 21% (standard atmospheric concentration) are referred to as *enriched-oxygen environments*. This distinction is important in that certain materials that do not burn at room air are able to burn in such conditions. For example, polyvinyl chloride–based materials used in endotracheal tubes, cords, and lines (even nasal cannulas) that do not burn in room air have been reported to burn at O_2 concentrations of 26% or greater.[10]

HOW DO WE PREVENT FIRES IN THE OPERATING ROOM?

You are already on the path toward becoming a steward of fire safety in the operating environment by reading this chapter! Awareness of the risk of fire in surgical setting is the most important part of the entire prevention strategy, as you must understand the risks associated with surgery prior to being able to develop a sound strategy for prevention and intervention should a fire occur. Aside from knowing the specifics regarding the equipment and materials in the OR, you should be familiar with your institutional policies regarding fire safety, and you should know where all fire extinguishers and fire exits are in your operating suite.[10] Many institutions have developed tools that not only assist in continuous learning they also serve as reinforcement strategies to heighten awareness (Figure 48.1).

COMMUNICATION

It is important to have clear lines of communication between all staff members. This can take the form of a *Fire Risk Assessment*[4] during the time-out process prior to starting a case and having direct communication between the anesthesiologist and surgeon as to when gases are being delivered or when surgical energy devices, lasers, or fiber-optic light sources are active and in use.[6,10] The Association of periOperative Registered Nurses (AORN) has developed a Fire Risk Assessment Checklist[4] (Table 48.1) that has been integrated into the time-out process in many institutions. In addition, anyone present in the operating room should speak up if he or she identifies a fire hazard. It is always better to catch and correct a potential hazard before it becomes an adverse event.

CONTROLLING HAZARDS IN THE OPERATING ROOM

You should be aware with the various fire hazards present in your operating room for each operation you perform. Anesthesiologists use algorithms such as the Anesthesia Patient Safety Foundation (APSF) Fire Prevention Algorithm[5,6] for assessing fire risk and determining the best way to mitigate the fire hazards associated with the delivery of oxidizing gases. Surgeons have implemented other strategies for assessing fire risks and mitigating hazards. These include elements of the preoperative timeout procedure designed to identify fire risk as

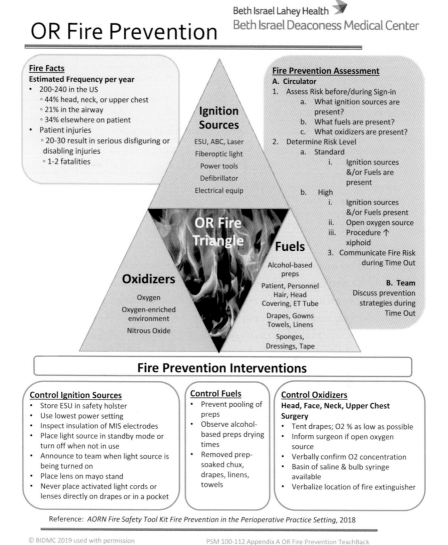

FIGURE 48.1 Operating room (OR) fire prevention. (Used with permission from Beth Israel Deaconess Medical Center, Boston, MA 2019 © BIDMC.)

well as targeted educational programs on how the different energy devices used in the operating room work. The Fundamental Use of Surgical Energy (FUSE) course gives an overview of these devices and how to operate them properly and safely, and it should be completed during your surgical residency.[11] All electrical

TABLE 48-1 AORN Fire Risk Assessment Checklist

		Yes	No
1	Is an alcohol-based skin antiseptic or other flammable solution being used preoperatively?		
2	Is the operative or other invasive procedure being performed above the xiphoid process or in the oropharynx?		
3	Is open oxygen or nitrous oxide being administered?		
4	Is an electrosurgical unit, laser, or fiber-optic light being used?		
5	Are there other possible contributors (eg, defibrillators, drills, saws, burrs)?		

AORN, Association of periOperative Registered Nurses.
Reprinted with permission from AORN Fire Prevention Assessment Tool. Retrieved from https://www.aorn.org/-/media/aorn/guidelines/tool-kits/fire-safety/2019-update/fire-prevention-assessment-tool.doc?la=en&hash=10AB5C936C8D084F381026166A1ED9A2

devices should be inspected regularly, and any devices with frayed or damaged cords should be sent for repair or replacement. Additionally, standard precautions should be used around electrical devices, such as keeping open fluids away from generators or outlets, and keeping flammable materials away from active energy devices.

The beginning of the operation is one of the most important times for minimizing fire hazards. When using alcohol-based skin preparations, care should be taken to minimize pooling on skin, collecting in skin folds, or saturating absorptive materials, as the liquid alcohol is the most prone to causing a large flame that will require extinguishing.[2,12] It should be clearly communicated to the circulating nurse when skin prep has been applied so that a three-minute timer can be started. Although 3 minutes has been determined to reduce the chance of fire, the risk of fire is not zero at 3 minutes, as was demonstrated in an ex-vivo study looking at fire rates with skin preparations at different time intervals on porcine skin.[2] Minimizing pooling and saturation of absorptive materials is paramount in reducing the likelihood of fire. These materials need to be removed prior to commencing the draping process.

To the untrained eye, draping the patient may seem like a mindless element to the operating room setup, but proper draping technique has tremendous implications in reducing fire hazards during surgery. Since supplemental oxygen and nitrous oxide are commonly used during surgery, limiting the entrapment of these oxidizing gases under the drapes or around a particular body part can reduce the chance that a fuel source will catch flame. If possible, use adhesive dressings across the upper chest and keep the face uncovered to prevent the entrapment of these gases.

WHAT HAPPENS IF THERE IS A FIRE?

If a fire happens during an operation, it is extremely important to not panic, as you likely have a patient under anesthesia and can cause more harm than good if a thoughtful fire management plan is not well-executed. Prior work on fire prevention has determined that preassigned tasks to different members of the surgical team are helpful in creating a coordinated, efficient effort to manage fires.[6,13] Because of the uniqueness of the operating room environment, the acronym RACE (rescue, alarm, confine, and extinguish) that is used in most environments for responding to a fire generally does not apply.[9] First, you should immediately cease using the ignition source, remove the fuel source from the surgical field, and extinguish the flame. While one team member is performing this task, another person (ideally the anesthesiologist) should immediately shut off the delivery of supplemental oxygen or nitrous oxide.[9] Fires that occur on the operative field should be extinguished first with the direct application of saline or by smothering with saline-soaked towels. Do not pat the fire, as this motion can encourage spreading.[9] If necessary, a CODE RED should be activated. For large fires that create health and safety hazards for staff and bystanders, an appropriate evacuation plan should be executed as well. As interest in emergency preparedness for in-hospital disasters continues to increase, some hospitals are doing full-scale exercise drills in operating room evacuation.[14] If you are offered an opportunity to participate in any type of disaster drill, you should seize the opportunity as a surgical resident. Another opportunity that you should consider taking advantage of given the opportunity is realistic fire drills. Full team simulations offer practitioners a safe realistic environment to experience the OR fire that we all hope we never see.[15]

Care should also be taken to inspect the patient for any burns. Sometimes burns are not immediately evident, especially when fires occur inside a body cavity or along the airway. Appropriately manage any burns that are identified, involving the appropriate surgeons and critical care specialists as necessary.

Lastly, all fires need to be documented and reported. Improper documentation will limit the institution's ability to correct any hazards and adjust any fire safety policies.

CONCLUSION

It is everyone's responsibility to ensure proper fire safety in the operating room. As a future surgeon, it is important to start forming the leadership skills necessary to guide the team safely through an operation to maximize therapeutic benefit and minimize harm. There are many additional resources at your disposal to further educate yourself on the safe operation of potentially hazardous materials, such as chemicals and energy devices. It is recommended that everyone in surgical training complete the FUSE course, which provides an in-depth overview of important energy devices used in most operations. We hope that you now have a better understanding of the fire hazards in the operating room and can use this information to perform surgery at your highest level in the safest way possible (Tables 48.2 and 48.3).

TABLE 48-2 Safety Tips in the Operating Room

Ignition source control	Electrosurgical unit (ESU, "Bovie")	■ Use cut/blend ■ Use the lowest power possible ■ Remove/dispose of active electrode when not needed ■ Keep in safety holster when not in use
	Light sources (laparoscopic light sources, headlamps, lighted retractors)	■ Inspect cables routinely ■ Light source should be on standby mode when not in active use ■ Never put the end of the light source directly on the drapes ■ Remove light sources from operative field when they are not in use
	Electrodes (ECG leads, defibrillator, or pacemaker pads)	■ Use correct size for patient and for energy supply ■ Use correct lubricants (should be stocked appropriately) ■ Precise placement of the leads ■ Make sure cables are connected properly before using
Oxidizer control	Setup	■ Limit covering face with drapes ■ Use adhesive drapes where possible ■ Dilute under-drape gases with room air if $FIO_2 > 30\%$
	Communication	■ Use direct, plain language ■ Clearly state when gases are being delivered and when energy devices are being activated
	Airway protection	■ ETT or LMA when supplemental O_2 or anesthetic gases are required ■ Use appropriate ETT or LMA when certain energy devices are in use (eg, laser-resistant ETT) ■ Air-O_2 blenders may reduce need for O_2 ■ Wet sponges around ETT cuff or in back of mouth during airway surgery
	Remove hazards	■ Evacuate surgical smoke ■ Suction O_2 from oral cavity when applying energy devices to airway operations

TABLE 48-2 Safety Tips in the Operating Room   (Continued)

Fuel control	Alcohol-based skin preparation	▪ Minimize pooling on skin or on absorptive surfaces (hair, towels, linens) ▪ Clearly communicate when prep has been fully applied ▪ Wait full 3 min prior to draping patient
	Drapes	▪ Minimize redundant drapes ▪ Clear surgical field of sponges and towels that are not in use
	Chemicals	▪ Keep flammable chemicals in sealed containers when not in use ▪ Do not store chemicals near energy devices

ECG, electrocardiography; ETT, endotracheal tube; FIO_2, fraction of inspired oxygen; LMA, laryngeal mask airway. Data from: AORN. Fire Prevention in the Perioperative Setting. Denver, Colorado; 2018. https://www.aorn.org/guidelines/clinical-resources/tool-kits/non-member-tool-kits/fire-safety-tool-kit-nonmembers and Kaye AD, Kolinsky D, Urman RD. Management of a fire in the operating room. J Anesth. 2014;28(2):279-287. doi:10.1007/s00540-013-1705-6 and O.I. Ahmed, MD, G. Sanchez, BA, K. McAllister, and PA, M. Girshin M. Fire Safety In The Operating Room. Anesth Patient Saf Found Newsl. 2013;(Spring-Summer):17. https://www.apsf.org/article/fire-safety-in-the-operating-room/ and Stewart MW, Bartley GB. Fires in the operating room: Prepare and prevent. Ophthalmology. 2015;122(3):445-447. doi:10.1016/j.ophtha.2014.08.049 and Daane SP, Toth BA. Fire in the Operating Room: Principles and Prevention. Plast Reconstr Surg. 2005;115(5):73e-75e. doi:10.1097/01.PRS.0000157015.82342.21 and Association of Perioperative Registered Nurses. AORN guidance statement: fire prevention in the operating room. AORN J. 2005;81(5):1067-75.

TABLE 48-3 Operating Room Fire Response Plan: Role-Specific Responsibility in an Airway Fire

Beth Israel Lahey Health ➤ Beth Israel Deaconess Medical Center		
OPERATING ROOM FIRE RESPONSE PLAN		
ROLE-SPECIFIC RESPONSIBILITIES IN AN AIRWAY FIRE		
Fire Category: Small Fire (Unable to put out by hand)		
Airway Fire	**Responsible Person**	**Action**
Example: The cuff of an endotracheal tube is ignited by sparks from laser.	Anesthesia Provider	1. Stop flow of oxygen. 2. Remove endotracheal tube. 3. Restore breathing with air (Ambu bag).

(Continued)

TABLE 48-3 Operating Room Fire Response Plan: Role-Specific Responsibility in an Airway Fire (Continued)

	Anesthesia Technician	1. Get new endotracheal tube. 2. Assist with airway management.
	Surgeon	1. Immediately stop source of ignition (ie, laser). 2. Assess patient injury.
	Scrub	1. Pour saline from back table onto fire or throw a wet towel on the ignited tube if the tube is still burning. 2. Push back table away from field.
	Circulating Nurse	1. Activate RED emergency call light (West campus only). 2. Dial 2-1212 and report fire in (exact location: West, Feldberg, Shapiro) O.R. #___. 3. Stat page for help. 4. Notify Floor Marshall. 5. File incident report.
	Resource Nurse/Floor Marshall	1. Pull fire alarm. 2. In collaboration with anesthesia, turn off oxygen shut-off valve outside of room. 3. Direct personnel to close all doors; unplug electrical devices if involved, get fire extinguisher if needed.
	Code Red Team	Responds immediately.

Extracted from *PSM 100-112 Fire Plan, Perioperative Services.* Beth Israel Deaconess Medical Center, Boston, MA; 2019 © BIDMC used with permission.

 PEARLS

1. Be sure to take note of all possible fire causes and take the necessary precautions, this includes laying down towels at the patient's side when prepping so that the flammable liquid prep does not drip or pool.
2. Should a fire occur, remove all materials that may be on fire, extinguish all materials on fire, control bleeding, and conclude the procedure as soon as possible. If emergent evacuation is necessary, place sterile towels or covers over the surgical site and evacuate the operating room expeditiously.
3. FUSE is an important course that is free to study and shed light into electrosurgery and its potential risks.

References

1. FDA. Consumer Update : FDA and Partners Working to Prevent Surgical Fires. https://www.fda.gov/ForConsumers/ConsumerUpdates/ucm282810.htm.
2. Jones EL, Overbey DM, Chapman BC, et al. Operating room fires and surgical skin preparation. *J Am Coll Surg*. 2017;225(1):160-165. doi:10.1016/j.jamcollsurg.2017.01.058.
3. ECRI Institute. Technology hazards for 2013 top 10 health. *Health Devices*. 2012;41(HIT HAZARDS):1-25.
4. AORN. *Fire Prevention in the Perioperative Setting*. Denver: Colorado; 2018. https://www.aorn.org/guidelines/clinical-resources/tool-kits/non-member-tool-kits/fire-safety-tool-kit-nonmembers.
5. OR Fire Safety Video – Anesthesia Patient Safety Foundation. https://www.apsf.org/safetynet/apsf-safety-videos/or-fire-safety-video/. Accessed July 23, 2018.
6. Kaye AD, Kolinsky D, Urman RD. Management of a fire in the operating room. *J Anesth*. 2014;28(2):279-287. doi:10.1007/s00540-013-1705-6.
7. Guglielmi CL, Flowers J, Dagi TF, et al. Empowering providers to eliminate surgical fires. *AORN J*. 2014;100(4):412-428. doi:10.1016/j.aorn.2014.08.003.
8. Ahmed OI, Sanchez G, McAllister K, PA M. Girshin M. Fire safety in the operating room. *Anesth Patient Saf Found Newsl*. 2013;(Spring-Summer):17. https://www.apsf.org/article/fire-safety-in-the-operating-room/.
9. Stewart MW, Bartley GB. Fires in the operating room: prepare and prevent. *Ophthalmology*. 2015;122(3):445-447. doi:10.1016/j.ophtha.2014.08.049.
10. Daane SP, Toth BA. Fire in the operating room: principles and prevention. *Plast Reconstr Surg*. 2005;115(5):73e-75e. doi:10.1097/01.PRS.0000157015.82342.21.
11. Jones S. Fundamental use of surgical energy (FUSE): an essential educational program for operating room safety. *Perm J*. 2017;(c):4-9. doi:10.7812/TPP/16-050.
12. Spruce L. Back to basics: preventing surgical fires. *AORN J*. 2016;104(3):217-224.e2. doi:10.1016/j.aorn.2016.07.002.
13. Association of Perioperative Registered Nurses. AORN guidance statement: fire prevention in the operating room. *AORN J*. 2005;81(5):1067-1075.
14. Hart A, Femino M, Sears B, Wolberg A, Cook CH, Gupta A. Have you "CORED" lately? A comprehensive operating room evacuation drill. *Am J Disaster Med*. 2018;13(4):239-252.
15. Keane J, Pawlowski J. Using simulation for OR team training on fire safety *AORN J*. 2019;109(3):374-378.

49

FUNDAMENTALS OF LAPAROSCOPIC SURGERY

BRIAN MINH NGUYEN, MD | STEVEN D. SCHWAITZBERG, MD, FACS

The Fundamentals of Laparoscopic Surgery (FLS) was designed by the Society of American Gastrointestinal and Endoscopic Surgeons (SAGES) as a web-based educational module designed to teach the physiology, fundamental knowledge, and technical skills required to perform basic laparoscopic surgery. The course was developed to improve the quality of care provided to patients undergoing laparoscopic surgery by setting standards for basic knowledge and technical skills required when performing laparoscopy. In order to assess proficiency, certification requires a hands-on skills assessment and a multiple-choice examination.

General surgery residents in the United States are required to pass FLS by the end of residency to be considered eligible for the General Surgery Qualifying Examination by the American Board of Surgery.

The course material consists of five modules and contains comprehensive information pertaining to the fundamental principles of laparoscopic surgery.

Module 1 (perioperative considerations) reviews basic laparoscopic equipment, energy sources, OR setup, patient selection, and preoperative assessment.

Module 2 (intraoperative considerations) includes topics such as anesthesia and patient positioning, establishment of pneumoperitoneum, trocar placement, physiology of pneumoperitoneum, and exiting the abdomen.

Module 3 (basic laparoscopic procedures) provides an overview of current laparoscopic procedures such as diagnostic laparoscopy, biopsy, suturing, and hemostasis.

Module 4 (postoperative care and complications) discusses how to care for postoperative patients and how to manage common complications.

Module 5 (manual skills training) provides an overview of the hand-on skills assessment and describes the tasks that will be tested, including peg transfer, precision cutting, ligating loop, extracorporeal knot tying, and intracorporeal knot tying.

INDICATIONS

The FLS course allows for learning and practicing laparoscopic techniques in a safe simulated environment without putting patients at risk.

The course was designed for any physician with exposure to laparoscopic surgery. This includes residents, fellows, and practicing board eligible/certified physicians in general surgery, gynecology, urology, or other programs that utilize laparoscopic surgery.

PEG TRANSFER

1. The goal is to transfer six rubber ring objects to the opposite side of the board, then back again to the original side of the board.
2. You will be given two Maryland dissectors, one peg board, and six rubber ring objects to complete this task.
3. Place all six objects on the side of the peg board that corresponds to your nondominant hand.
4. Start by picking up a single object with a grasper in your nondominant hand and transferring it in midair to the grasper in your dominant hand.
5. Carefully place the object on the opposite side of the board. There is no importance given to the color of the object, nor the order in which they are transferred.
6. Once all the objects have been transferred, grasp one of the previously transferred object with the dominant hand first, transfer it to the nondominant hand, and place it on the original side of the board.

7. If an object is dropped within the field of view, you can pick it up with the grasper that it dropped from and continue the task.
8. If the object falls outside the field of view, you may not retrieve it.
9. Time begins when you touch the first object and ends upon the release of the last object.
10. You have a maximum of 300 seconds to complete the task.

NOTES

1. To minimize your time, try picking up the next object in one hand while simultaneously placing the previous object on the opposite side.
2. It is important to complete the task with both speed and accuracy without compromising either of them. A dropped peg out of the field of view may prove costly even with a fast time.

PRECISION CUT

1. The goal of this task is to cut a circle along the black line as accurately as possible.
2. You will be given a Maryland dissector and a laparoscopic scissors to complete this task.
3. A 4 × 4 piece of gauze with a premarked circle is secured with one jumbo clip secured to the Velcro with the open edge inside the clip and the folded edge closest to you secured by two alligator clips, which are attached to the trainer box.
4. The clips should be adjusted so that the gauze is pulled taut and suspended slightly above the surface of the trainer.
5. Start by cutting through the border of the cloth to gain access to the circle and carefully cut along the black line.
6. Continue working your way around the circle until it is completely excised.
7. Penalties are assessed for any cuts deviating from the line, be it inside or outside of the black line.
8. If the gauze comes out of the jumbo clip during the task, you must continue to complete the task without reaffixing the gauze.
9. Time begins when the gauze is touched and ends when the marked circle is completely cut out.
10. You have a maximum of 300 seconds to complete the task.

NOTES

1. You can use the grasper and scissors in either hand and can switch hands at any time during the procedure.
2. The cloth that is provided will be two-ply, but only the top layer that includes the black line will be scored. You can cut as much or as little of the bottom layer as you like. You may find it easier to cut only the top layer.
3. It is helpful to provide counter tension with the Maryland dissector to assist in cutting the circle as accurately as possible, but be aware that too much tension may cause the gauze to fall out of the large clip, making the task significantly harder to complete.

LIGATING LOOP

1. The goal of this task is to place a pretied ligating loop around the provided mark on the middle appendage of the foam organ.
2. For this task, you will be provided one grasper (choice of Maryland dissector or one with a locking/ratcheted handle), one pair of laparoscopic scissors, and a pretied ligating loop.
3. A red foam organ with appendages is fixated to a large clip attached to the trainer box.
4. Place the loop around the indicated line on the appendage.
5. Once the loop is around the appendage, break off the end of the plastic pusher on the outside of the trainer.
6. Slide the pusher rod down to secure the knot on the mark.
7. Once the knot is completely synched down, remove the grasper and use the laparoscopic scissors to cut the suture, completing your task.
8. You will be penalized for any deviation of the knot from the mark on the foam appendage or if the knot is not secured to properly in the appendage.
9. Timing begins when either the grasper or loop material is visible on the monitor and ends when you have cut the end of the loop material inside the trainer.
10. You have a maximum of 180 seconds to complete this task.

NOTES

1. FLS allows using either one or two hands to cinch down the ligating loop. Mastering the two-handed technique will allow you to maintain tension to assure accuracy of placement. The use of a locking grasper will allow you to use the two-handed technique.
2. Do not break off the end of the plastic pusher prior to beginning the task.

SUTURE WITH EXTRACORPOREAL KNOT TYING

1. The goal of this task is to place a long suture through the two preformed marks on a Penrose drain and place three single throws of a knot extracorporeally using a knot pusher, closing the slit on the Penrose drain.
2. For this task you will be given two needle drivers (or choice of one needle driver and one Maryland dissector), a knot pusher (open or closed), a 2-0 silk suture measuring either 90 or 120 cm in length, and a pair of laparoscopic scissors.
3. A Penrose drain, with two premarked targets and a slit through the middle, is secured with Velcro to a suture block, which is secured the floor of the trainer box.
4. Insert the needle by grabbing it by the suture (not the needle) and inserting it through the trocar. Make sure the tail of the stitch remains on the outside of the trocar.
5. Load the needle onto the needle driver and then drive the needle through the two black dots on the Penrose drain. This can be done in one motion or more.
6. Grab the suture and remove through the same trocar that it was inserted.
7. Throw the first knot of a square knot and use the knot pusher to push the knot down toward the Penrose drain, while pulling up on the stitch with the opposite hand.
8. Then perform the second knot of the square knot, and push the knot down in a similar fashion.
9. After three knots have been placed, use the laparoscopic scissors to cut both ends of the suture near the knot, completing your task.
10. Penalties are assessed for any deviation of the suture material from the two marks on the Penrose drain, for not properly closing the slit of the drain, and for a knot that slips or unravels with applied tension.
11. If the Penrose drain is avulsed or separated from the suture block, you automatically fail the task.
12. Timing begins when the first instrument is visualized on the monitor and ends when both ends of the suture or cut inside the trainer box.
13. You have a maximum of 420 seconds to complete the task.

NOTES

1. Depending on the testing center, the type of knot pusher may vary so make sure you are familiar with various types of knot pushers prior to your test date.

2. Remember, the needle cannot be inserted through the trocar if loaded in the needle driver, so it must be inserted by grasping the suture close to the needle, but not the actual needle itself.

3. Be careful not to avulse the Penrose drain when pulling the suture through the drain as this will result in an automatic failure of the task. You can use the other instrument as a pulley to minimize tension on the drain while pulling the suture through an out the trocar.

4. The ends of the suture may be cut separately or together, and there is no importance given to the length of the tails.

SUTURE WITH INTRACORPOREAL KNOT TYING

1. The goal of this task is to place a short suture though the two preformed marks on a Penrose drain and place three throws of a knot intracorporeally, closing the slit in the Penrose drain.

2. For this task you will be given two needle drivers, one 2-0 silk suture cut to 15 cm, and a pair of laparoscopic scissors.

3. A Penrose drain, with two premarked targets and a slit through the middle, is secured with Velcro to a suture block, which is secured the floor of the trainer box.

4. Insert the needle by grabbing it by the suture (not the needle) and inserting it through the trocar.

5. Load the needle onto the needle driver and then drive the needle through the two black dots on the Penrose drain. This can be done in one motion or more.

6. Regrab the needle and pull the stitch through leaving a short tail.

7. Perform an instrument tie with the two needle drivers. The first throw is a double throw, or surgeon's knot. Make sure to loop the suture twice before grabbing the tail and pulling through. You may start tying with either hand.

8. Switch the needle into the opposite hand and perform another throw of the knot.

9. Switch the needle back to the original hand and perform the last throw of the knot.

10. After three knots have been placed, use the laparoscopic scissors to cut both ends of the suture near the knot, completing your task.

11. Penalties are assessed for any deviation of the suture material from the two marks on the Penrose drain, for not properly closing the slit of the drain, and for a knot that slips or unravels with applied tension.

12. If the Penrose drain is avulsed or separated from the suture block, you automatically fail the task.
13. Timing begins when the first instrument is visualized on the monitor and ends when both ends of the suture or cut inside the trainer box.
14. You have a maximum of 600 seconds to complete the task.

NOTES

1. Remember, the needle cannot be inserted through the trocar if loaded in the needle driver, so it must be inserted by grasping the suture close to the needle, but not the actual needle itself.
2. Be careful not to avulse the Penrose drain when pulling the suture through the drain as this will result in an automatic failure of the task. You can use the other instrument as a pulley to minimize tension on the drain while pulling the suture through an out the trocar.
3. The ends of the suture may be cut separately or together, and there is no importance given to the length of the tails.

 PEARLS

1. Although there may be more than one way to perform certain tasks in clinical practice (ligating loop, intracorporeal knot tying), FLS provides a proven safe approach to learning basic laparoscopic skills.
2. You residency program will likely provide you access to FLS trainer boxes. Even if not required in your surgical subspecialty, ask your leadership about accessing this effective curriculum.
3. For residents taking the FLS examination, it is important to allow adequate time to complete the examination and receive your test results in order to register for the American Board of Surgery (ABS) qualifying examination.

50

LAPAROSCOPIC CAMERA NAVIGATION

BRIAN MINH NGUYEN, MD | JORDAN R. GUTWEILER, MD, FACS

Surgical scopes have been around for centuries, with evidence of examples dating back to 70 AD. This ancient relic consisted of a hollow tube used to look into hard-to-visualize areas and were later adapted to include magnification and illumination. The laparoscope has evolved into a complex surgical instrument that has the ability to zoom in and out, adjust focus, see around angles, and project onto a large monitor for an optimal visual experience.

There are many different types of laparoscopes. Laparoscopes come in a variety of sizes, ranging from 1.9 to 12 mm, but the 5 and 10 mm laparoscopes are by far the most common sizes used.

Laparoscopes are also designed with varying viewing angles, ranging from 0° to 70°, which allows visualization of structures from a variety of angles and around corners. A 0-degree laparoscope offers a straight, panoramic view of the surgical field. An angled laparoscope, often a 30- or 45-degree laparoscope, allows for visualization around corners and can be rotated in different directions to provide the best view of a structure from all angles. By changing the angle of the camera, the laparoscope can be repositioned, allowing for more room to manipulate other laparoscopic instruments during surgery. An angled lens provides a narrower field of view and may be less bright compared to a nonangled laparoscope.

The laparoscopic camera is a crucial aspect of laparoscopic surgery and provides visualization of the abdomen or chest. You may be asked to navigate the camera during laparoscopic cases. This job is extremely important, because in laparoscopic surgery, the surgeon can only see what is being shown to him/her.

INDICATIONS

The use of a laparoscope is required for all laparoscopic or thoracoscopic procedures.

TECHNIQUES

SETUP

The laparoscope needs to be connected to a camera and a light source. Once connected, the light source should be turned on and the picture needs to be white-balanced. This is often calibrated using a piece of white gauze. The light intensity, focus, screen capture, white balance, and zoom can be adjusted by using either the control buttons on the camera or through the central control panel. The control buttons should be oriented upward. Any deviation from this will change the horizon and tilt the picture, altering the surgeon and assistant's perception of anatomy.

INSERTING THE LAPAROSCOPE

Depending on the size of the laparoscope, it must be inserted through the corresponding sized trocar. Smaller laparoscopes can be inserted through larger trocars, but not vice versa. When inserting the laparoscope through one of the trocars, make sure the lens is focused and free of debris. Also, make sure that the trocar is free of debris, and if needed, the trocar can be cleaned with a dedicated trocar cleaner or gauze. You should be familiar with how to disassemble the trocar to clean its lumen. To prevent the lens from fogging up in the abdomen, the laparoscope can be warmed in saline or an antifog solution can be used on the lens.

NAVIGATING THE LAPAROSCOPE

When operating the laparoscope, you will be asked to look in a variety of directions. In order to look a certain direction, the stem of the laparoscope should be moved in the opposite direction. This is because the patient's abdominal wall acts as a fulcrum to the laparoscope which serves as a lever. For example, if the surgeon asks you to look up at the abdominal wall, you would tilt the handheld stem of the laparoscope down. To look left, you move the stem to the right.

USING AN ANGLED SCOPE

In order to change the direction of the laparoscope, the laparoscope is rotated while maintaining a steady horizon. Conventionally, the laparoscope is designed so that the light post that is attached to the stem of the laparoscope is oriented in the opposite direction of the angle. Therefore, in order to look in a certain direction, the light port should be oriented in the opposite direction. For example, in order to look to the right of the surgical field, the light source should be pointed to the left.

NEXT STEPS

As your familiarity with the surgical procedure evolves, you may start to anticipate the next steps of the operation and adjust the camera accordingly without requiring prompting.

COMPLICATIONS

POOR VISUALIZATION

This can be due to a variety of things. If there is debris on the lens, remove the laparoscope and remove the debris. If there is debris on the trocar, use a dedicated trocar cleaner, and if not available, gauze or a sterile cotton swab to clean the inside of the trocar. If the lens is foggy, this can be due to a relative difference in temperature between the laparoscope and the abdomen. To prevent this, you can prewarm the laparoscope with warmed saline or use an antifog solution on the lens.

INJURY TO INTRA-ABDOMINAL STRUCTURES

Avoid direct contact between the lens and intra-abdominal structures, because the lens can become very hot and cause thermal injury.

It is also safe practice to watch instruments as they are inserted and removed from the abdomen so that intra-abdominal structures are not stabbed when inserting sharp instruments or pulled through a trocar upon removal of the instrument.

OPERATING ROOM FIRE

Although rare, it has been estimated that over 600 operating room fires occur annually in the United States. If the light source is left on and the laparoscope is rested on the surgical drapes, the drapes can burn and catch fire. To avoid this, the light source can be turned on standby when the camera is not in use. Remember that the laparoscope is still hot for several minutes after turning off the light source; never rest the end of the laparoscope on the surgical drapes or anything flammable!

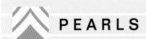 **PEARLS**

1. Always try to keep the surgeon's instruments in the center of the field of view. As the instruments move, so should the field of view.
2. When inserting and removing instruments from the abdomen, it is good practice to keep those instruments in view to avoid inadvertent injury to intra-abdominal structures.
3. When the light source is turned on, the tip of the laparoscope can become hot and can cause thermal injury. Make sure to keep the tip away from direct contact with intra-abdominal structures. Never rest the tip of the camera on the surgical drapes when not in use, as this is can pose a fire risk.

Suggested Readings

1. Brackmann MW, Andreatta P, McLean K, Reynolds RK. Development of a novel simulation model for assessment of laparoscopic camera navigation. *Surg Endosc.* 2017;31(7):3033-3039.
2. Franzeck FM, Rosenthal R, Muller MK, et al. Prospective randomized controlled trial of simulator-based versus traditional in-surgery laparoscopic camera navigation training. *Surg Endosc.* 2012;26(1):235-241.

51

FUNDAMENTALS OF ENDOSCOPIC SURGERY

DANIEL A. HASHIMOTO, MD, MS | ERIKA K. FELLINGER, MD, FACS

Endoscopy is a core component of general surgery, thoracic surgery, and otolaryngology practice. This chapter will focus on both upper and lower gastrointestinal (GI) endoscopy for a variety of indications. The Fundamental of Endoscopic Surgery (FES) program,[1] created by the Society of American Gastrointestinal and Endoscopic Surgeons (SAGES), is a test of knowledge and skill in flexible GI endoscopy that has set a benchmark of proficiency for surgeons (Figure 51.1). The cognitive knowledge portion of the examination consists of a multiple-choice examination administered online. The skill portion of the examination is performed on a virtual reality simulator and involves five tasks that assess the following skills: (1) scope navigation, (2) loop reduction, (3) mucosal inspection, (4) retroflexion, and (5) targeting. Validation of this examination was based on the performance of experienced endoscopists (defined as those having performed >100 upper and lower endoscopies) and those of novice endoscopists.[2] It is a requirement for certification of endoscopic proficiency and for general surgery board certification from the American Board of Surgery.[3]

405

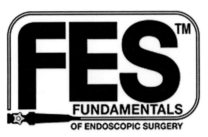

FIGURE 51.1 Fundamental of Endoscopic Surgery (FES) program logo. (Reprinted with permission from the Society of American Gastrointestinal and Endoscopic Surgeons.)

FES is hosted on the 3DSystems GI Mentor endoscopic simulator (Figure 51.2), a virtual reality endoscopy simulator that has been the subject of multiple studies assessing construct validity.[4-6] Recent research has demonstrated that proficiency-based training can improve pass rates on the FES examination.[7-9] Completing and passing FES reliably indicates basic competency and safety in upper and lower endoscopy for surgeons. Proficiency and efficiency in endoscopy are gained over time with increasing volume and monitoring of quality indicators in early practice. The FES-certified endoscopist must be able to perform basic therapeutic interventions as part of the endoscopic procedure including biopsy, polyp removal by hot or cold snare, injection for tattooing and saline lift of lesions, or other indication. It is not appropriate to perform endoscopy solely for visual inspection without having the ability to intervene therapeutically if needed. Endoscopists should be able to recognize abnormal pathology.

INDICATIONS FOR ENDOSCOPY

UPPER ENDOSCOPY

Upper endoscopy includes esophagoscopy, esophagogastroscopy, and esophago-gastroduodenoscopy. There are numerous indications for patients to undergo initial endoscopy of their upper GI tract and include

- Failure of PPI therapy
- Failure of *Helicobacter pylori* treatment with persistently elevated *H. pylori* titer
- Anemia

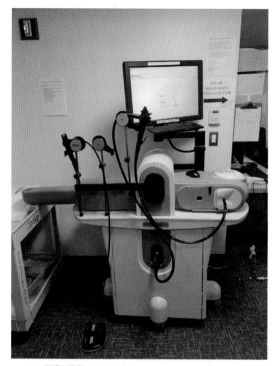

FIGURE 51.2 The GI Mentor simulator.

- GI bleeding (including hematemesis, hematochezia, melena)
- Weight loss >10 pounds in 3 months
- Dysphagia or odynophagia
- Upper GI obstruction
- Suspected GI neoplasm
- Mucosal irregularities seen on radiologic imaging

Furthermore, once initial endoscopy is performed, there are also indications for which a patient should undergo routine surveillance. These include but are not limited to

- Familial polyposis: every 1 to 2 years
- Esophageal varices after sclerotherapy or banding: every 6 to 8 weeks
- Gastric and esophageal ulcer: every 6 weeks until healed
- Barrett esophagus
  - Low risk (<3 cm, no dysplasia): every 2 years

- Moderate (>3 cm, circumferential): yearly
- High risk (low-grade dysplasia): every 6 months

Upper endoscopy can also be therapeutic in nature. Procedures that can be performed via upper endoscopy include sclerotherapy, banding, or injection of bleeding esophageal or gastric varices; endoscopic retrograde cholangiopancreatography (ERCP) for alleviation of choledocolithiasis, gallstone pancreatitis, or stenting of common bile duct strictures; stenting of the esophagus; and even surgical procedures such as per oral endoscopic myotomy (POEM) for achalasia.

There are also a number of procedures which depend on the endoscopic approach. Percutaneous endoscopic gastrostomy (PEG) is one of the most common.

LOWER ENDOSCOPY

There are similarly numerous possible indications for lower endoscopy (ie colonoscopy, sigmoidoscopy, proctoscopy).

Colon cancer screening guidelines include the following:

- For patients with average colorectal cancer risk (average risk patients are those without a personal history of colorectal cancer, inflammatory bowel disease, or certain polyps; a family history of colorectal cancer; a hereditary colorectal cancer syndrome; and a personal history of radiation to the abdomen or pelvis for a prior cancer)[10]:
  - Colonoscopy or other screening mechanism beginning at the age of 45 years with repeat colonoscopy at 10-year intervals
- For patients with a first-degree relative with colorectal cancer or adenoma and age of onset older than 60 years:
  - Colonoscopy at 40 years of age with repeat at 10-year intervals
- For patients with a first-degree relative with colorectal cancer or adenoma and age of onset younger than 60 years:
  - Colonoscopy at 40 years of age or 10 years before age of onset in relative, whichever is younger, with repeat colonoscopy at 5-year intervals
- For patients with familial adenomatous polyposis (FAP), which is an autosomal dominant inactivation mutation of APC gene that is expressed as adenomatous polyposis of the colon with progression to colorectal cancer:
  - Screening with upper and lower endoscopy in teenage years
  - These patients will ultimately require prophylactic colectomy to avoid colorectal cancer

- For patients with hereditary nonpolyposis colorectal cancer (HNPCC), an autosomal dominant mutation in DNA mismatch repair that conveys increased risk of cancer:
  - Colonoscopy beginning at the age of 20 years or 10 years before age of onset of colorectal cancer in youngest relative with repeat colonoscopy at 1 to 2-year intervals

  Other indications for colonoscopy include the following:

- GI bleeding
- Unexplained alterations in bowel habits, including prolonged constipation or diarrhea
- Abnormal imaging findings in the colon or rectum
- Assessment of prior colonic anastomoses

Surveillance colonoscopy is typically indicated for patients with colorectal cancer and adenomas/polyps found on screening (frequency is based on the type and number of polyps identified) and for patients with inflammatory bowel disease.

STEPS

Informed consent for endoscopic procedures must be done diligently and should include at minimum the following points: risk of bleeding, return to the endoscopy suite to control bleeding, risk of perforation, need for surgery to repair perforation, and missing a lesion, even with a good preparation.

For both upper and lower endoscopy, the endoscope is held in the left hand to provide control over the scope with the dials (Figure 51.3).

UPPER ENDOSCOPY

Patients do not have to undergo a bowel preparation for upper endoscopy; however, patients should be NPO (nil per os) for 6 to 8 hours prior to undergoing their endoscopy. Upper endoscopy can be performed without sedation, with sedation, or under general anesthesia, depending on the situation and the patient. If usage of electrosurgical energy is anticipated, a grounding pad (ie dispersive electrode) should be placed on the patient.

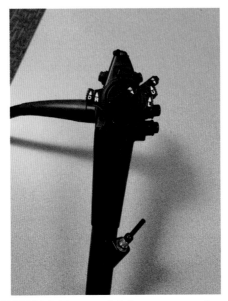

FIGURE 51.3 The typical dials seen on an endoscope.

To perform an esophagogastroduodenoscopy, the following steps are recommended:

1. The patient should be positioned in the left lateral decubitus position with the head slightly elevated. If the endoscopy is being performed for upper GI bleeding, the patient can be placed in the right lateral decubitus position to facilitate emptying of blood from the fundus of the stomach.
2. The endoscope is inserted into the patient's mouth, preferably under direct visualization, through a bite block. The scope tip should be deflected downward using the large dial. The scope is then advanced along the posterior hypopharynx as the patient swallows, while the endoscopist pushes the scope into the upper esophagus.
3. The endoscope is then advanced through the esophagus with care being taken to examine the entire mucosa circumferentially.
4. The gastroesophageal junction, marked by the Z-line (Figure 51.4), should be noted and examined for changes such as Barrett esophagus or hiatal hernia.
5. The stomach is then entered. The gastric rugae (Figure 51.5) provide visual confirmation that the stomach has been entered. Insufflation of the stomach will allow greater visualization of the gastric mucosa as the rugae smooth out.

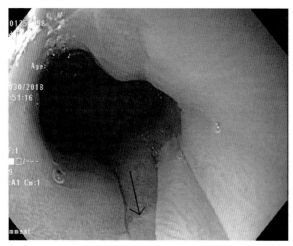

FIGURE 51.4 The Z-line or squamocolumnar junction (black arrow) that denotes the gastroesophageal junction.

6. The endoscope is then further advanced toward the pylorus, often seen at the 1 or 2 o'clock position on the endoscope screen if proper orientation of the scope has been maintained.
7. The endoscope is carefully passed through the pylorus into the duodenum.

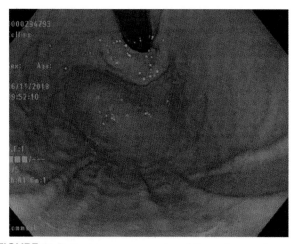

FIGURE 51.5 Gastric ruggage as viewed through an endoscope.

8. The bulb of the duodenum is examined before proceeding around the superior angle of the duodenum to inspect the ampulla of Vater.
9. Biopsies of the duodenum can be taken as necessary.
10. The scope is then withdrawn from the duodenum and back into the stomach to inspect the antrum and body.
11. The large dial of the endoscope is turned backward to deflect the tip of the endoscope up and into a J-shape. This allows visualization of the gastroesophageal (GE) junction in a retroflexed view.
12. The endoscope is then rotated 360° to allow visualization of the entire GE junction.
13. Biopsies of the stomach can be taken as necessary.
14. The scope is then straightened and withdrawn back into the esophagus and out of the patient's mouth, as the lumen is desufflated.

LOWER ENDOSCOPY

For lower GI endoscopy, a bowel preparation is needed to maximize visualization of the mucosa. Bowel preparations can be isosmotic (safer for patients with hepatic failure, renal failure, or congestive heart failure) or hyperosmotic (smaller volume of fluid to ingest but with higher risk of creating fluid and electrolyte imbalance). Sigmoidoscopy can be performed with or without sedation. Colonoscopy can be performed with sedation or general anesthesia, depending on the patient and situation.

To perform colonoscopy, the left hand is used to control the dials, insufflation, suction, and irrigation, while the right hand is used to drive the shaft of the scope. Two-handed techniques can also be used as needed. Steps for colonoscopy include the following:

1. The patient is placed in the left lateral decubitus position or in the supine, frog-leg position. If the colonoscopy is being performed through a stoma, the patient is laid supine.
2. Every colonoscopy should begin with visual inspection of the anus and a digital rectal examination.
3. The lubricated colonoscope is introduced via the anus into the rectum. It is then advanced upwards into the sigmoid colon.
4. Insufflation is used as needed for visualization.
5. The scope should be maintained as straight as possible to increase control.

6. The sigmoid colon is the most tortuous element of the colon, and redundant sigmoid colon can make it difficult to navigate loops. Techniques such as torqueing the shaft of the scope clockwise and counterclockwise can help navigate loops and turns.
7. The splenic flexure can sometimes be recognized by assessing for cardiac pulsation that is transmitted through to the colon.
8. The transverse colon can be recognized by the triangular shape of the colonic walls. These are due to the taenia coli lining the colon.
9. The hepatic flexure is often recognized by a bluish shadow on the mucosal wall from the liver.
10. The cecum can be identified by the presence of the appendiceal orifice, the ileocecal valve, or the crow's foot confluence of the taenia coli.
11. As the scope is withdrawn, the mucosa of the entire colon is inspected carefully for polyps and other lesions.
12. Snares and forceps can be utilized to perform biopsies and polypectomies as needed.
13. The dentate line demarcates the upper two-thirds and lower third of the anal canal.

Additional tips, tricks, and demonstrations can be found by taking the free online FES didactic curriculum at www.fesdidactic.org.

COMPLICATIONS

Complications that can occur during or after upper GI endoscopy include sedation- or anesthesia-related cardiopulmonary complications (eg arrhythmia, myocardial infarction, stroke, hypotension, hypoxia, bronchospasm, etc), aspiration, bleeding, perforation, pancreatitis (if undergoing ERCP), and even death. Signs of upper GI perforation include cervical crepitus, substernal chest pain, abdominal pain, and peritonitis.

For lower GI endoscopy, complications are similar and include cardiopulmonary complications, bleeding, perforation with peritonitis, and death. For lower endoscopy, half of all perforations will require operative intervention for further management.

PEARLS

1. For upper endoscopy, internal and external rotation of the endoscope can help turn the tip of the scope without further turning of the dials. For colonoscopy, gentle and strategic palpation of the patient's abdomen—in combination with positional changes—can facilitate passage of the endoscope around tight turns and twists in the colon.
2. Procedures with the highest risk of bleeding include sphincterotomy, polypectomy, dilation, PEG tube placement, fine-needle aspiration, laser ablation and coagulation, and variceal treatment.
3. Nonthermal techniques to control bleeding include submucosal injection, band ligation, placement of endoscopic clips, and balloon tamponade. Thermal techniques include monopolar or bipolar cautery and argon plasma coagulation (APC). Care should be taken when using monopolar cautery, as it has the highest risk of causing full-thickness injury and perforation to tissue.

References

1. Surgery FoE. *Fundamentals of Endoscopic Surgery* [Surgical Fundamentals Online web site]. 2002-2018. Available at http://fesdidactic.org/. Accessed June 28, 2018.
2. Vassiliou MC, Dunkin BJ, Fried GM, et al. Fundamentals of endoscopic surgery: creation and validation of the hands-on test. *Surg Endosc.* 2014;28(3):704-711.
3. ABS , ed. *Flexible Endoscopy Curriculum for General Surgery Residents.* American Board of Surgery; 2014.
4. Bar-Meir S. Simbionix simulator. *Gastrointest Endosc Clin N Am.* 2006;16(3):471-478, vii.
5. Buzink SN, Koch AD, Heemskerk J, et al. Acquiring basic endoscopy skills by training on the GI Mentor II. *Surg Endosc.* 2007;21(11):1996-2003.
6. Fayez R, Feldman LS, Kaneva P, et al. Testing the construct validity of the Simbionix GI Mentor II virtual reality colonoscopy simulator metrics: module matters. *Surg Endosc.* 2010;24(5):1060-1065.
7. Franklin BR, Placek SB, Gardner AK, et al. Preparing for the American Board of Surgery Flexible Endoscopy Curriculum: development of multi-institutional proficiency-based training standards and pilot testing of a simulation-based mastery learning curriculum for the Endoscopy Training System. *Am J Surg.* 2018;216(1):167-173.
8. Hashimoto DA, Petrusa E, Phitayakorn R, et al. A proficiency-based virtual reality endoscopy curriculum improves performance on the fundamentals of endoscopic surgery examination. *Surg Endosc.* 2018;32(3):1397-1404.
9. Ritter EM, Taylor ZA, Wolf KR, et al. Simulation-based mastery learning for endoscopy using the endoscopy training system: a strategy to improve endoscopic skills and prepare for the fundamentals of endoscopic surgery (FES) manual skills exam. *Surg Endosc.* 2018;32(1):413-420.
10. Smith RA, Andrews KS, Brooks D, et al. Cancer screening in the United States, 2018: a review of current American Cancer Society guidelines and current issues in cancer screening. *CA Cancer J Clin.* 2018;68(4):297-316.

52

FUNDAMENTAL USE OF SURGICAL ENERGY

DANIEL A. HASHIMOTO, MD, MS | DANIEL B. JONES, MD, MS

Surgical energy is a key component of modern surgical practice and can come in many forms ranging from monopolar and bipolar current to ultrasonic energy. Although surgical energy is used multiple times a day in operating rooms across the world, the physical properties underlying surgical energy are often poorly understood.

In the operating room, a few common terms are used frequently to describe a wide range of electrosurgical energy events or properties. Perhaps the most common use you will encounter is the word "Bovie." Dr William Bovie was a Harvard engineer who demonstrated electrosurgical cautery to Dr Harvey Cushing in 1926. Dr Cushing successfully used cautery in an operation to limit bleeding, and Bovie's name is now used as a verb in operating rooms through the United States to refer to the act of applying cautery.[1] However, there is more to cautery and electrosurgical energy than merely "burning" tissue to prevent or stop bleeding.

The **Fundamental Use of Surgical Energy (FUSE)** curriculum and examination was designed to inform clinicians, nurses, and technicians on best practices in the use of electrosurgical, ultrasonic, and other energy devices in the operating room for safe use in patients (Figure 52.1).[2] There are three major

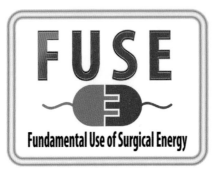

FIGURE 52.1 Fundamental Use of Surgical Energy logo. (Reprinted with permission from the Society of American Gastrointestinal and Endoscopic Surgeons)

categories of electrosurgery: (1) cautery describes the destruction of tissue by passive transfer of heat from a heated instrument, (2) radiofrequency electrosurgery is the conversion of electromagnetic energy into kinetic then thermal energy, and (3) ultrasonic electrosurgery utilizes a piezoelectric transducer to vibrate a blade to generate heat. In this chapter, you will learn the basic terminology, principles, and techniques required to understand the electrosurgery you will encounter in the operating room.

The FUSE curriculum expands on each of these types of electrosurgery, and additional in-depth explanations of concepts with video is available in the free online curriculum from SAGES at www.fusedidactic.org.

BASIC TERMS IN ELECTROSURGERY

To better understand principles of safe surgical energy use, one must first understand the terminology used to describe the physical phenomena underlying electricity. Current (I) refers to the flow of electrons and is measured in amperes (A). Direct current (DC) is that in which the polarity and flow of electrons remain constant while in alternating current (AC), electrons oscillate and result in no net flow of electrons. Voltage (V) is the force needed to push charge along a circuit, and, not unexpectedly, is measured in volts. Impedance or resistance (R) refers to the degree to which the circuit resists electron flow and is measured in ohms. When thinking about surgery and tissue, tissues that are hydrated (ie, have ions) have lower impedance than tissues with a lower water content, such as fat or scar tissue. Thus, current will flow less readily through high-impedance tissues. Energy, measured in joules, is the ability of force to do work, whereas power (P) is the amount of energy expended per unit of time (measured in watts).

Current density is an important concept to understand in surgical energy. It is defined as the amount of current over the area in which that current is applied (A/cm^2). It is important to note that current density is directly proportional to the applied power and inversely proportional to resistance. Therefore, high current density at the tip of a monopolar current electrode can be used to quickly heat and vaporize tissue. Lower current density can be used to coagulate tissue. Tissue heating can be mathematically described as current density squared; thus, the same amount of current over a large area may have less of an effect than that applied over a small area.

CELLULAR EFFECTS OF ELECTROSURGERY

The physical properties and terms described earlier can be utilized to create specific desired effects on tissue to assist surgeons in performing safe operations. The effects of electrosurgery on tissue are occurring largely at the cellular level. Thus, while many surgeons will refer to any act of using cautery as "cauterizing" or "bovie-ing" tissue, there are specific actions occurring at the cellular level depending on the type and amount of current being applied.

Vaporization occurs when the intracellular temperature rapidly elevates to 100°C, generating steam that causes cellular rupture through cell expansion. This is often achieved through use of the "Cut" setting on monopolar instruments. *Desiccation* describes dehydration of the cell through a thermally damaged cell wall (45°C-100°C) and can be achieved with either monopolar or bipolar current. *Coagulation* or "white coagulation" occurs from protein denaturation (50°C-100°C) and is used to obtain hemostasis through vessel coaptation.

Fulguration or "black coagulation" occurs through superficial protein coagulation via carbonization and organic molecular breakdown (>200°C). It requires modulated high-voltage waveforms typically produced by the "coagulation" output of the electrosurgical generator and a "no touch" technique. It is most effective for superficial coagulation of superficial, capillary, and small arteriolar bleeding (ie, "ooze"). *Carbonization* refers to the breakdown of molecules to sugars and the creation of an eschar.

COMMON ELECTROSURGICAL ENERGY INSTRUMENTS

The electrosurgical energy unit converts the low frequency and voltage output from the wall into the high-frequency, high-voltage output needed for electrosurgery (Figure 52.2). It allows for control over the power delivered to a

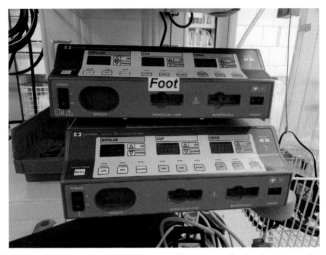

FIGURE 52.2 An electrosurgical unit can provide current for both monopolar and bipolar cautery. If using monopolar cautery, a dispersive electrode must be plugged into the "Patient" slot.

handpiece (monopolar or bipolar instrument) and allows for adjustments to the duty cycle. The duty cycle refers to the proportion of time that a waveform is generated in a given amount of time. For example, the "cut" output has 100% duty cycle with relatively low voltage. The "coag" output, on the other hand, has an interrupted, high-voltage duty cycle that is active on average 6% of the time.

Monopolar instruments have an active electrode (often a penlike device as in Figure 52.3), as well as a dispersive electrode that attaches to the patient (away from the surgical field) to disperse current and prevent thermal injuries. Bipolar instruments are often forcep-like instruments where the two electrodes are within the surgical field and current passes across a small area.

Radiofrequency ablation (RFA) is used to coagulate large areas of tissue. It is often utilized for patients who are palliative or poor surgical candidates or have masses that are deemed unresectable. Although there are many different instrument systems for RFA, the underlying principle involves application of alternating current at a high frequency (375-500 kHz) to heat tissue.

Ultrasonic energy devices use piezoelectric transducers to convert electrical to mechanical energy via vibration of a blade between 23 and 55 kHz to generate heat. These devices can be used for mechanical cutting or to achieve coagulation. Because heat is generated through mechanical energy, it is important to remember that the ultrasonic blade can retain residual heat that can unintentionally burn tissue.

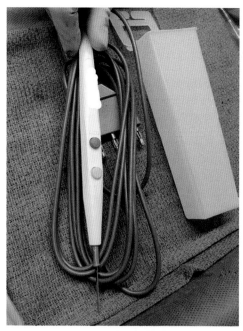

FIGURE 52.3 Monopolar cautery instrument (often referred to as a "Bovie pen"). The yellow button is the "Cut," whereas the blue button is "Coag." When not in use, the instrument should be housed in the plastic holster to prevent accidental activation of the instrument and thermal damage.

COMPLICATIONS

The most common complication of electrosurgical energy is thermal injury or burn. This can occur through a number of mechanisms depending on the type of electrosurgical energy being used.

For any type of energy, one must always consider the potential damage that can occur from the active electrode. Inadvertent activation of the active electrode or ultrasonic instrument can injure tissue. Direct extension injuries can occur when another portion of tissue is directly in contact with the target tissue (such as when two structures are immediately adjacent to one another or adhered to one another with adhesions/scar). One should also inspect the cables used for any instrumentation, as breaks in the insulation can cause current to escape and burn tissue unintentionally. Breaks in insulation are often small holes, leading to high current density and current transmission at the escape site.

Direct coupling occurs when the active electrode is in contact with a second instrument that can then act as a conductor to transmit current to other tissue.

This can occur, for example, if an active electrode comes into contact with a retractor, which then conducts current to skin edges. Sometimes, surgeons will use direct coupling to their advantage to transmit current to different target tissue intentionally.

One common site of thermal injury is at the site of the dispersive electrode. Remember that the dispersive electrode's large area helps to reduce current density and thus limit the risk of injury. Partial detachment of the dispersive electrode can cause burns at the site as the area is reduced and current density increases. Modern systems now use split dispersive electrodes to monitor impedance to two pads, stopping the supply of current if one becomes partially detached.

Burns can affect the surgeon as well as the patient. Use of high voltages can overcome the insulating capacity of the surgical gloves. Furthermore, there is decreased glove resistance with time and exposure to saline (ie, sweat). Also, the residual heat from ultrasonic instruments can burn the surgeon just as easily as it can the patient.

 PEARLS

1. In monopolar electrosurgery, the dispersive electrode has a large area specifically to reduce current density and risk of causing a burn to a patient. Furthermore, the dispersive electrode does not collect the current.
2. Understanding the difference between "cut" and "coag" mode and their setting is important as the tissue effect is variable and allows you to accomplish different tasks.
3. Ultrasonic energy instruments can cause injury even if the instrument is not active through residual heat.

References

1. O'Connor JL, Bloom DA, William T. Bovie and electrosurgery. *Surgery*. 1996;119(4):390-396.
2. Committee FUSE. *Fundamental Use of Surgical Energy*. 2002-2018. Available at: http://www.fusedidactic.org. Accessed June 26, 2018.

53

DO IT YOURSELF LAPAROSCOPIC TRAINER

CARA B. JONES | DENISE W. GEE, MD

Traditional laparoscopic box trainers play an important role in laparoscopic training but can be expensive and difficult to transport. Lower-cost trainers can be easily created from common household materials. These Do It Yourself (DIY) trainers are cost-effective and more mobile. In addition, they can be specifically created to incorporate basic laparoscopic surgical principles such as fulcrum effect, utilize basic laparoscopic instruments, and help learners practice the Fundamentals of Laparoscopic Surgery (FLS) skills. Below, we describe the Twelve Pack Box Trainer, a DIY trainer constructed from a 12-pack soda box and a smartphone functioning as both the laparoscopic camera and operative screen.

MATERIALS REQUIRED

1. Twelve-pack soda box
2. Box cutter or scissors
3. Scrap cardboard

4. FLS pegboard + six triangles or suture block
5. Two laparoscopic graspers
6. Duct tape
7. Small heavy object
8. Ruler
9. iPhone 6 (or similar smartphone)

TRAINER CONSTRUCTION

1. Gather materials listed earlier (Figure 53.1).
2. Using a box cutter, cut a semicircle into the soda box. This semicircle should be 8 to 9 inches wide at the bottom. Use the side with the hand hold gap and make sure not to cut onto the top or bottom side of the box. This will be the side of the box facing AWAY from the surgeon (Figures 53.2 and 53.3).
3. Remove soda cans through the opening created in step 2 (Figure 53.4).
4. If the bottom or top is cut too thin near the top on the box, reinforce this side with duct tape. This is to ensure structural integrity. Put the box to the side for later (Figure 53.5).

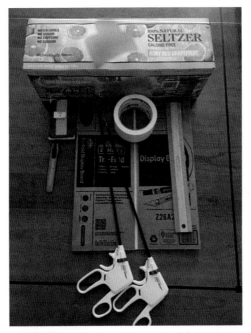

FIGURE 53.1 Materials required for TPBT.

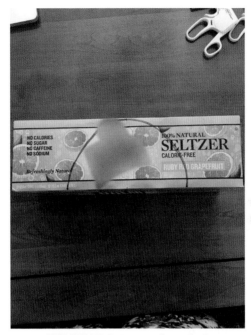

FIGURE 53.2 Semicircle marked.

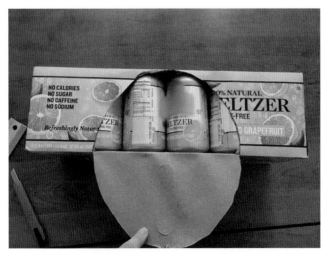

FIGURE 53.3 Semicircle cut.

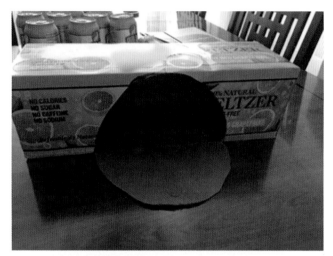

FIGURE 53.4 Soda cans removed.

5. Take scrap cardboard and cut two pieces that measure 5 inches wide by 14 inches long (Figure 53.6).
6. Take one piece of the prepared cardboard and mark at 2, 7, and 9 inches from the short end (Figure 53.7).

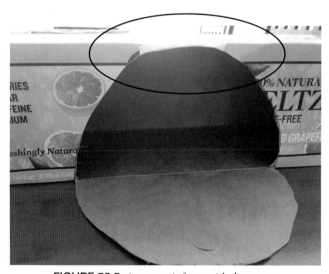

FIGURE 53.5 Area to reinforce with duct tape.

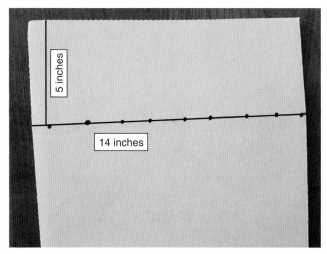

FIGURE 53.6 Scrap cardboard for creating two 5" x 14" rectangles.

7. With slight pressure, use the box cutter to cut superficially the depth of the cardboard at each of these measurement sites to make a foldable edge (be careful not to completely divide the cardboard) (Figure 53.8).
8. Repeat steps 5, 6, and 7 with another piece of cardboard.
9. Fold each cardboard piece to make two rectangles and use duct tape to secure (Figure 53.9).

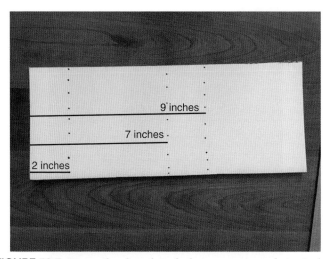

FIGURE 53.7 Prepared carboard marked at two, seven, and nine inches.

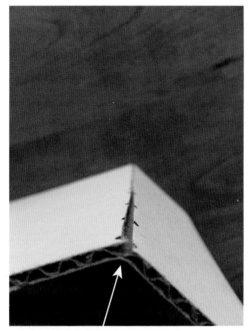

FIGURE 53.8 Cardboard scored to make a foldable corner.

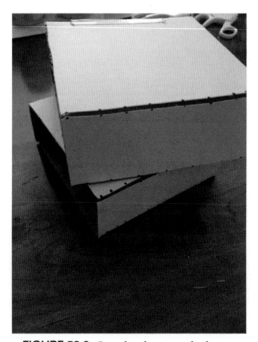

FIGURE 53.9 Completed rectangular boxes.

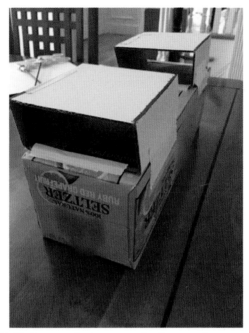

FIGURE 53.10 Rectangular boxes taped to bottom of empty 12-pack box.

10. These two cardboard rectangles will act as a lift to provide approximately 2 inches of height to your trainer. Tape the 5-inch base of the cardboard rectangles to the bottom of the empty 12-pack box (Figures 53.10-53.12).

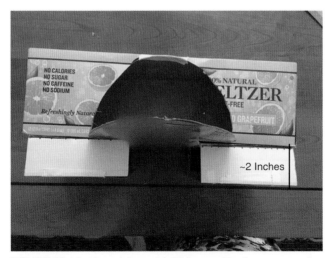

FIGURE 53.11 12-pack box with lift boxes affixed as seen on edge.

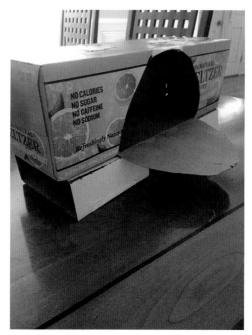

FIGURE 53.12 Box with lifts, set upright.

11. If the height still seems too short or too high, choose the appropriate table height on which the trainer sits.
12. Cut two holes approximately 6 inches apart on the center of the top of the trainer, about the size of a fingertip (Figure 53.13).

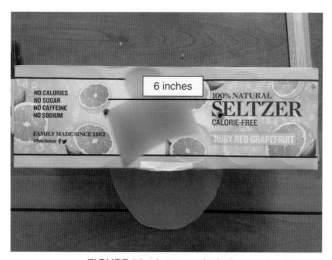

FIGURE 53.13 Layout for holes.

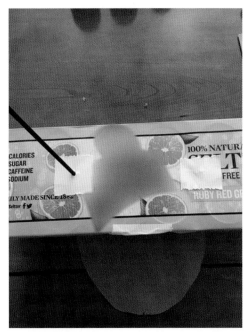

FIGURE 53.14 Holes reinforced with tape.

13. Place duct tape over the holes for reinforcement and poke holes through the tape with the laparoscopic graspers (Figures 53.14 and 53.15).
14. Attach an 11 by 7 ½-inch piece of cardboard at the front base of the trainer. Attach the pegboard to this platform (Figures 53.16-53.18).
15. Take another piece of cardboard, and trace the outline of an Iphone (or similar smartphone) (Figures 53.19 and 53.20).
16. Cut out this outline, and mark the middle of the longest edge. Centered on the long edge, cut out a piece 1 inch in depth, width matching the width of the cell phone. This will be the phone support (Figures 53.21-53.24).
17. Cut a slit in the top of the trainer, about an inch from the front edge, wide enough to accommodate the phone rest (Figure 53.25).
18. Insert the phone support and secure with tape (Figures 53.26-53.28).
19. Position phone on rest so that the pegboard is visible on the phone screen. Adjust accordingly, adding more tape above or below the cardboard phone rest as needed.
20. Insert the graspers, and make sure that there is not any obstruction from the inserted phone rest. If there is, cut the cardboard underneath and resecure with tape.
21. Put a small heavy object inside the trainer to weigh it down and provide stability (Figure 53.29).
    The finished project is shown in Figures 53.30 and 53.31.

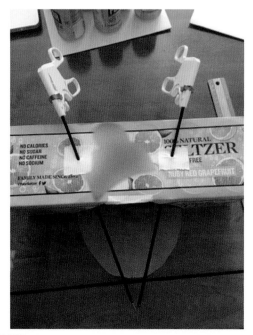

FIGURE 53.15 Laparoscopic graspers passed through holes.

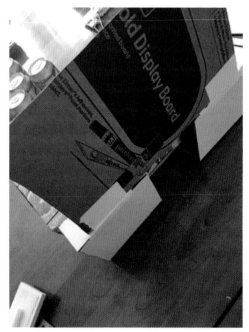

FIGURE 53.16 11" x 7.5" piece of cardboard attached to the front base of the trainer, shown from bottom side.

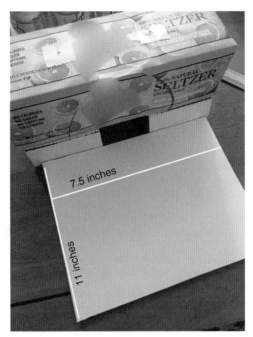

FIGURE 53.17 11" x 7.5" piece of cardboard attached to the front base of the trainer, shown from front.

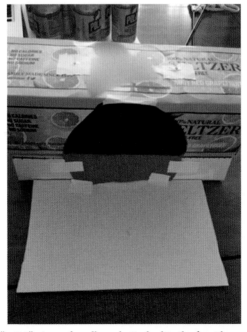

FIGURE 53.18 11" x 7.5" piece of cardboard attached to the front base of the trainer, shown from front and with semicircle window open.

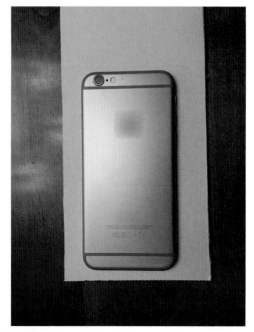

FIGURE 53.19 Smartphone on cardboard for tracing.

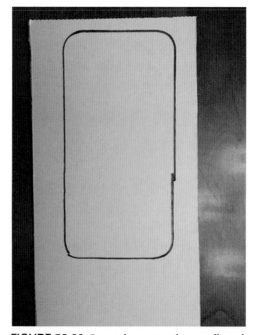

FIGURE 53.20 Smartphone traced on cardboard.

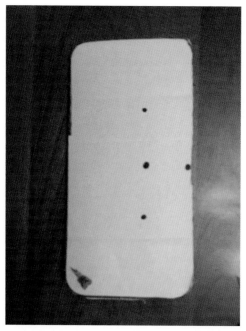

FIGURE 53.21 Cardboard cut to smartphone outline, center of long edge located.

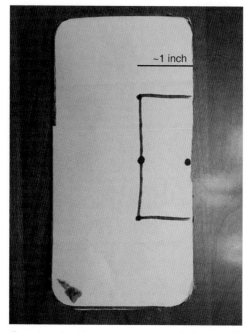

FIGURE 53.22 Cardboard marked for cutting to one inch depth and width of smartphone.

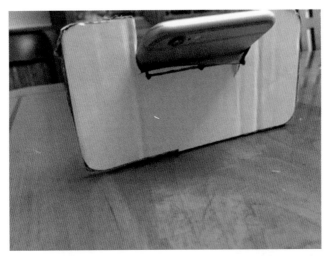

FIGURE 53.23 Phone supported by cardboard, viewed from side.

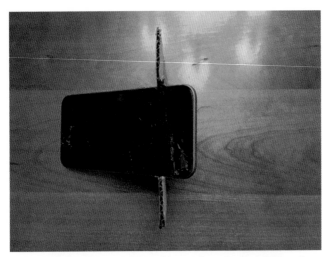

FIGURE 53.24 Phone supported by cardboard, viewed from above.

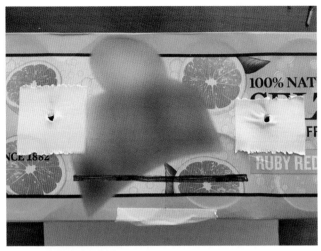

FIGURE 53.25 Slot cut in top for phone support.

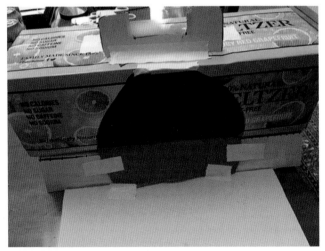

FIGURE 53.26 Phone support taped in place, viewed from front.

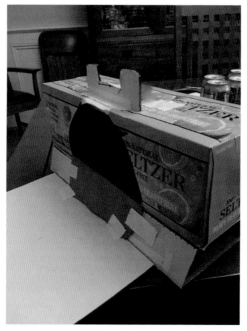

FIGURE 53.27 Phone support taped in place, viewed at angle from front.

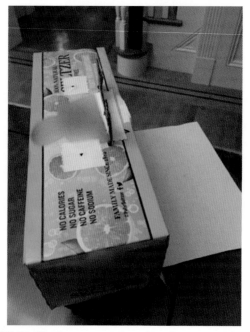

FIGURE 53.28 Phone support taped in place, viewed from side.

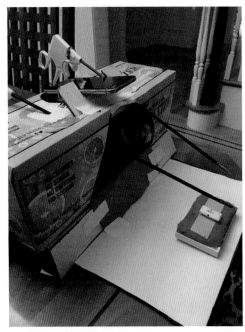

FIGURE 53.29 Assembled trainer with object inside for ballast.

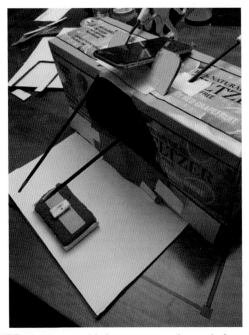

FIGURE 53.30 Assembled trainer, viewed at angle from front.

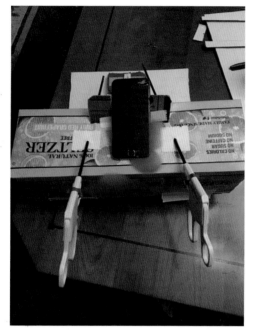

FIGURE 53.31 Assembled trainer, viewed from above.

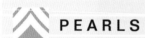 **PEARLS**

1. In a preliminary study, 10 residents were asked to perform the Peg Transfer task on both the standard FLS trainer and the DIY Trainer for a total of four repetitions. The DIY trainer was more difficult for residents to use compared with the FLS trainer likely because of the small size of the smartphone screen.

2. However, the DIY trainer was cost-efficient and effective in simulating the effects of laparoscopy and half of the residents indicated that they would be willing to use it as a take home simulator.

3. This provides a unique opportunity to practice and hone your skills outside the simulation center.

Suggested Reading

1. Jones CB, McKinley S, Valle CValle, et al. A Pilot study of laparoscopic performance on a DIY low cost laparoscopic trainer. Abstract presentation. SAGES Annual Meeting 2018, Seattle, WA.

54

INTRODUCTION TO ROBOTIC SURGERY

MOHAMAD RASSOUL ABU-NUWAR, MD | OMAR YUSEF KUDSI, MD, MBA, FACS

The development of the current robotic surgery systems was funded by the Defense Advanced Research Projects Agency and National Aeronautics and Space Administration. They were intended to perform surgery from long distances via console during remote deployments. The technology that led to the creation of the *da Vinci* system was initially licensed from IBM, MIT, and SRI International. The first robotic surgery performed using da Vinci was in 1998 in Europe for cardiac surgery (coronary artery bypass graft). Since then, five generations of robots have become commercially available. Currently, there are more than 4000 robotic systems (*da Vinci*, intuitive) installed worldwide and over 4 million procedures have been performed by surgeons since inception (Figures 54.1 and 54.2).

In regards to competition, TransEnterix, Inc. entered the market with their first Senhance system in 2017. Titan Medical, Inc. is in the process of entering the market with their SPORT robotic platform. Google has collaborated with Ethicon and formed Verb Surgical Inc. in the process of designing a digital surgical platform. There are numerous other companies in the process of entering the market, such as Medtronic and Cambridge Medical Robotics, in the near future.

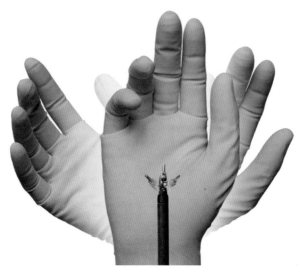

FIGURE 54.1 Endowrist instrument mimicking hand articulation. (With permission from Intuitive Surgical.)

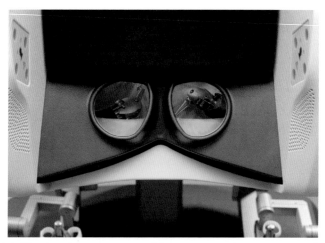

FIGURE 54.2 The view the surgeon sees while operating at the surgeon console. (With permission from Intuitive Surgical.)

THE DA VINCI PLATFORM

The system is based on three components: (1) the patient-side cart, (2) the surgeon-side cart also known as surgeon console, and (3) the vision cart. The *da Vinci* platform utilizes stereoscopic three-dimensional endoscope and near infrared imaging technology Firefly to help in the assessment of tissue perfusion and identification of anatomical structures after injection of indocyanine green. There is a large arsenal of advanced wristed instrumentations (Figure 54.3), such as vessel sealer, monopolar scissors, bipolar graspers, staplers with SmartClamp, and wristed suction irrigation device. Industry has taken collaboration to the next level by integrating the *da Vinci* technology with the operating table TruSystem 7000dV (TRUMPF Medezin System, Germany). Such option enables repositioning of the operating room (OR) table without the need to redock the robotic arms (patient-side cart).

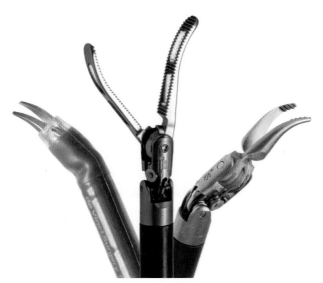

FIGURE 54.3 A close-up view of the da Vinci Xi System instruments. (With permission from Intuitive Surgical.)

SURGEON-SIDE CART (SURGEON CONSOLE)

The surgical console is similar to the pilot cockpit, as it includes the master controllers, central touchpad, foot-switch panel, 3D HD stereo viewer, and right and left pods. As the technology continues to evolve, surgeons are being able to adjust and control more features from the touchpad, such as controlling the brightness, adjusting monopolar and bipolar energy. The surgeon despite being outside the sterile field is able to operate four robotic arms while comfortably seated. The technology enables seamless translation of the surgeon's hand, wrist, and finger into precise, filtered real-time movement of wristed instruments. Such translation could be adjusted according to the operating surgeon preference. Clutch buttons enable surgeons to disengage the master controllers from the robotic instruments thus enabling repositioning without any robotic arm movement to ensure proper ergonomics (Figures 54.4 and 54.5). In regards to stereo viewer the surgeon has advanced features such as multi-image mode, which displays, for example,

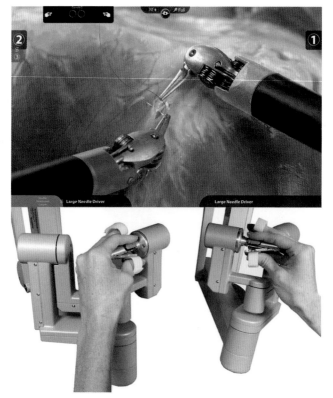

FIGURE 54.4 Surgeon siting at the console. (With permission from Intuitive Surgical.)

ultrasound image along the image of the surgical field, which is as well visible to all OR personnel. Lastly, the existing surgeon console has no haptic feedback, which is a topic of debate as many are able to compensate with visual feedback.

PATIENT-SIDE CART

The patient-side cart allows the robotic instruments and camera to be introduced with tremor stabilization into the surgical field. The patient-side cart consists of four robotic arms that allow for humanlike maneuvers. Their design enables 7° of freedom, mimicking full articulation of human wrist allowing for dexterity in minimally invasive surgeries. All robotic arms are covered with sterile drapes and equipped with adapters to facilitate mounting or exchanging any of the instruments (Figures 54.6-54.8).

The robotic cannulas are metallic as they offer a sturdy replacement to ensure they withstand the forces from the robotic arms. They are reusable with disposable rubber stoppers and come in two lengths, 11 and 16 cm, for patients with higher body mass index. The cannulas are marked by three black stripes (two thin and one thick) toward their end. When inserting the cannula, a single thin

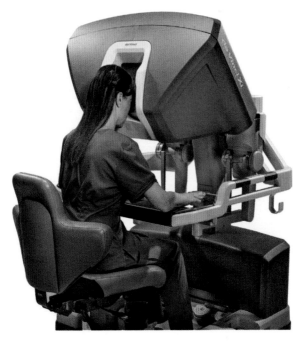

FIGURE 54.5 Surgeon's hands on the console controls and a view of the operative screen. (With permission from Intuitive Surgical.)

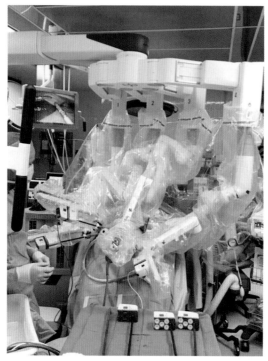

FIGURE 54.6 Patient cart docked with sterile drapes and operating instruments.

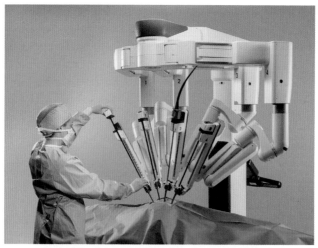

FIGURE 54.7 An operating room staff assisting in robotic surgery next to the patient cart. (With permission from Intuitive Surgical.)

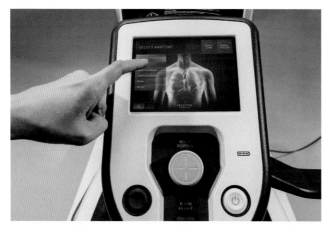

FIGURE 54.8 The user interface on the back of the patient-side cart. (With permission from Intuitive Surgical.)

stripe should be visualized intraperitoneally. The thick band should ideally be at the abdominal wall musculature and is the ports "remote center." This is a fixed point of axis along which the robot will use this port, its purpose is to minimize trauma to the abdominal wall through pulling and pushing. A distance of 20 cm from the target anatomy provides an excellent visual field and is recommended.

Docking refers to attaching the robotic ports to the patient-side cart. With reference to port placement, it is advised to have 6 to 8 cm between each port to offer adequate working space for the robotic arms and avoid collision. The latest patient-side cart has the target feature where the (+) sign is positioned on top of the camera port. After attaching one robotic arm to a cannula and inserting the endoscope, the point of interest is identified visually followed by pressing the targeting button, which in turn repositions all four robotic arms into a proper position allowing for docking/attaching of the remaining arms. Obviously, surgeons should be able to trouble shoot and optimize the joint angles before scrubbing out and sitting on the surgeon console.

VISION CART

The vision cart contains the system's central connect hub, touchscreen monitor, enabling OR personnel to control the system and watch the surgery as well (Figure 54.9). The touchscreen monitor has a feature of drawing, enabling teachers to draw and provide instructions to their trainees. There are speakers and microphone to facilitate clear communication with the

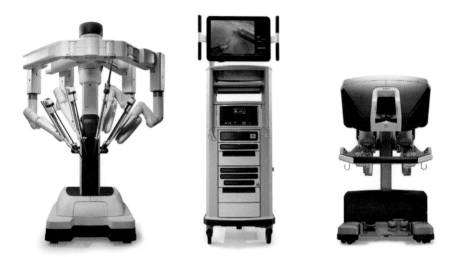

FIGURE 54.9 Surgeon console, vision cart, and patient cart. (With permission from Intuitive Surgical.)

operating surgeon on the console. The cart contains as well the electrosurgical generator and space for additional attachments such as video recorders and pressure flow control devices. During surgery the hub is connected to the internet through ethernet cable; such connection facilitates troubleshooting when calling customer service. A proper OR design should be considered upon deploying the three carts with their connecting wires to ensure patient safety and efficient work flow.

TRAINING

As robotically assisted surgery continues to grow and expand, we can expect the field to continue to evolve. Currently available at many centers, it is becoming incorporated into the training of attendings, fellows, and residents. Unlike other specialties in surgery there is no curriculum or set pathway to become certified in robotic surgery. Industry, however, offers a curriculum of their own that takes trainees through a stepwise fashion to attain their certification. As time progresses a curriculum is sure to develop.

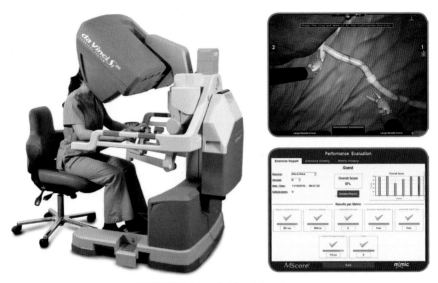

FIGURE 54.10 da Vinci simulator.

Training progresses systematically through four phases. Phase one starts off with review of the education material, including lectures explaining the system hardware and software with digital assessment (Figure 54.10). It includes also a beginner training on the robotic simulator (the peg transfer, walking a ring along a rail, suturing, etc.). Phase two includes review of surgical videos and additional simulator experience. Phase three has a focus on hands-on skills with a dry lab followed by animal lab, finally ending in phase four in which the trainee needs 10 cases as first assistant where she/he docks the robot and 20 cases as operating surgeon where they performed >50% of the case. Teaching console is an additional surgeon console that enables both surgeons to exchange control and collaborate in a more efficient and effective way.

Simulation continues to develop with the recent addition of procedure-specific options such as inguinal hernia repair. Finally, we truly believe that, to have successful robotic programs, there is need to develop and implement proper robotic team training to ensure patient safety and avoid prolonged unnecessary operative expense.

PEARLS

1. Robotic surgery has many benefits to offer the surgeon, including elimination of tremors, greater range of motion, and ergonomic controls.
2. When docking the robot, it is important to include at least 6 cm distance between ports and 20 cm between the camera port and the target anatomy and place the cannula in the appropriate location so that the remote center axis is accurate.
3. As a trainee, access to the robot may be limited. It falls upon you to make the effort to find a suitable time and place to train. This may be very rewarding if you can demonstrate confidence and knowledge in basic robotic skills.

55

WORK LIFE BALANCE

STEPHANIE K. SERRES, MD, PhD | ALLEN D. HAMDAN, MD

INTRODUCTION

Work life balance, although difficult during residency, is very possible to achieve. The balance will likely fluctuate based on your year in training, the time of the year, and the specific rotation.

Most residents are able to do at least one activity outside of work well during residency. For instance, some residents focus their efforts on running and are able to train for marathons in their free time. Other residents have children, and use their time outside of work for parenting. No matter what you decide to use your free time for, you will inevitably go through phases of having more or less balance. Enjoy the times when you have more balance, and focus on working hard through the times you are missing balance. You cannot be or do everything, but you can be or do anything.

In general, as a resident it is useful to delegate as much as possible. If able to do so financially, pay for someone to do your housekeeping, laundry, grocery shopping, and so on. This will free up those precious free minutes to do something you actually enjoy. When you have a golden weekend, try to get out of town to have a mini vacation. Be protective and measured with the time outside of work.

HEALTH

Protect it. Sleep when you can. Eat regular balanced meals. This requires some planning. Keep doctor and dentist appointments. Do something physical you like, from running to basketball. Consider yoga and/or meditation to get your mind off the rigors of work.

SIGNIFICANT OTHERS AND SPOUSES

For those with a significant other or spouse, good communication is key. Having realistic and aligned expectations are paramount in making a relationship work during residency. Having a supportive significant other who understands the rigors of the job and can support you through it is invaluable. The process is a difficult journey for them as well. Review your schedule with your significant other so they know what your rotations are and which rotations will have longer hours. This allows them to have realistic expectations. Also, make sure they are aware of days when you are on call or may be taking late cases to the operating room so they are not surprised or disappointed. Encourage them to have activities that they do on their own so they are not entirely reliant on you to be available for their social life. Communicate when you are having a bad day. It is better to say, "I've had a difficult day so I am quiet" than to be sullen and snap at them. Plan small things that you know you can make, and keep your promise.

FAMILY AND FRIENDS

Family and friend relationships can be challenged during residency, but these relationships remain important in supporting you through a challenging but rewarding time in your life. It is important to set expectations early. Make sure that those around you know how your schedule works, and help them to have realistic expectations of your availability. Use travel time during either walks or drives from work in the evenings to call friends and family. Even if you have only 15 minutes to touch base, it will keep you connected to your life outside of work.

CHILDREN

Having children presents a unique challenge to surviving a surgical residency. It is important to remember that quantity of parenting does not equal quality parenting. Just because you have less hours per week with your child, does not mean that you cannot be the perfect parent. It is, however, important to use your time wisely. The free time you have can be used for quality interactions that will be meaningful to both you and your child/children. Mentorship on how to balance being a surgeon and a parent is crucial.

The following are some suggestions:

- Use videoconference technology such as Facetime as a means to see your children while you are in the hospital on call.
- Use whatever combination works for you to cover the hours of residency—au pair, day care center, in-home daycare, nanny, or even a spouse of a coresident who stays home who wants extra income.
- Be willing to pay someone to perform household tasks, such as emptying the dishwasher or doing laundry to free up your time. This will enable you to spend quality time with your child.
- Do not forget that your children will be proud of you once they are old enough to understand your job.
- Your kids will remember love, effort, and your presence. They will not remember that Mom missed one soccer game if you try to attend as many as possible. You will always feel worse than they do about missing events.

PREGNANCY

As the numbers of female residents in surgical residencies increase, the numbers of women becoming pregnant during residency is bound to increase. When/if you become pregnant, it is important to speak with your program director as early as you are comfortable to address scheduling. When considering maternity leave, consider that you are allowed to extend training if the ACGME is petitioned.

During pregnancy, it is important to take care of yourself maintaining hydration and nutrition and making sure to attending prenatal appointments. In surgery, we tend to forgo life necessities such as food and water for the sake of the job. However, during pregnancy, you have to remember that your baby is a patient too, and taking care of your baby is also critical. Carry water with you and eat healthy snacks often. Do not forget to avoid radiation, and always wear wrap around lead. It is also important to avoid other workplace exposures that could be teratogenic.

BREASTFEEDING

Breastfeeding is another difficult challenge while in surgical residency, but it is possible. Pumping can typically be done discretely while doing work. One can go to a designated breastfeeding room, office, locker room, or call room. Many residents have chosen to pump in shared work rooms, while rounding or during educational sessions. These have all been done before. It ultimately depends on your level of comfort in where you wish to pump.

- Consider joining Dr. Milk on Facebook for additional suggestions and support.
- Do not wash pump parts in between pumping sessions. Instead place them in a refrigerator for the next session. These can be washed at the end of the day.

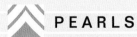 **PEARLS**

1. Communication is key in your interpersonal relationships. Be sure to communicate your schedule and set expectations regarding your work schedule and free time.
2. No parent has a perfect life. Parents with normal hours still have difficulty with balancing home life, and those who decide to be stay-at-home parents have difficulties with balancing other aspects of their life.
3. Remember that there are significant benefits to both baby and mom with breastfeeding. If you decide to breastfeed, it is perfectly acceptable to make breastfeeding a priority and ask your program for the resources and time to do so.

56

FINANCIAL LITERACY FOR SURGICAL RESIDENTS

RASHI JHUNJHUNWALA, MD, MA | ALOK GUPTA, MD

INTRODUCTION

It is well known that physicians are not great at managing finances. We are not taught basic finance concepts in medical school and residency, and very few physicians take the time to understand these topics well. Doctors know it, lenders and investment companies know it, and often times physicians end up losing out on opportunities to increase their financial security in the long term as a result. This is an important aspect of our livelihood. It is important for medical students and residents to make an effort to learn about these concepts.

In this chapter, we will go over the fundamentals of financial literacy for physicians. It is important to note that, just like in medicine, there are often many correct ways to approach each topic. We will present a few varying opinions as well as some resources to explore as you investigate how to manage your financial health. We hope this chapter will serve as a good primer for most novices. If you are particularly savvy on financial literacy, you may find the resources at the end of the chapter useful.

In general, everything can be split into two buckets—debt management and wealth management. Although early on it seems as though most of what you need to know falls into the first category, it is important to have a general sense of both sides of the coin. We will start off with debt management and then shift to wealth management.

DEBT MANAGEMENT

BUDGETING

Most medical students and residents are in a significant amount of debt with relatively high expenses and limited cash inflow. Residency, especially surgical residency, can be long. You are likely aware of nonmedical careers in which compensation begins much earlier, and at a higher salary than residency. However, as you start residency and continue to progress in your training, the salary does go up incrementally. And yes, although a career in medicine is uniquely rewarding and overall offers incredible financial stability and job security, *early* high compensation is not one of its big draws. We work in a system of delayed financial gratification. It is important to budget in all stages of your professional life, but especially in this phase during residency.

"Expense creep" can severely affect your debt and the amount of money you can save at the end of each pay period. This is a singularly important concept. As your salary increases, it is easy to convince yourself that you deserve an Uber rather than the bus, or the extra bottle of wine, or extra legroom on your cross-country flight. And yes, it is true that these luxuries may be very well deserved. But, although these expenses are not in and of themselves exorbitant, the extra 10% to 20% per purchase comes directly out of your bottom line for the month. These expenses add up quickly. Yes, it is important to treat yourself with things that add value to your daily experience, but expense creep is real, and you should be mindful of it. One approach is to decide what things are important for you to splurge on and *specifically* what you will forgo to make that possible.

One way to minimize the impact of expense creep is to make yourself a budget. You do not have to adhere to it down to the dollar if that becomes too stressful, but it is important to have a general sense of your posttax income, your fixed expenses (rent/mortgage, car payments, gas, groceries, utilities), and how much money you have left over. The money that remains after you pay your fixed costs is called your "discretionary income." This is the money that you can spend on things like going out to eat, vacations, or shopping—and also the money that you can put into a savings account or toward a credit card balance. Obviously, the more discretionary spending you do the less you have to save. Writing out the numbers in a budget spreadsheet or using an online tool is a great way to get a sense of how you want to approach this balance and avoid expense creep.

One simple framework to adjusting your spending habits is to base your plan around how much money you have. If you have no money, like many residents, then plan to minimize your credit card debt, purchase things on sale, and minimize your overall costs. This is damage control mode. If you have a moderate amount of money, like many who chose medicine as a second career or those with spousal income, start by paying off your highest-interest loans first. Save the rest of your cash and avoid expense creep and luxury items. If you have a true surplus of money due to gifts or a large inheritance, pay off your high-interest-rate loans completely and bank the rest.

CREDIT

Your credit score is an indication of your trustworthiness and your ability to responsibly handle money. It is extremely important to have good credit. If you treat your credit with respect by paying your bills and loans on time and keeping your debt burden low, you will enjoy the rewards of having good credit for years to come. You will obtain lower interest rates on your mortgages and credit cards, require lower down payments, and be able to purchase more expensive cars for the same cost. If you do not have good credit, you will pay a premium for being thought of as "untrustworthy," even after you have high income as an attending surgeon. So the first priority is to fix your credit. You can check your credit annually with each credit bureau without it affecting your score, so it is worth checking each one in some sort of regular rotation so you can keep track of how you are doing and petition to get mistakes removed if there are any.

There are hard checks and soft checks on your credit score. Having too many hard checks in a calendar year has the potential to negatively affect your score. Hard checks are common for things like mortgage applications or to open a new credit card. If you use an app or credit tracking service to look up your score, or if you request your score through the credit bureaus annually, these count as soft checks and have minimal impact. As such, if you are planning on applying for a loan or a mortgage with multiple banks, it is worthwhile to have the banks check your score in a short amount of time; this may count as the same hard check.

The main factors that negatively affect residents' credit scores are late credit card payments, opening up too many credit cards, and carrying a high balance on your credit cards relative to your credit limit. Each can count against you on your credit score and can stay on your record for 7 years. So, even one late bill payment that you pay off 2 months late can negatively affect you over half a decade later. Being mindful of these seemingly little things can go a long way to creating and maintaining good credit.

CREDIT CARDS

There is often a lot of confusion about how to manage credit cards. In general, it is wise to have one or two good credit cards that give you at least 2% rewards, have a low or no annual fee, and potentially have specific savings related to travel or other benefits that make sense for you and your lifestyle. Some people prefer having hotel rewards, others prefer airline miles, and others just want cash back. It is important not to fall for gimmicks that credit cards try to sell you, like 0% APR for the first 18 months or a free t-shirt. Generally speaking, it is not worth the free t-shirt! If you tend to carry a credit card balance, you should be paying attention to the interest rate that follows the promotional period. There are many websites that can help you compare credit cards and choose one that is best for your spending patterns. Having a credit card for a long period of time that is in good standing, meaning you are not carrying a large balance and you make your payments on time, can be beneficial to your credit, as it shows that you are have been responsible with payments over that entire duration. Thus, it is important to pick a card that has benefits over a long period of time.

Ultimately, the most important thing you can do with your credit card is to keep your balances below 30% of your credit limit and pay your bills on time. These two actions help improve your credit score, which is the end goal. Ideally, avoid carrying a balance on your card from month to month. This sometimes is not possible, especially during residency or when you have a numerous expenditures in a short period of time, but at the very least you should be paying your minimum balance on the card every month without fail.

LOANS

Many people graduating from medical school have loans, from college, medical school, or both. Depending on your career goals, your potential spousal income, and your other assets, there are varying approaches to paying down or paying off your loans.

Initially, your goal as a resident will likely be to lower your monthly payment as much as possible given your low monthly income. Most federal loans automatically default to low monthly payment over a long repayment period. You can find more information about the specific plans on the federal student loans website. Plans like these are often the only practical choice for residents. Remember, though, that interest continues to accrue and the total repayment amount is much more over a 25- to 30-year loan term than the same loan paid over 10 years with a higher payment. Paying as little as possible every month sounds great and may be your only feasible option, but it is worth looking into the big picture of how much you will be paying back in total.

Often, loan consolidation comes into play as a way to decrease your monthly payment as well as your interest rate to decrease your total loan payment. This can be a good option, with some caveats. If you are counting on loan forgiveness programs like the Public Service Loan Forgiveness (PSLF) program, you cannot consolidate your loans to private banks. Additionally, certain loan types, like Perkins loans, are not included in PSLF, and as such consolidating your loans to include Perkins loans will disqualify you from those programs. Depending on your interest in applying for loan forgiveness programs, it is worth your while to thoroughly investigate the terms of the forgiveness programs before consolidating. Remember, there are plenty of forgiveness programs for which surgeons are eligible! You do not have to be a primary care doctor practicing in a rural area to reap the benefits.

There are varying schools of thought on whether you should pay down your loans as much as possible once you finish training. Depending on the type of student loan you have and whether you consolidate your loans, your interest rates may be lower than other debts you carry, like a mortgage or a car loan. As a general rule of thumb, it is best to pay off your highest interest debts first. In your individual situation, this needs to be balanced against paying down loans quickly to reduce your total payment over time.

WEALTH MANAGEMENT

BUYING VERSUS RENTING

This is a very nuanced and personalized topic that has to take into consideration your personal, career, and family goals, as well as more basic parameters like the cost of living in your city and the duration of your residency. Surgery residents are often good candidates for buying property because of the sheer length of training, sometimes 7 years. If you end up staying in the same city for fellowship, this can stretch out even longer. On the other hand, if you are in a shorter residency program in a city with a high cost of living, the transaction cost of buying (and later selling) a property may outweigh the benefits of earning equity.

There are numerous benefits to owning your home. First, home equity is a large part of a surgeon's financial stability. Your equity in a property is the difference between its fair market value and your outstanding balance on the mortgage. Most real estate increases in value over time, and your loan balance typically decreases as you make payments toward the principal. So your equity should rise over time. This is the major benefit of buying over renting. Second, there are tax benefits that you may gain from owning your home, but these can vary greatly based on your state, especially with the new Internal Revenue Service (IRS) tax code enacted in 2018. Equity can also be thought of as an asset and can be used as the down payment on your next home or as a home equity line of credit (a cash loan you take against your house) to be used for a variety of things.

There are some downsides to owning your home. The upfront cost of down payment is often the barrier to entry for most residents. Closing costs (which often can be pricey) and taxes can add up to a substantial amount, but many of these costs can be rolled into your mortgage payment. Your new home may also require maintenance, renovations, or repair. There is no landlord or superintendent to call when your dishwasher floods your kitchen!

Renting is another great option, especially for the short term, if you are unable to buy a home, or if it does not make sense in your individual situation. Renting is easier and cheaper. And often you can land a nicer apartment for the same amount in rent versus mortgage. There are much lower upfront costs and often promotional rent rates. And do not worry, your career as a surgeon is predictive of strong financial stability in the future, and you can purchase your first home once you finish your training.

If you decide to purchase a home, one hot topic is that of physician loans. These are great loans that let young physicians get in the game without a large down payment. Lenders know that physicians are generally a low-risk population as we have fairly good job security and the expectation of a steady increase in income. Physician loans often lower the required down payment to 5% to 10% (from 20% on a traditional loan) and in some cases to zero down payment. These loans also often drop the otherwise required private mortgage insurance that can be costly month to month. A lower down payment often means a higher monthly payment but can help you afford your first home and begin building equity earlier.

LIFE AND DISABILITY INSURANCE

With regards to life insurance, the most important thing to think about is whether you need it. If you have dependents, like a spouse or children, who are relying upon your income, then you should strongly consider it. However, if you do not have dependents or others depending upon your earnings, you might not need to invest in life insurance at this point. If you do plan on obtaining life insurance, consider buying "term" life insurance rather than "whole life" or "universal" life insurance. Although insurance retailers might urge you to buy whole life insurance, they are often much more expensive. At this stage of your career, you are unlikely to have enough wealth to benefit from the potential advantages of those types of policies.

Another thing to keep in mind about life insurance is that certain types of loans pass on to your family in your absence, namely, private loans. Government loans do not pass on to your family. If you have a consolidated private loan, keep this in mind when accounting for how much life insurance you may want to purchase.

Accidental death and dismemberment is an additional insurance policy that augments your life insurance policy. For example, if you were to die in a car crash, this additional policy would add to your life insurance, so your family or dependents would receive an additional compensation.

Disability insurance is another type of insurance that essentially continues to disburse 60% to 80% of your monthly salary in the case of an unexpected event that renders you unable to continue working in your current position. The most important aspect of disability insurance for surgeons or other proceduralists is the "own occupation" clause. Most disability insurance policies allow you to file a claim *only if* they suffer a loss of income. In other words, if you are not able to continue in your job as a surgeon but are able to gain employment as a consultant, you are not able to make a claim on your disability insurance because you have not suffered a loss in your income. The "own occupation" clause specifically states that you have to no longer be able to make money ONLY within your own specialty. So if you have a freak garbage disposal accident and lose your hand and cannot operate, you can still generate an income as a consultant and simultaneously submit a claim under your disability insurance. The thing that you are insuring under an "own occupation" clause is your ability to operate. This is a really important concept for surgeons. Although your residency program is unlikely to offer this option to you, it is worth looking into independently, especially as you move toward the end of training.

Disability insurance can be costly. Here is an analogy that helps put that cost into perspective. If you are told that a black box exists that can pay up to 80% of your income in the event of your inability to work, how much would you be willing to pay for that black box?

FINANCIAL PLANNING AND INVESTING

Finally, we will tackle the expansive topic of investments, planning for retirement, and developing long-term wealth. This chapter is not mean to offer robust financial advice, which is very personal and very situation dependent, but rather to provide a framework within which to think about these topics. These subjects seem relatively futuristic for most starting residents, but it is always judicious to keep them in the back of your mind as you plan for life after residency. Most importantly, save, save, save. There are many ways to do this. You may have heard the saying that a penny saved is a penny earned. The truth is that a dollar saved is MORE than a dollar earned, because a dollar earned is taxed.

Most employers offer either a 401K or a 403B as a retirement investment plan. These have some nuanced differences but for practical purposes are very similar. Importantly, if your employer offers to match your contribution, for example, if they agree to match 100% for every dollar you contribute up to the first $2000 a year, you should put in the full amount and get a free $2000. This money is pretax, and you get a 100% return on investment on the money right away. This is better than paying off your credit card, or mortgage, or student loans. This should be your number one bucket for where your salary goes, and you should put in the full amount your employer matches even if it means adding a little debt elsewhere. However, if your employer does NOT match contributions to the 401K/403B, then you should revert back to paying off your highest interest loans or credit card balances first. It does not make sense to earn 7% in investments while paying 18% in credit card debt.

Another good long-term investment option for residents is investing in a Roth IRA. In a traditional IRA, pretax dollars accrue value over time and gains are taxed upon withdrawal from the account at retirement. However, a Roth IRA allows posttax dollars to be invested into the account and the money is then not taxed when it is withdrawn at retirement. This is great for residents, as they are often in lower-income brackets than they will be as retiring surgeons. It is worth discussing this with a financial advisor or accountant because there is an income limit per household that determines eligibility and benefit from a Roth IRA, and this may vary depending on whether your spouse has a higher income that pushes your household into a higher bracket. This Roth IRA option can be especially beneficial if your hospital does not match your contributions into a retirement account. It may make sense to max out your Roth IRA first, then make contributions to your 401K/403B accounts. Also consider exploring the "back door Roth" if your household income is higher than a typical resident salary. As of this writing, it is a good option once you have maxed out your traditional 401K/403B contributions.

Ultimately, keep in mind that wealth is made by saving, not by earning. Net worth is what builds wealth. If you earn a huge income but save none of it, your net worth (and quality of life in retirement) is likely much lower than someone who saves a large portion of their modest salary.

HIGHER-LEVEL ASSET AND WEALTH MANAGEMENT

Once you have paid off your high-interest loans, contributed to a retirement account, and made decisions about housing and other high-yield investments, congratulations! It is now time to start thinking about planning for your family's future and protecting your assets.

If you have children or are planning for children, a 529 plan is a college savings account that accrues interest. They are linked to states, but you are not obligated to participate in the 529 plan for the state in which you live. For example, if you live in Massachusetts, you are able to sign up for the Utah 529 plan. Some states offer tax benefits for participating in your in-state 529. Some credit cards will also put 1% of your spending back into a 529 account for you instead of giving you cash back. This is not the best way to contribute to these kinds of accounts, but it allows for an easy way to contribute if you are otherwise unable to do so.

Investing in mutual funds, protecting your investments and assets, and establishing trusts are complex topics. We recommend finding and hiring a TRUSTWORTHY financial planner. Often, hospitals will allow vendors to come speak about financial planning with residents. Although these sessions are useful in learning about options and basic vocabulary, it is important NOT to let the fox in the henhouse! The planners at these sessions are often paid to recruit you rather than look out for your best interests. Ideally, you should find a financial planner who is paid by you rather than by a company who is incentivizing them to sell their product.

TIME

Remember that time is your most valuable commodity. You should spend your time excelling as a resident, reading to build your knowledge base, and working hard to build your technical skills. You should also strive to have a healthy work life balance, which is fortunately more possible than a few decades ago. Remember to not waste time doing things that do not add value to your life. Consider outsourcing time-consuming tasks, as possible. For example, it may be only a bit more expensive to outsource your laundry than to use the coin-operated machines in your apartment building.

CONTRACT NEGOTIATION

When you are finishing your training and negotiating your first job, you should strongly consider hiring an attorney to review your contract. This is even more true outside major academic medical centers. An attorney can help you look for problems and help you negotiate salary, benefits, moving expenses, signing bonuses or loan repayment, and protected time.

 PEARLS

1. Financial literacy is crucial for surgeons, and although we are traditionally not very savvy at managing our debt and wealth, there are resources listed at the end of this chapter that can be helpful in learning more about how to manage money as a physician.
2. To manage your debt effectively, try to make (and largely stick to) a monthly budget, preserve your credit, be smart with your credit cards, and manage your loans in a way that is effective.
3. On the wealth management side, buy a house if that makes sense for your situation, maximize your life insurance and buy "own occupation" disability insurance, focus on saving, and hire a financial planner for helping with investments. Most importantly, learn how to protect your time and your assets.

Resources

1. The White Coat Investor (book by Dr. James Dahle) and associated website, www.whitecoatinvestor.com.
2. www.YNAB.com.
3. www.bankrate.com.
4. https://www.nytimes.com/interactive/2014/upshot/buy-rent-calculator.html.
5. Personal Capital App.
6. www.mint.com.
7. www.investopedia.com.

57

RESIDENT AS TEACHER

MARIAM F. ESKANDER, MD | TARA S. KENT, MD, MS

Teaching is an expectation during residency, but few have had formal training in medical education or adult learning theory. Fortunately, teaching, like other skills, can be taught and, if practiced and refined, becomes a habit and a regular part of your daily routine.

This chapter will distill the components of a "Resident as Teacher" course into an easy-to-read format, as well as provide some basic principles to help you step into your new role as a teacher, both of medical students and of your colleagues.

At our institution, we include a discussion about the resident's role as teacher and a crash course on effective teaching at our medical student Surgical Boot Camp, as well as during our intern practical skills curriculum, and reinforce these ideas with an annual session at our mandatory resident didactics, attended by residents of all levels.

Medical student teaching awards are presented to one junior and one senior resident every rotation based on medical student evaluations. In addition, residents choose one senior resident to receive a teaching award at an end-of-year ceremony.

A "RESIDENT AS TEACHER" CURRICULUM

ADULT LEARNING PRINCIPLES

1. Adults relate new knowledge to prior and current experiences.
   a. Create a link between what you are teaching and a clinical case or patient you are seeing.
   b. Build on what the learner already knows.
2. Adults need to understand the relevance of what they are learning.
   a. Make your teaching practical.
   b. Whenever possible, move your teaching to the bedside.
   c. Be clear with your learning goals and objectives and why they are important.
3. Adults like to be engaged and actively solving problems.
   a. Structure your discussion around a case. Encourage learners to defend their differential diagnosis or treatment plan. Probe their underlying thought process and rationale.
   b. Ask higher-order questions such as "how?" and "why?"

THE ENVIRONMENT

Many of the tips in this chapter work only if the teacher creates an environment that is safe for learning. Build a relationship with your team. At the very least, know your medical students' names and interests. Create a transparent "culture of error" in which you approach mistakes as learning opportunities. Be intellectually honest yourself: admit when you do not know the answer and encourage the team to look it up and contribute to your collective knowledge.

FEEDBACK

Good teachers give feedback—continuously—not just formative feedback at the end of a rotation. Feedback is less useful if it is vague and delayed from the event. Deliver specific, actionable feedback as soon as possible after an event. Make sure to point out and reinforce good behaviors as well.

CLINICAL TEACHING

Use the five-step "Microskills" model, first published by Neher et al., as a framework:

1. Get a commitment
   a. "Priya, what do you think is going on with this patient?"
2. Probe for supporting evidence
   a. "What about this patient and her data make you think she has cholecystitis? What else did you consider?"
   b. "Why do people get gallstones?"
   c. "What are some sequelae of gallstone disease?"
3. Teach general rules
   a. "Biliary colic is recurrent and self-limited. Patients with cholecystitis will have had pain for many hours and will be tender on exam. Ultrasound typically shows stones, pericholecystic fluid and gallbladder wall thickening."
4. Reinforce what was done right
   a. "You kept your differential broad for epigastric pain and asked about risk factors for gastritis. Not every patient with epigastric pain has a gallbladder problem."
5. Correct mistakes
   a. "I would not order a CT scan in a patient with suspected cholecystitis. Sometimes you won't see the gallstones because they are isodense to bile. Ultrasound is the gold standard diagnostic test."

BEDSIDE ROUNDS/TEACHING

This is an opportunity to teach both team members and patients.

1. Choose appropriate patients, and if possible, advise the patient before rounds.
2. Assign roles within your team. Who will speak? Who will examine the patient?
3. Take advantage of teachable moments. Does the patient have a positive Murphy sign? Point it out!
4. Communicate the plan to the patient and team. Demystify medical jargon so the patient can participate. Ensure the patient knows each individual's roles, for example, student or resident.
5. Debrief with your team outside the patient's room.

PROCEDURAL TEACHING

1. Prepare in advance.
   a. Review the objectives, equipment, relevant anatomy, and potential complications with the learner.
   b. Assess the learner's level of experience.
   c. Refer the learner to simulation videos and reading material.
2. Demonstrate the procedure, narrating each key step and its rationale.
3. Have the learner practice the procedure, preferably in a simulated environment initially, verbalizing each step.
4. Manage expectations before moving bedside. Let learners know you will be giving them pointers as they work and may need to show them a technique by briefly taking over. If the patient is awake, be careful not to say anything that would make the patient uncomfortable.
5. Debrief after the procedure. What did the learner do well? What can the learner do differently next time?

INTRAOPERATIVE TEACHING

1. Before the case:
   a. Set goals along with the learner. Discuss his/her experience with this type of case. What are your expectations?
2. During the case:
   a. Teach specifically to the goals you set.
   b. Provide frequent verbal feedback.
   c. Emphasize anatomical landmarks.
   d. Verbalize operative judgment and decision-making.
   e. Use unexpected errors as teachable moments.
   f. Promote graduated responsibility, moving the learner toward independence.
   g. Allow the learner time to struggle safely.
3. After the case:
   a. Debrief while you are closing incisions. What level of competence did the learner achieve? What specific skills should he/she should work on and how?

CONCLUSION

How you treat your patients and colleagues leaves a lasting impression on medical students and can influence a student's decision to go into surgery. Model respectful and compassionate behavior, no matter how stressful your day.

Finally, ask learners how you can be a better teacher and act upon that feedback. Learning how to teach is an iterative process: your skills will improve as you hone your style.

PEARLS

1. Know your audience. Ask your students what rotations they have completed thus far. Ask what they would like to get out of this rotation and to reflect on their strengths and weaknesses at this point in their training. Help them achieve their goals! Be clear with your expectations for the rotation and for each task.

2. Have one to two teaching points that you would like your students to get out of every interaction. Do not inundate them with new information. Have your students do most of the thinking and talking. Avoid long lectures.

3. Give a learner time to think of the answer to your question. When in a group, ask the question first then call on a person to answer it, not the other way around. People tend to zone out when they know they are not the person in the spotlight.

Resource

1. Newman L, Tibbles C, Atkins K, et al. *Resident-as-Teacher DVD Series.* MedEdPORTAL Publications; 2015. Available at https://www.mededportal.org/publication/10152.

Suggested Readings

1. Brodsky D, Smith CC. Educational perspectives: a structured approach to teaching medical procedures. *NeoReviews.* 2012;13:e635-e641.
2. Busch KM, Keshava HB, Kuy S, Nezgoda J, Allard-Picou A. *Teaching in the OR: New Lessons for Training Surgical Residents.* Bulletin of the American College of Surgeons; 2015. Available at http://bulletin.facs.org/2015/08/teaching-in-the-or-new-lessons-for-training-surgical-residents/.
3. Gonzalo JD, Chuang CH, Huang G, Smith C. The return of bedside rounds: an educational intervention. *J Gen Intern Med.* 2010;25(8):792-798.
4. Neher JO, Gordon KC, Meyer B, Stevens N. A five-step "Microskills" model of clinical teaching. *J Am Board Fam Pract.* 1992;5;419-424. Available at http://www.jabfm.org/content/5/4/419.full.pdf+html?utm_medium=referral&utm_source=r360.
5. Patton K, Morris A, Çoruh B, Kross E, Carlbom D, Thronson L. *Teaching to Teach Procedures: A Simulation-Based Curriculum for Senior Residents or Fellows.* MedEdPORTAL Publications; 2014. Available at https://www.mededportal.org/publication/9997/.
6. Smith C, Ricotta D. The resident as teacher. *N Engl J Med.* 2016;360. Available at https://resident360.nejm.org/content_items/1969.
7. Timberlake MD, Mayo HG, Scott L, Weis J, Gardner AK. What do we know about intraoperative teaching?: a systematic review. *Ann Surg.* 2017;266(2):251-259.

58

ACGME PROFESSIONALISM

EMILIE B. D. FITZPATRICK, MD

Within the current culture of medical education, professionalism is widely embraced as an integral component of physician education and practice. It is a fundamental element for providing safe and effective patient care. The literature has shown that patients are more satisfied with, more likely to trust, and more likely to follow through with treatment recommendations of physicians who display professionalism. Unprofessional physician behavior is the most common cause for patient complaints and increases the likelihood of medical malpractice claims.[1] We also know that physician professionalism influences patient safety.

In 2008, the Joint Commission issued a Sentinel Event Alert regarding the impact of unprofessional behavior on patient care and outcomes. This warning states that "intimidating and disruptive behaviors can foster medical errors, contribute to poor patient satisfaction and to preventable adverse outcomes."[2] Disruptive surgeon behavior in the operating room (OR) (ie, degrading comments, throwing instruments, sexual harassment) has also secured its own place of distinction in the literature. Not surprisingly, these behaviors are shown to inhibit effective exchange of information among physicians, patients, and staff; have a negative impact on surgical team morale; and reduce team collaboration.[3] Although these findings may seem obvious, it is important to recognize that the very existence of such studies reflects a much broader cultural shift in the value of medical professionalism. The paternalistic approach to patient care (and tolerance for scalpel throwing) is now a thing of the past; patient-centered care in an environment of professionalism is the new, improved standard.

PROFESSIONALISM IN PHYSICIAN TRAINING

Although professionalism has always been an inherent core value in medicine, the incorporation of professionalism training into physician education remains a relatively new concept. Since William Halsted pioneered the concept of the modern surgical residency in the 1880s, surgical training has been structured around four fundamental competencies: medical knowledge, patient care, practice-based learning, and improvement.[4] As the residency model evolved over generations, eventually becoming competency-based, nationally standardized curriculum of today, these elements have continued to form the basis of surgical training. For decades, all trainees have been required to prove mastery of a broad surgical knowledge base and technical skillset through the use of objective standardized assessment tools (ie, in-service and board certifying examinations). In contrast, an entire *century* passed before surgical trainees were officially obligated to demonstrate professionalism and the ability to communicate effectively with other humans. True story.

This is not to say that surgeons, or physicians as a whole, have historically been unprofessional. Humanistic qualities and professional behavior have always been implied expectations of a good physician. But they were also viewed more as innate characteristics than as skills that could (or should) be taught. It was assumed that physicians-in-training would assimilate these professional qualities and interpersonal skills through role modeling.[5]

THE ACGME STANDARD

As of 2002, the Accrediting Council on Graduate Medical Education (ACGME) and Residency Review Committee mandated that every residency program include six core competencies within the curriculum: (1) patient care and procedural skills, (2) medical knowledge, (3) practice-based learning and improvement, (4) interpersonal and communication skills, (5) professionalism, and (6) systems-based practice. Although maintaining the original foundational elements of Halsted's model, residents were now required to receive specific training in communication skills and professionalism.

The ACGME requirements for resident professionalism are as follows:

- "Residents must demonstrate a commitment to carrying out professional responsibilities and an adherence to ethical principles.
- Residents are expected to demonstrate:
  - compassion, integrity, and respect for others;
  - responsiveness to patient needs that supersedes self-interest;
  - respect for patient privacy and autonomy;
  - accountability to patients, society and the profession; and,
  - sensitivity and responsiveness to a diverse patient population, including but not limited to diversity in gender, age, culture, race, religion, disabilities, and sexual orientation."[6]

Thus, the community of medical/surgical educators has been faced with the challenge of converting the intangible concepts of "professionalism" and "interpersonal communication" into tangible, teachable skills. This has been a considerable focus of research in the past 2 decades. The use of standardized patients and objective structured clinical exams is an example of one modality that is well suited for developing these skills.[7]

DEFINING PROFESSIONALISM

There are three fundamental principles at the core of medical professionalism(1): primacy of patient welfare,(2) patient autonomy, and(3) social justice. Professionalism serves as the basis of the social contract between the medical community and the greater society.

But what, precisely, is professionalism? Is it a behavioral standard? A set of moral or ethical values? Is it an innate humanistic quality? Can it even be "taught"?

Some assert that "professionalism" and "humanism" are distinctly different concepts. Professionalism refers to the observable behaviors or actions used by physicians to fulfill their obligation to patients and society. It is a "way of doing," a code of conduct, based on the three fundamental principles noted earlier. On the other hand, humanism is a "way of being." It is an inherent conviction regarding ones' obligations to others and is manifested by qualities such as altruism, duty, integrity, respect for others, and compassion. In this view, "humanism provides the passion that animates authentic professionalism."[8]

The concept of professionalism includes cognitive, behavioral, ethical, and social components.[9] Thus, it eludes a universal, succinct definition. In context of surgical education and the ACGME standard, to be "competent" in professionalism, trainees must adhere to the three fundamental principles, follow ethical standards, show personal integrity and accountability, and display both humanistic qualities and respectful behaviors.

A group of expert faculty and educational leaders at the University of Southern California (USC) department of surgery set out to develop a framework for professionalism within their own institution. They generated an inclusive list of professionalism attributes and then combined these attributes into 11 categories, formulating a comprehensive framework for professionalism. The categories include respect, altruism, practice-based improvement, clinical competence, interpersonal skills, accountability, ethics/legal, education, appearance, cultural competence, and leadership.[10] What is notable is that the other five ACGME core competencies all appear, in some form, within this framework. This highlights the fact that professionalism is a prerequisite for meeting all of the goals of residency education.

GUIDELINES FOR PROFESSIONALISM

Several medical societies have published specific guidelines for physician professionalism; the American Medical Association created a declaration of professional responsibility in 2001[11]; a charter of medical professionalism was published by the American Board of Internal Medicine, the American College of Physicians, and the European Federation of Internal Medicine in 2002[12]; and the American College of Surgeons (ACS) published a code of professional conduct in 2003.[13] Although all are based on the same fundamental principles, there is some variation in how professionalism is defined within each specialty. The following responsibilities are included in the ACS code of professional conduct:

- "Serve as effective advocates of our patients' needs
- Disclose therapeutic options, including risks and benefits
- Disclose and resolve any conflict of interest that might influence decisions regarding care
- Be sensitive and respectful of patients, understanding their vulnerability during the perioperative period
- Fully disclose adverse events and medical errors
- Acknowledge patients' psychological, social, cultural, and spiritual needs
- Encompass within our surgical care the special needs of terminally ill patients
- Acknowledge and support the needs of patients' families

- Respect the knowledge, dignity, and perspective of other health care professionals
- Provide the highest quality surgical care
- Abide by the values of honesty, confidentiality, and altruism
- Participate in lifelong learning
- Maintain competence throughout our surgical careers
- Participate in self-regulation by setting, maintaining, and enforcing practice standards
- Improve patient care by evaluating its processes and outcomes
- Inform the public about subjects within our expertise
- Advocate for strategies to improve individual and public health through communication with government, health care organizations, and industry
- Work with society to establish just, effective and efficient distribution of health care resources
- Provide necessary surgical care without regard to gender, race, disability, religion, social status, or ability to pay
- Participate in educational programs addressing professionalism."[13]

PRACTICAL TIPS: HOW TO BE THE MODEL OF PROFESSIONALISM AS A SURGICAL INTERN

Understanding the concept of professionalism, and knowing the ACGME standard, is obviously a necessity for all physicians-in-training. However, how do you apply this to your day-to-day life as an individual surgical intern?

In this section, we will highlight specific categories and attributes of professionalism (borrowing from the USC framework) that are most pertinent at this level and offer advice on how to demonstrate professionalism as a surgical learner.

Respect: *interdisciplinary, patient autonomy, patient confidentiality, allied health, colleagues.*

- It really goes without saying, but there is never an excuse for disrespect or rudeness. Ever. Treat everybody with respect (patients, coworkers, staff, nurses, ancillary services).
- Patients will get frustrated, and some will take their frustration out on you. Acknowledge their feelings, apologize when necessary, and keep your cool. Never raise your voice or use sarcasm with patients.
- Even if someone is treating you disrespectfully, it does not give you the right to do the same in return.

- If you overreact or say something inappropriate, recognize it and apologize.
- Do not get frustrated with nurses who page to ask you patient care questions, regardless of how unimportant or ill-timed you believe the question is. Do not sound annoyed over the phone, even if you are.
- As you advance in training and take on the role of leading other interns/medical students/residents, treat the folks below you with respect. Remain humble—do not get an ego.
- Public shaming is poisonous and counterproductive.

Accountability: *Reliability*

Recall the proverb: "For want of a nail the shoe was lost. For want of a shoe the horse was lost. For want of a horse the rider was lost. For want of a rider the message was lost. For want of a message the battle was lost. For want of a battle the kingdom was lost. And all for the want of a horseshoe nail."

Interns—YOU are the nail. Embrace it. Be the nail.

- Be on time, all the time.
- If you are running late, let your team know as early as possible to allow redelegation of patient care responsibilities. It happens to everyone from time to time, but habitual tardiness is never acceptable.
- If there are extenuating circumstances that require you to miss a scheduled shift, make sure you communicate this to your supervising chief resident, staff, or program director. Remember that they are accountable for you. It is never ok to just "not show up."
- Give thorough patient hand-offs between shifts. Sloppy hand-offs inevitably result in balls being dropped, and the patients are the ones who will ultimately suffer for it.
- At first, you will be painfully inefficient in your attempts to triage and carry out your many tasks. *The importance of keeping checklists cannot be understated!* Get in the habit early. Write down plans for each patient, item by item. Make a separate "master checklist" help with prioritizing. As the day goes on, refer back to your checklist, adding items, and making sure all of your boxes are checked. If your supervising resident or staff is relaying patient care plans or delegating tasks to you, and you are not actively writing this information down, you are probably wrong.
- The act of writing an order does not guarantee that the thing you order will actually happen. Make sure to communicate directly with nurses, especially if something needs to be done ASAP. If it seems to be taking longer than usual, check in and figure out why. When your senior asks you why something did not get done, the answer should never be "I don't know why – but I wrote the order!"

- Avoid complacency. Maintain a baseline level of paranoia. Assume that at any given moment you are probably forgetting to do something. Therefore, refer to your checklist.
- Be a compulsive "number checker." You should be tracking the vitals, ins and outs, labs, and events throughout the day. Try to avoid last-minute surprises before afternoon rounds or signing out.
- Keep your seniors updated throughout the day, especially when they are in the OR for long periods. You are the eyes and ears of the team. Go seek them out, give them status updates, and see if there is anything that needs to be done.

Altruism: Nonjudgmental, caring, civic minded, dedicated, compassionate, patient advocate, integrity/honesty.

- Integrity first—do the right thing, all the time. For your patients and for your teammates.
- Never lie. Seems like a no-brainer, but at some point you will be asked a hard question about something you should know but do not, something you should have done but failed to do, or something you decided to do but should have known better. If you are caught in a lie, even once, your integrity will be permanently demolished. You can never recover from that.
  - Always be an advocate for your patients, even if it requires a little extra leg-work. A simple task on your part, such as a phone call, can sometimes save a lot of time and hassle for the patient. If a patient is encountering difficulty getting in to see his or her primary care manner, or scheduling an outpatient study, this is an easy one for you to help facilitate.

Practice Improvement: self-awareness, self-reflection, recognizes limits, manages emotions, admits mistakes, response to criticism, aware of biases, motivation to improve.

- Self-awareness and self-reflection are not easy skills for everyone. Practice these skills. Learn to be introspective. Ask yourself at the end of every day what you could have done better.
- Recognize your limits:
  - As a brand new intern, strive for independent *thought*, not independent *action*. You may think you are showing initiative by doing something you were not specifically instructed to do, but assume there is a reason you were not asked to do it. Remember that you do not know what you do not know.

- If you are not sure how to do something correctly, or you are uncomfortable performing a task independently, speak up. You might feel "dumb," but your pride is not a priority.
- If a patient is doing poorly, "load the boat" early. Call your senior resident—they can help care for the patient, and this takes the onus off you.
- Much like self-awareness, emotional management skills are not evenly distributed. Know where you are on the spectrum at baseline.
  - Remember there is never an excuse to take out your emotions on other people. Do not get angry, do not lash out.
  - Learn how your mind tends to react in an extreme situation. Recognize if you have a tendency to "freeze up," and take advantage of simulation-based training to learn to manage high-stress situations. It takes time, experience, and deliberate practice to improve any skill. This applies to emotional regulation as well.
- Learn to handle criticism well. Avoid defensiveness, explanations, and excuses. Even if you feel it is unfair or unwarranted, handle it with tact. If the criticism comes in the "destructive" form, figure out the underlying teaching point (what you did wrong, how you could have done better) and let the negativity roll off your back. Develop a thick skin.
- Demonstrate motivation to improve by actively seeking out feedback. Prepare well for your cases and conferences. Read about every case you are assigned, bring questions to your staff the day before, and ask for specific feedback at the end of the case.

Interpersonal Skills: Effectively communicates (information gathers, effective listening, transmits key information, giving bad news), works well within a team, fosters relationship development, approachable.

- Always be a team player, and take care of your teammates. If things are slow on your team, but the intern on another team is drowning, lend a hand. Avoid the temptation to "pass the buck" to the next person on call as the end of your shift approaches. Get as much done as you can, and set that person up for success.
- Be helpful on rounds and in the OR, without being asked.
  - When rounding with the team: have a few basic supplies on hand (scissors, gauze, tape); familiarize yourself with the medical supply room (you will definitely be sent in search of supplies); learn where the light switches are; grab gloves for your chief resident/staff; move bedside tables out of the way; help with taking down dressings; cover the patient after the examination.

- In the OR: assist with transferring the patient; move the stretcher out of the room; grab extra blankets/pillows if needed; make sure safety straps and sequential compression devices (SCDs) are in place; help with clipping and cleaning up hair. Scrub in on other residents' cases and be an asset: have scissors in your hand when sutures are being tied; learn how to suction without obstructing the view; retract like a pro. If you prove your worth, you will be called when extra hands are needed.
- Give organized, efficient presentations on rounds. Disorganized presentations are hard to follow, and information gets lost in translation.

Appearance:

- Dress appropriately and know what is expected at your institution (inpatient and outpatient settings).
- Although you will often feel completely disheveled, try not to appear that way. If you look like a mess, this will not inspire patients to have confidence in your abilities as a surgeon. Wear a clean white coat, buttoned up. Tuck in your scrub shirt.
- When presenting at the podium: stand up straight, project your voice, and speak with confidence. Do not slouch or fidget. Rehearse ahead of time if you need to. Practice maintaining your poise, in spite of inner turmoil.

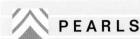 **PEARLS**

1. Own your mistakes. Never try to cover up an error, pass the blame onto someone else, or try to fake ignorance. Use every mistake as a learning opportunity, and never make the same mistake twice.
2. Convince your chief resident early on that you are dependable by *being* dependable. Complete every task that you are given, and if you do not understand something, clarify it early on so you can do it correctly. Follow up on results. Make sure plans are implemented.
3. From day one, invest in building rapport with everyone around you. Get to know the nurses on the ward and in the OR by name. Make connections with providers on other services and departments (radiology and GI especially). Forming these relationships will open up doors for you along the way and make your daily work more rewarding.

References

1. ACGME Outcome Project: Advancing Education in Medical Professionalism. Available at: http://www.usahealthsystem.com/workfiles/com_docs/gme/2011%20Links/Professionalism%20-%20Faculty%20Dev..pdf. Accessed 20 July 2018.
2. Joint Commission. Behaviors that undermine a culture of safety. Sentinel Event Alert 40. Available at https://www.jointcommission.org/sentinel_event_alert_issue_40_behaviors_that_undermine_a_culture_of_safety/.
3. Deptula P, Chun M. A literature Review of professionalism in surgical education: suggested components for development of a curriculum. *J Surg Educ.* 2013;70(3):408-422.
4. Imber G. *Genius on the Edge: The Bizarre Double Life of Dr. William Stewart Halsted.* New York, NY: Kaplan Publishing; 2010.
5. Hochberg MS, Kalet A, Zabar S, et al. Can professionalism be taught? Encouraging evidence. *Am J Surg.* 2010;199:86-93.
6. Accreditation Council for Graduate Medical Education. Common program requirements. Available at http://www.acgme.org/Portals/0/PFAssets/ProgramRequirements/CPRs_2017-07-01.pdf.
7. Hochberg MS, Berman RS, Kalet A, et al. The professionalism curriculum as a cultural change agent in surgical residency education. *Am J Surg.* 2012;203:14-20.
8. Cohen JJ. Viewpoint: linking professionalism to humanism: what it means, why it matters. *Acad Med.* 2007;82:1029-1032.
9. Hultman CS, Connolly A, Halvorson EG, et al. Get on your boots: preparing fourth-year medical students for a career in surgery, using a focused curriculum to teach the competency of professionalism. *J Surg Res.* 2012;177(2):217-223.
10. Sullivan ME, Trial J, Baker C. A framework for professionalism in surgery: what is important to medical students? *Am J Surg.* 2014;207:255-259.
11. American Medical Association. Declaration of professional responsibility. Available at http://www.ama-assn.org/resources/doc/ethics/decofprofessional.pdf.
12. ABIM Foundation; ACP-ASIM Foundation; European Federation of Internal Medicine. Medical professionalism in the new millennium: a physician charter. *Ann Intern Med.* 2002;136:243-246.
13. ACS, Task Force on Professionalism. Code of professional conduct. *J Am Coll Surg.* 2004;199:734-735.

INDEX

Note: Page numbers followed by "f" indicate figures and "t" indicate tables.

A

Abdominal radiograph
    free fluid *versus* abscess, 102, 104, 104f
    ileus *versus* obstruction, 102, 103f
ABG test. *See* Arterial blood gas
    (ABG) test
Absorbable suture, 333
ABW. *See* Actual body weight (ABW)
Accrediting Council on Graduate Medical
    Education (ACGME) standard,
    470–471
Acetaminophen, 61, 66
ACGME standard. *See* Accrediting Council
    on Graduate Medical Education
    (ACGME) standard
ACS code. *See* American College of
    Surgeons (ACS) code
Actual body weight (ABW), 132
Acute transfusion reactions, 84, 85t–86t
Admission orders
    ADC VAANDIMLS system, 244–246
    brief plan writing, 244
    computerized admission order sets,
        243–244
    electronic medical record systems, 244
    indications, 244
    patient history, 244
    problem-based framework, 243, 246
Adson forceps, 316, 316f
A-FIB. *See* Atrial fibrillation (A-FIB)
Albumin, 38–39, 133
Albuterol, 30
Alcohol-based scrub, 303
Alginates, 204
Allowed amount, 263
Alprazolam, 29
Altered mental status (AMS), 157–159
American College of Surgeons (ACS) code, 472
Aminoglycosides, 45

AMS. *See* Altered mental status (AMS)
Analgesic medication, 29
Anesthesia Patient Safety Foundation (APSF)
    Fire Prevention Algorithm, 386
Angiotensin-converting enzyme
    inhibitors, 30
Ankle stirrup splint, 211, 213f
Anterior urethra, 194
Antiemetics, 31
Antihypertensives, 30
Antimicrobial dressings, 204
Antiplatelet agents, 32
Appendicitis, 49
APSF Fire Prevention Algorithm. *See*
    Anesthesia Patient Safety
    Foundation (APSF) Fire
    Prevention Algorithm
Army-Navy retractors, 322, 327f
Arterial blood gas (ABG) test, 146–147
    complications, 219
    equipments, 216–217, 216f
    indications, 215
    needle insertion, 217
    needle removal, 218–219
    pulsatile blood return, 218
    radial artery palpation, 217
Aspirin, 31
Association of periOperative Registered
    Nurses (AORN) Fire Risk
    Assessment Checklist, 386, 388t
Atelectasis, 99–100, 100f
Atrial fibrillation (A-FIB), 112, 113f, 164–166
Atrial flutter, electrocardiogram (EKG),
    112, 113f
Atrophic vaginitis, 128
Augmentin, urinary tract infections (UTIs), 43

B

Baclofen, surgical pain management, 62
Balfour retractor, 328, 329f
Balloon port, 194
Basic metabolic panel (BMP), 140

479